P

Dental Restorations

Protocols for
Predictable Aesthetic Dental Restorations

Irfan Ahmad

BDS, The Ridgeway Dental Surgery, Middlesex, UK
Active member European Academy of Esthetic Dentistry

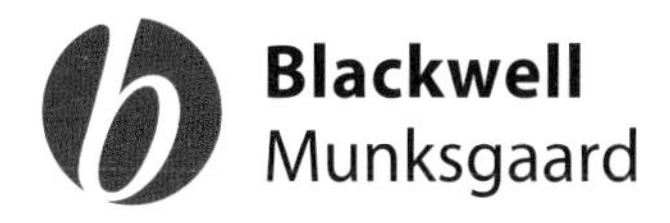

Blackwell Munksgaard, a Blackwell Publishing Company,
Editorial Offices:
Blackwell Publishing Ltd, 9600 Garsington Road, Oxford OX4 2DQ, UK
Tel: +44 (0)1865 776868
Blackwell Publishing Professional, 2121 State Avenue, Ames, Iowa 50014-8300, USA
Tel: +1 515 292 0140
Blackwell Publishing Asia, 550 Swanston Street, Carlton, Victoria 3053, Australia
Tel: +61 (0)3 8359 1011

First published 2006 by Blackwell Munksgaard

ISBN-13: 978-14051-1820-0
ISBN-10: 1-4051-1820-2

Library of Congress Cataloging-in-Publication Data
Ahmad, Irfan, BDS.
Protocols for predictable aesthetic dental restorations / Irfan Ahmad.
p. cm.
Includes bibliographical references and index.
ISBN-13: 978-1-4051-1820-0 (pbk. : alk. paper)
ISBN-10: 1-4051-1820-2 (pbk. : alk. paper)
1. Dentistry–Aesthetic aspects. 2. Prosthodontics. I. Title.
[DNLM: 1. Esthetics, Dental. 2. Dental Restoration, Permanent.
3. Dental Restoration, Temporary. WU 100 A286p 2006]
RK54.A46 2006
617.6′9–dc22
2005024528

A catalogue record for this title is available from the British Library

Set in 10 on 12pt Sabon
by SNP Best-set Typesetter Ltd., Hong Kong
Printed and bound in Spain
by GraphyCems, Navarra

The publisher's policy is to use permanent paper from mills that operate a sustainable forestry policy, and which has been manufactured from pulp processed using acid-free and elementary chlorine-free practices. Furthermore, the publisher ensures that the text paper and cover board used have met acceptable environmental accreditation standards.

For further information on Blackwell Publishing, visit our website:
www.dentistry.blackwellmunksgaard.com

Note: the author is an invited lecturer for many dental organisations but has no financial interests and no formal links with any of these organisations.

Contents

Dedication

To my wife and soul companion, Samar, and my son Zayan.

Foreword

I have always thought that any teacher of beauty, including cosmetic dentistry, should have an artistic "eye." In my opinion, Irfan Ahmad falls within this requirement. The first time I saw him lecture I was quite impressed with his understanding and attention to all that is classified as esthetic. So, it is appropriate that Dr Ahmad has authored *Protocols for Predictable Aesthetic Dental Restorations*. His approach to basic and advanced principles of esthetics is well grounded. Although each of us may have our own way of doing a particular procedure we should nevertheless realize that there is more than one way to achieve the same goal and therefore Dr Ahmad's unique approach to problems is well worth our attention. His stunning photography is both creative and educational, making step-by-step procedures easier to comprehend. All too often we see self-styled clinicians who both lecture and write as if they originated every single technique they show and with little or no evidence to back up their claims. Therefore it is refreshing to see that Dr Ahmad relies on evidenced-based principles to back up his artistic talent. The uniqueness of our profession is that we are not all "clones," each of us has his or her own "tricks" or technique to accomplish a common goal – that of pleasing the patient and achieving both a functional and an esthetic result. Thus it is both refreshing and a true learning experience to discover Dr Ahmad's unique way of how to accomplish his esthetic goals.

It has been over thirty years since I wrote the first edition of *Esthetics in Dentistry*. This was the very first comprehensive textbook describing esthetic techniques both as an entity as well as a vital part of interdisciplinary dentistry. Working with specialists for virtually all disciplines of dentistry, this concept has now been finally accepted into what we consider the prevailing standard of care in both diagnosis and treatment planning.

Dr Ahmad understands this concept and thus he spends most of his text dealing with the details of how he, and we, should be achieving greater success with all ceramic crowns and bridges. Just as I did in my first text, Dr Ahmad devotes a chapter to each of the essential six steps to a successful restoration. There is an important lesson in spending an entire chapter on each step, and that is not only to learn new tips on being more efficient and seeing if another method is better than the one you currently use, but also that each of the steps is a separate entity. This helps us constantly remember to spend an adequate amount of time with attention to detail, so that in the end we will have done our very best in each phase of the restoration. It is this attention to detail that can make the difference between an ordinary and an **extra**ordinary restoration. Dr Ahmad knows this difference and I am so pleased he chose to share that "difference" with all of us.

Roland E. Goldstein, DDS

Preface

The aim of this book is to furnish the clinician with knowledge for providing aesthetic dental restorations that are virtually indistinguishable from natural teeth. Dental aesthetics is intangible, influenced by the wishes of the patient, experience of the clinician, and the artistic and technical skills of the ceramist. Aesthetics lies in the murky twilight between art and science. Art is not enough to create aesthetic restorations, while science alone is inadequate for pleasing results. However, the clinical protocols necessary for aesthetic restorations are tangible, relying on biological concepts combined with scientific research. Using the health, function and aesthetic (HFA) triad, the clinician and ceramist can deliver prostheses that are durable and harmonise with surrounding soft and hard tissues. The appearance of dental restorations is subjective: one person's *Xanadu* may be another's *Inferno*. Aesthetics is a passion, not a craft, and one that has to be sought rather than taught. According to Carl Jung, '*A man who has not passed through the inferno of his passions has never overcome them*'.

The layout of the book is a chronological clinical journey, starting with treatment planning and ending with cementation. The intervening chapters between these start and end points transport the reader through successive stages for providing aesthetic dental restorations. Most chapters commence with scientific rationale and finish with clinical practice, applying theory to a practical scenario. Whilst the learning curve at times seems onerous, once mastered the techniques can be expedited for making aesthetic restorations that are predictable, functional and long lasting. Furthermore, the systematic approach adopted in this book gains patient gratitude and creates clinical satisfaction.

I am indebted to Ronald Goldstein, who is undoubtedly regarded as the pioneer of aesthetic dentistry. The two people who have spurred me on: Bernard Touati and Nitzan Bichacho, as well as eminent clinicians who have helped, directly or indirectly, with this project, including Avishai Sadan, Gerard Chiche, Markus Blatz, Tom Trinkner, William Liebenberg, Alan Gluskin, Homa Zadeh, Fereidoun Daftary, Stefano Gracis, Mauro Fradeani, Douglas Terry, Stephen Hancocks, Rafi Romano, Galip Gürel, Alan Sidi, Eric van Doreen, Youval Elyat, Ervin Weiss, Nitzan Fuhrer, Ilan Gilboa, members of the European Academy of Esthetic Dentistry and Dentology study group, especially Sanjay Sethi, who founded Dentology five years ago for like-minded clinicians.

My special thanks to Stephen Chu for his support and friendship, and whose bestselling book on colour has been the inspiration for Chapter 4 of this book. I would also like to express my gratitude to the ceramists whose talents are featured through this publication, including Willi Geller (Maestro), Gerald Ubassy, Jason Kim, Paul Sturridge, Jean Marc Etienne, John Hubbard and David Korson. My dear friends Karl Theis, Magnus Persson, Ann-Louise Holding, Hina Halai, Sital Patel, Bob Muggleston, my father, Mansur Ahmad, late mother Bilqis Bibi, aunty Razia Khanum and sisters Ayesha and Samina. I am also thankful to Omowunmi Braithwaite for her kindness and compassion, and for being there when my wife and I most needed her.

Finally, I am grateful to Caroline Connelly and all the staff at Blackwell Publishing for their hard work and efficiency in making this project a reality.

Irfan Ahamd

1 Treatment planning – assessment, planning and treatment

Treatment planning involves applying learned didactic scientific knowledge to clinical realities. To achieve this goal, a systematic approach is necessary, using the acronym APT (assessment, planning and treatment) (Fig. 1.1). Aesthetic treatment, unlike other forms of dental care, requires a radically different approach. For example, the protocol for endodontic treatment is infection removal and subsequent sealing of the canal(s), requiring little or no input from the patient. In fact, the patient is usually oblivious to the treatment modality, and is only aware of resolution of symptoms. Aesthetic treatment on the other hand, is highly subjective, with active patient participation. The colour, form and characterisation of anterior aesthetic restorations are open to scrutiny by the patient, family and friends. The clinician therefore has to adopt a different protocol to meet these challenges for avoiding disagreements and unsatisfactory outcomes.

In order to execute aesthetic treatment successfully, the following items are prerequisite:

- Time
- Aptitude
- Knowledge
- Skills
- Experience
- Patience

Without these qualities, aesthetic treatment is neither possible nor successful. To achieve these objectives, use of a systematic approach, such as APT, maximises success and minimises failures.

Assessment

Assessment begins with an initial consultation, which is a mutual evaluation between the patient and clinician. This appointment generates revenues below the clinician's usual hourly rate, but is worthwhile in the long run. The initial encounter is predominantly psychological, the clinician determining the patient's persona, emotional make-up and needs, and the patient assessing his/her confidence of the dental team, as well as the ambience of the dental practice. The clinician's approach should be empathetic and sincere, rather than dismissive and authoritarian, since this meeting will determine whether a satisfying dentist–patient relationship is possible.[1] Because aesthetic treatment is protracted, often

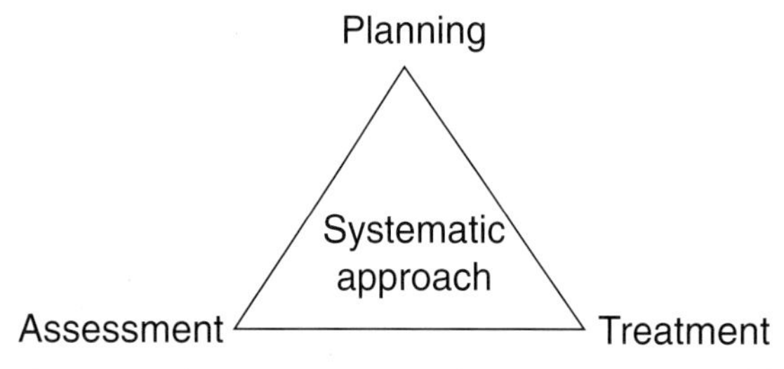

Figure 1.1 The APT (assessment, planning, treatment) model for a systematic approach to treatment planning.

involving a multiphase treatment plan, mutual respect should be established and maintained throughout the entire period. If mutual respect and rapport are not forthcoming, therapy is destined to failure, irrespective of clinical skill and support of the dental team.

The subsequent appointment is much longer, involving information gathering using a variety of examinations. More than one appointment may be necessary to gather information, requiring referral to a hospital or specialist clinics for specific diagnostic tests. The information-gathering process is divided into histories, examination and technological tests. Of course, not every item is necessary for every patient, depending on prevailing symptoms. Below is a proposed list, together with salient points for each item.

(1) Histories:
- Medical history – diabetes, immune response compromises, medication
- Risk history – medical (xerostomia, diabetes, immunosuppression), genetic (periodontal disease and caries), community (cultural, lifestyle priorities), fluoride (demographic), status (socio-economic, education), environmental (occupational hazards), disabilities (Down's syndrome, epilepsy), habits (smoking, betel nut chewing, poor plaque control)
- Nutritional history – diet, gastric regurgitation, bulimia
- Dental history – attendance, previous treatment, records from former or referring dentist, phobias, dental priorities, oral hygiene

(2) Examination:
- Verbal – initial consultation (listening and evaluation to determine patient's chief complaint as well as gauging persona, expectations and wishes)
- Visual:
  - Extra-oral: facial symmetry, facial contours, labial grooves and fissures, skeletal profile, muscular spasms, lymph nodes, speech
  - Aesthetic: smile line, degree of gingival exposure during a smile, degree of tooth exposure at rest and during a smile, tooth form, colour and texture
  - Intra-oral: soft tissue lesions. Tongue size and breathing pattern due to enlarged tonsils causing pharyngeal airway obstruction and tongue thrust may compromise anterior restorations. Caries, periodontal biotypes and bioforms, width of attached gingiva, edentulous ridge configuration according to the Misch classification[2], dental arch shape (anterior–posterior and lateral), imbrications and spacing, interocclusal clearance (checking for over-eruption, displacement of condyles, alveolar bone loss due to previous extractions, tooth wear (erosion, attrition, abrasion, abfraction), fractured teeth using transillumination
  - Occlusal assessment: centric occlusion (CO), centric relation (CR), lateral guidance, anterior guidance, horizontal and vertical overbite, Curve of Spee and Wilson, eccentric contacts, bruxism, failed restorations
- Tactile – muscle palpation, temporomandibular joint (TMJ), fremitus, tooth percussion (endodontic evaluation)
- Written – document verbal and visual finding. Use questionnaire(s) for ascertaining patient's aesthetic expectations. These forms should enquire about which aspect of aesthetic treatment is important to the patient, e.g. colour, shape, alignment of the teeth, etc.

(3) Technological tests:
- Articulated study models with jaw relation records
- Articulators and jaw movement/registration analysers
- Diagnostic wax-ups (Figs. 1.2 & 1.3)
- Radiographs (current and from previous or referring dentist)
- Photographic documentation (intra-oral and 35 mm cameras)
- Scans: computerised tomography (CT) scan, linear tomography, or interactive CT for assessing adequate bucco-lingual width and length of alveolar ridge for implant placement (Figs. 1.4 & 1.5); and magnetic resonance image (MRI) for suspected TMJ arthropathy
- Shade analysis: visual, digital, visit to ceramist (see Chapter 4)
- Instrumental/chemical caries and periodontal detection
- Pulp vitality tests (thermal and electrical)
- Bacterial and biopsy tests

Planning

Having completed the initial consultation, necessary histories, examinations and tests, the next stage is planning. The planning phase involves diagnosis, risk assessment, evidence-based decision making and presenting treatment proposals to the patient.

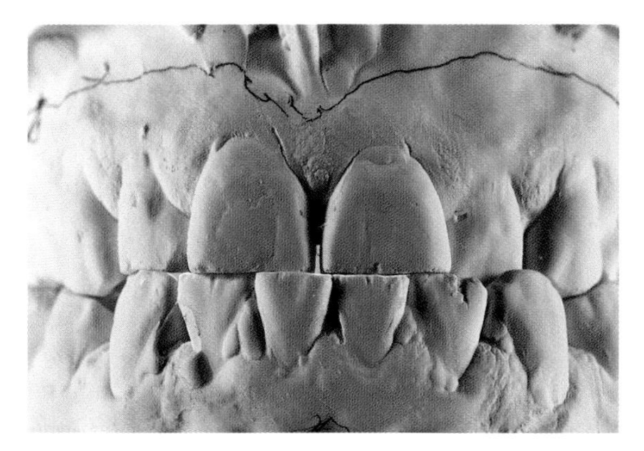

Figure 1.2 Pre-operative study casts showing reduced vertical dimension.

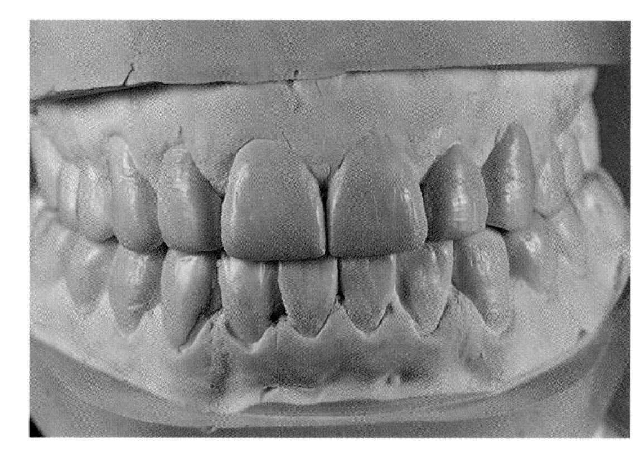

Figure 1.3 Diagnostic wax-up for proposed increase in occlusal vertical dimension for patient in Figure 1.2 (laboratory work by Gerald Ubassy, France).

Diagnosis

Before a diagnosis can be established, the clinician has to integrate all the pieces of information in a coherent and logical manner, not unlike a jigsaw puzzle, creating a picture of the patient's medical and dental status. Depending on the clinician's experience, relevant data is highlighted, while less important information is relegated, allowing commencement of the diagnostic process.

Diagnosis is the premise of planning, preceding any prescribed treatment. It is not limited merely to current symptomatic signs, but incorporates aetiology of the prevailing pathology.

A definitive diagnosis is essential before commencing therapy. For example, repairing a fractured tooth or crown with a replacement restoration is insufficient. The underlying cause of why the tooth or crown fractured is essential if the repair is to be successful (Fig. 1.6). Factors such as occlusal abnormalities, periodontal disease, endodontic status, etc. require investigation so that aetiology is defined and treated, before repair is instigated.[3]

Risk assessment

Currently, most risk assessment by clinicians is highly subjective, leading to inconsistencies and

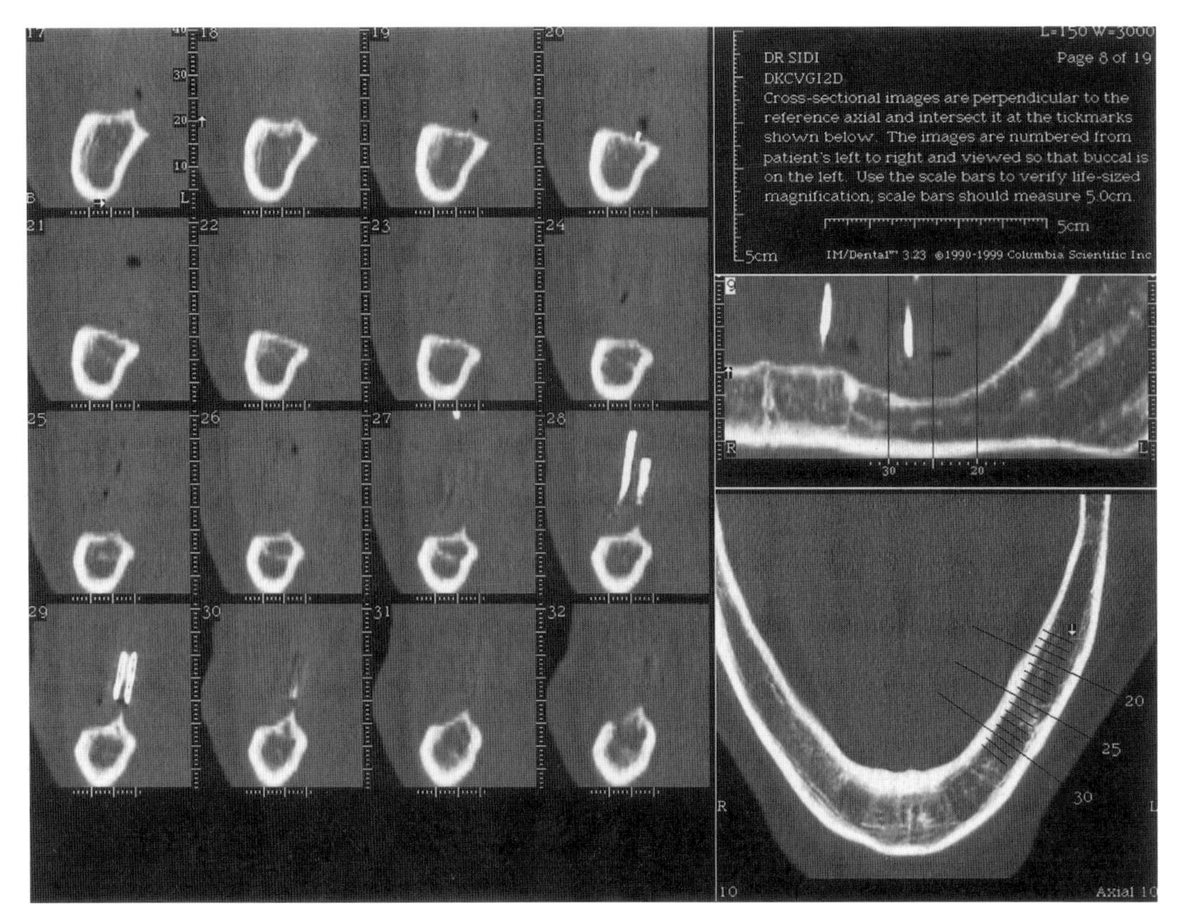

Figure 1.4 CT scan showing insufficient bone for endosseous implant placement (image courtesy of Dr Alan Sidi, UK).

inaccuracies. This usually results in underestimating disease severity, and necessitates more complex and costly treatment later. The aim of risk assessment is to tailor treatment plans individually according to a patient's dental profile, thereby moving away from a 'repair model' to a 'wellness model'. This will discourage disease recurrence and encourage long-term oral health.

Many studies have cited that the two major dental diseases, caries and periodontal disease, are preventable. This assertion is based on identifying and reducing risk, and implementing appropriate preventive measures.[4] For example, the diagnosis of severe periodontal disease does not imply a high risk of periodontal disease. Diagnosis assesses current clinical findings, while risk assesses or predicts future disease patterns. This is because traditional diagnosis is two-dimensional (2D) (clinical examination and radiographs), which indicate disease severity. The third dimension, risk assessment, is omitted. A three-dimensional (3D) diagnosis for periodontal disease incorporates the following (Fig. 1.7):

- Clinical examination and findings
- Radiographic assessment
- Risk prediction

Using a 2D diagnosis, all patients will be prescribed the same treatment, irrespective of risk. However, when individual patient risks are incorporated in a 3D diagnosis, the treatment plan differs for each patient, even though the 2D diagnosis is identical. Periodontal risk factors are crucial when considering implants or aesthetic prostheses. For low-risk patients, simple

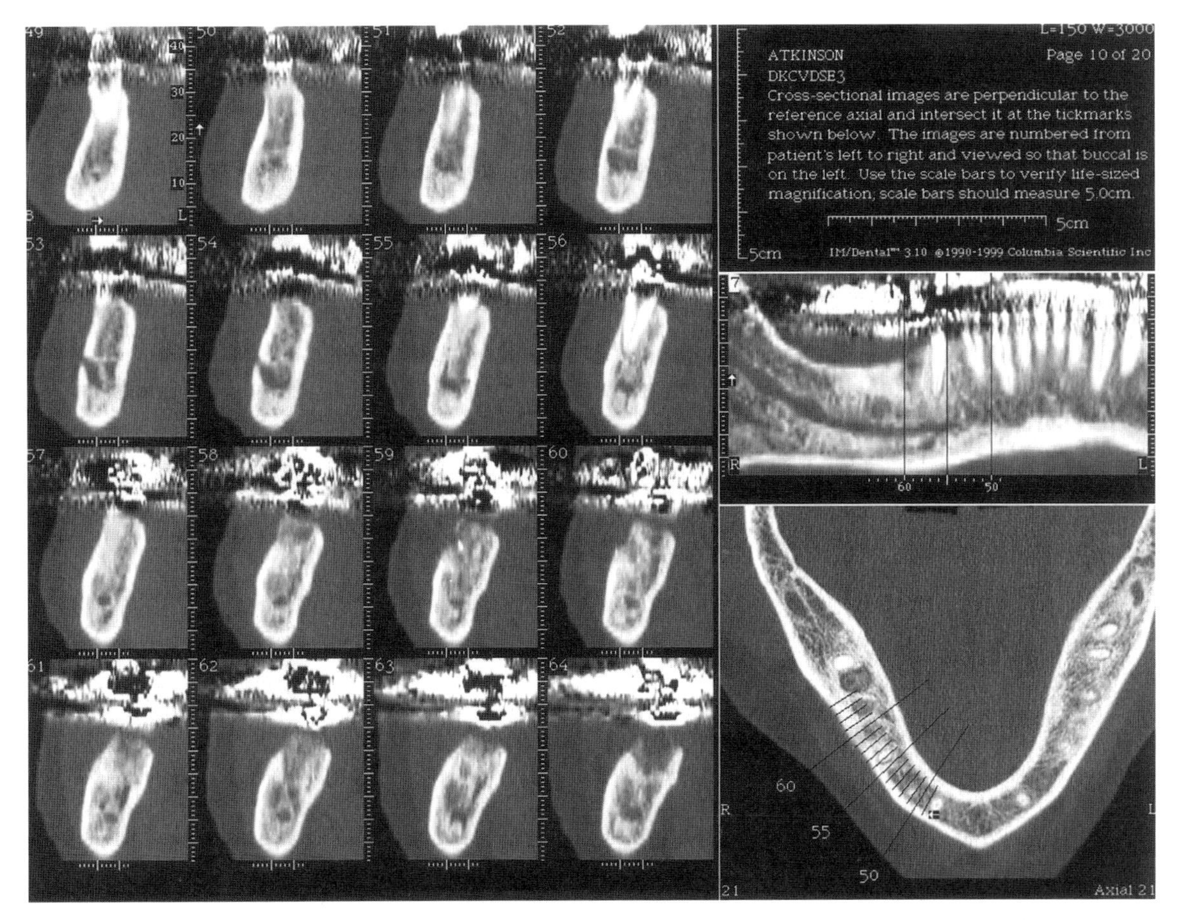

Figure 1.5 CT scan showing adequate bone for endosseous implant placement (image courtesy of Dr Alan Sidi, UK).

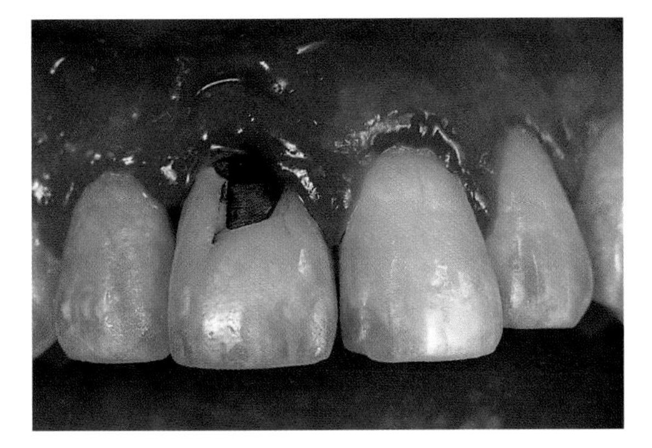

Figure 1.6 De-lamination of veneering porcelain on a metal–ceramic crown.

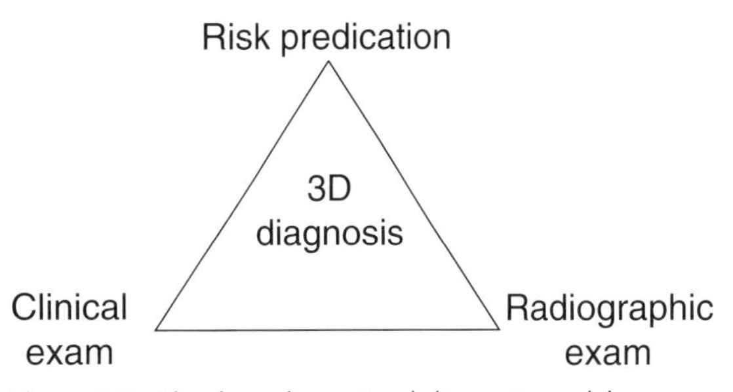

Figure 1.7 The three-dimensional diagnosis model.

prophylactic procedures are sufficient, and the probability of success of aesthetic restorations or implants is high. This is not the case with moderate- to high-risk periodontal patients, who require extensive periodontal therapy and more frequent recalls ensuring that periodontal health is established and maintained. In the latter, patients should be informed that unless their periodontal status is maintained, aesthetic restorations or implant longevity may be severely compromised.

The next question is how predictably and accurately to assess risk. A recent study shows that only 20% agreement was evident among expert clinicians, indicating that inter-evaluator assessment is unreliable. The clinical significance is that either over or under-treatment is prescribed depending on the opinion of the examiner.[5] A quantitative analysis using the Previser Risk Calculator has been proposed, which accurately predicts risk of periodontal disease, from a scale of 1 (low risk) to 5 (high risk). This test uses the latest computer technology and has been clinically evaluated over a 15-year period. As well as assessing risk, the test also provides a rating for current disease status from 1 (periodontal health) to 100 (severe generalised periodontitis). [6] This objective evaluation is a step towards the clinician being able to modify treatment according to risk, achieve and maintain periodontal health, and prevent future complex and costly therapies. This quantitative analysis is a paradigm shift from a repair to a wellness model.

Evidence-based decision making and treatment

Historically, dentistry was far ahead of medicine with regard to implementing preventive measures for caries and periodontal disease. These prophylactic interventions were underpinned by nearly four decades of scientific research and clinical trials. However, today the profession is so enamoured with technology that it has shed the solid scientific platform in favour of spurious marketing claims. Inventive materials and devices are readily embraced, endorsed by charismatic lecturers, and used on patients without evidence of long-term clinical success. Many 'opinion leaders' that lecture frequently at dental symposia reiterate a particular point of view, which may or may not be evidence-based. An opinion that is repeated perpetually eventually becomes the truth, irrespective of its validity.

There is nothing wrong with this approach as long as delegates are informed beforehand that the speakers are expressing their empirical experience, not scientifically proven rules and guidelines. As stated below, clinical experience forms a part of an evidence-based approach. Added to this are peer and media pressure, castigating those who prefer the traditional scientific approach as archaic or old-fashioned. However, sometimes faith is not enough, and seeing or reading anecdotal case studies are insufficient for sound clinical decision making.[7]

Viewed from a manufacturer's perspective, dental companies are keen to introduce novel products and make profits, which indirectly filter back to the profession in sponsorship for educational symposia. Furthermore, research is onerous, expensive and protracted, and by the time the results are published, the product may be obsolete, often replaced by a newer version. This vicious cycle is then repeated and perpetuated.

The scientific approach, although utopian, hampers innovation and technological advancement. Many new technologies have faced problems before a reliable product eventually emerges. Ultimately, it is the dentist, not the manufacturer, who is responsible for clinical decision making that impacts on patients' treatment. If things go wrong, the patient is unlikely to blame the manufacturer for the failure. Therefore, the onus is on the dentist to choose appropriate materials, backed by evidence-based research, to avoid rebuke or professional negligence litigation in the event of failure. Evidence-based treatment[8] is succinctly summarised as a combination of (Fig. 1.8):

- Clinical erudition
- Sound scientific research
- Patients' needs and wants

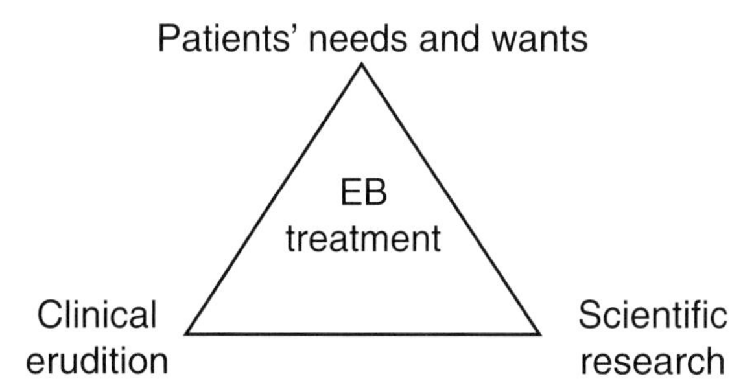

Figure 1.8 Components of evidence-based (EB) treatment.

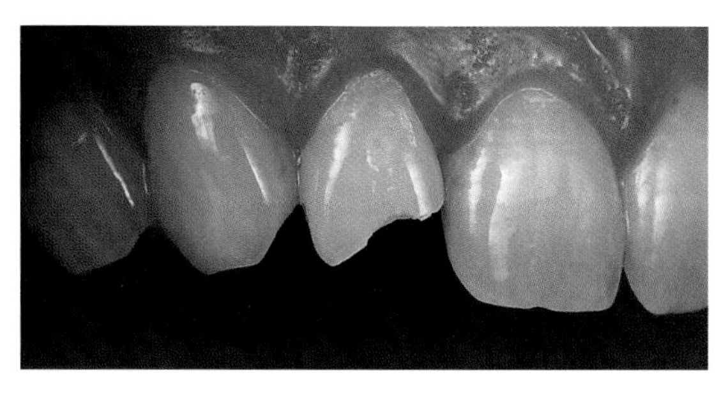

Figure 1.9 External trauma resulting in a fractured right maxillary lateral incisor.

Performing successful treatment is a combination of evidence-based information, clinical judgement and personal experience. It is this combination, rather than just one factor, which ensures validity and successful outcomes. Each factor requires scrutiny. Evidence-based information relies on randomised clinical trials as the gold standard, not merely a single anecdotal case study relying on chance events. Clinical judgement relies on reading appropriate literature and attending reputable symposia. Finally, personal experience, although invaluable, should not shroud or bias decision making. What works for one patient, is not a universal therapy for every patient.

Choosing the most appropriate treatment for a given clinical finding is influenced by the three components of evidence-based therapy: clinical erudition, sound scientific research and patients' needs and wants. For any given predicament, there are many solutions that yield the desired result. However, each modality should be assessed according to risks and, eventually, benefits.[9] For example, an accidental fracture of the maxillary incisor has the following treatment options (Fig. 1.9):

(1) Restore with a direct composite filling:
  - Benefits – minimally invasive, immediate, economical
  - Risks – technique-sensitive bonding procedures, future staining of composite, microleakage leading to endodontic involvement and compromised aesthetics, requiring replacement fillings and possible root canal therapy (RCT)

(2) Restore with indirect ceramic prosthesis (veneer or full coverage crown):
  - Benefits – excellent aesthetics using an all-ceramic restoration
  - Risks – highly destructive, technique-sensitive procedures, possible endodontic involvement due to tooth preparation trauma, use of a skilled (and therefore costly) ceramist to match a single crown with adjacent teeth, protracted, expensive, porcelain fracture due to improper clinical or laboratory protocols

(3) Extraction and immediate replacement with endosseous implant and implant supported crown:
  - Benefits – immediate, avoids future endodontic complications
  - Risks – surgical involvement, possible unpredictable soft and hard tissue healing with compromised aesthetics, use of a skilled (and therefore costly) ceramist to match a single crown with adjacent teeth, protracted, expensive

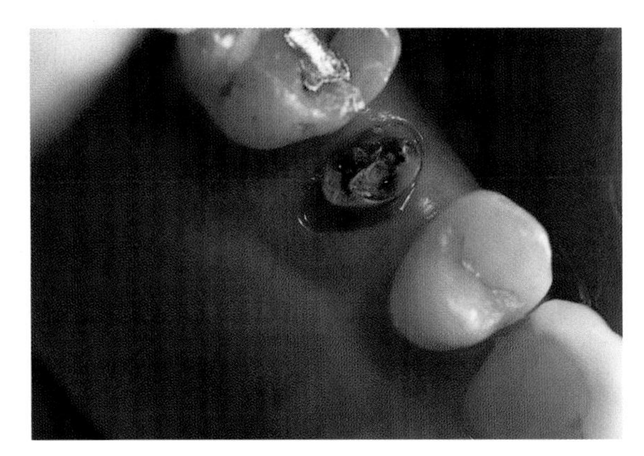

Figure 1.10 Fractured crown on root-filled second premolar.

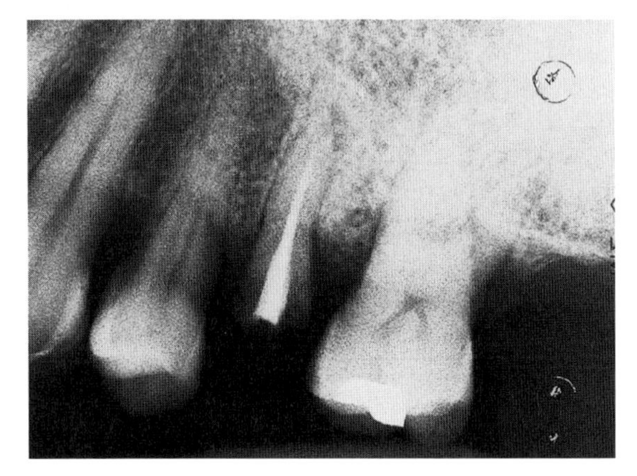

Figure 1.11 Radiograph of tooth in Figure 1.10 showing a thin root cross section and periapical radiolucency.

Another example is a fractured crown at the cervical margin, on a root-filled premolar with periapical radiolucency but no active suppuration (Figs. 1.10 & 1.11). The treatment options are:

(1) Re-RCT with intra-radicular support and replacement crown:
- Benefits – established clinical protocols for treatment modalities
- Risks – further trauma from re-RCT and post placement to an already weakening, delicate root, relapse of re-RCT, compromised retention for definitive crown and protracted treatment plan

(2) Apicectomy with intra-radicular support and replacement crown:
- Benefits – retrograde filling without inflicting trauma to delicate root from re-RCT
- Risks – shortening of root, resulting in poor root-to-crown ratio, compromised retention for definitive crown and protracted treatment plan

(3) Crown lengthening or orthodontic extrusion to increase retention and resistance form for definitive crown in conjunction with options (1) or (2):
- Benefits – exposure of root surface for definitive crown margin placement
- Risks – shortening of root, resulting in poor root-to-crown ratio and protracted treatment plan

(4) Extraction and immediate replacement with endosseous implant and implant supported crown:
- Benefits – expedient, predictable, but requires surgical experience and expertise
- Risks – surgical involvement. Local anatomy must be suitable with sufficient quality and quantity of soft and hard tissue volume for success

The patient opted for the last proposal. Firstly, the costs of all the options were similar. Secondly, the bone and soft tissue anatomy were conducive for successful immediate implant placement with immediate temporarisation, including sufficient bone apical to root apex primarily for stability, adequate mesial-distal implant-to-tooth distance of 1.5 mm and occlusal clearance (Figs. 1.12–1.16).

Arriving at the most appropriate treatment plan involves clinical findings and a definitive diagnosis, risk assessment, followed by an evidence-based approach (clinical erudition, sound scientific research and patients' needs and wants). Using evidence-based decision making and treatment planning maintains professional competence and competitiveness for delivering high quality, predictable treatment. When using an evidence-based approach, it is important to appreciate that this principle is not dogmatic but

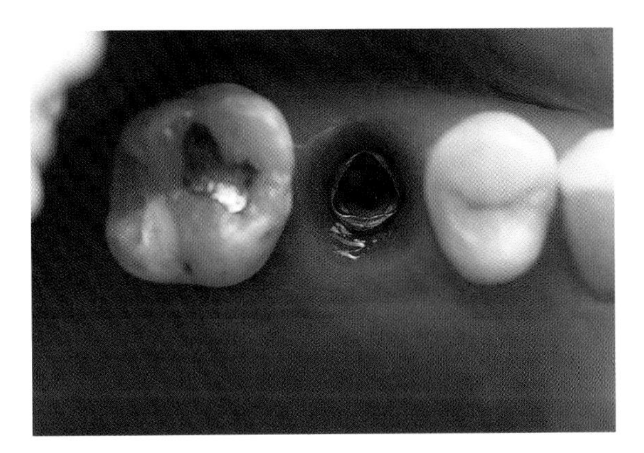

Figure 1.12 Immediate placement of implant fixture (Replace Select, Nobel Biocare) following atraumatic extraction.

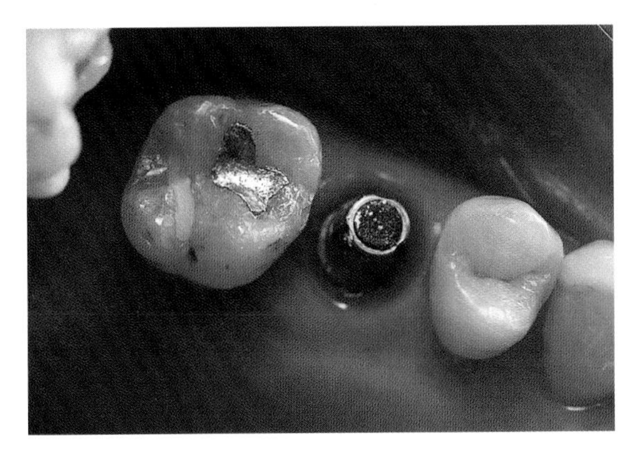

Figure 1.13 Abutment with occlusal plug prior to immediate provisionalisation.

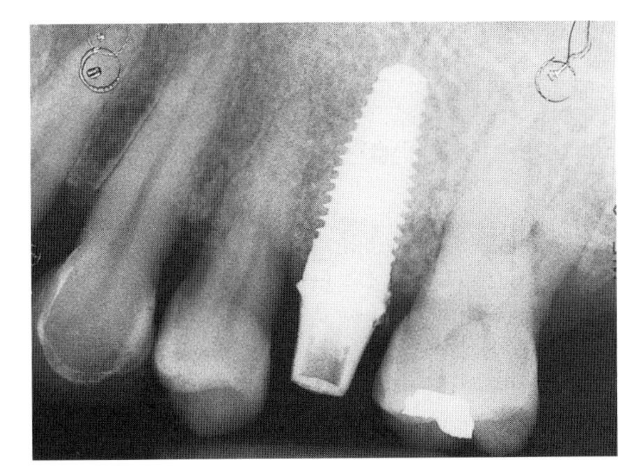

Figure 1.14 Four-month radiograph showing osseointegration.

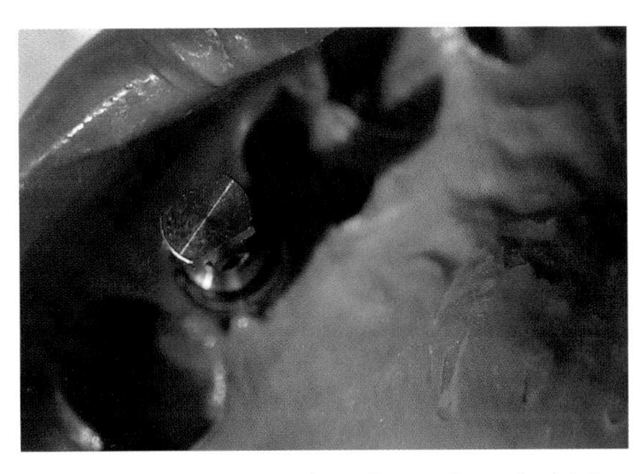

Figure 1.15 Impression with implant analogue for fabrication of definitive crown.

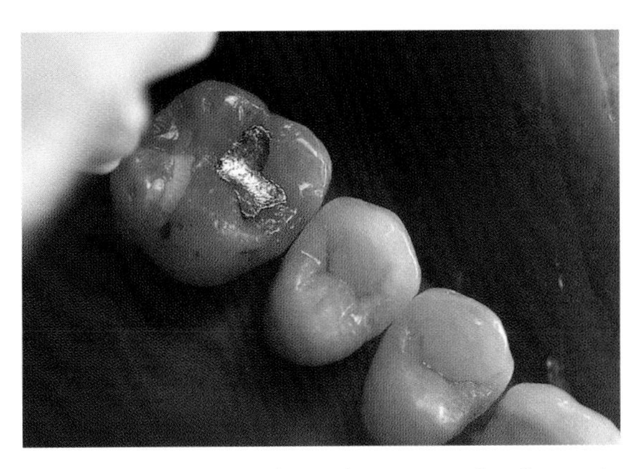

Figure 1.16 Cemented implant-supported all-ceramic crown (compare with Figure 1.10).

pragmatic, incorporating clinical experience as well as respecting patients' preferences and desires.[10]

Presenting treatment plan proposals to the patient

A treatment plan is a proposal, not a military procedure. In fact, treatment can change due to a myriad of reasons, including the patient's ambivalence, prevailing clinical presentations, unforeseen complications, financial burdens, etc. At the onset, it is the clinician's duty to convey the flexibility and fluidity of the proposed treatment, indicating that as treatment

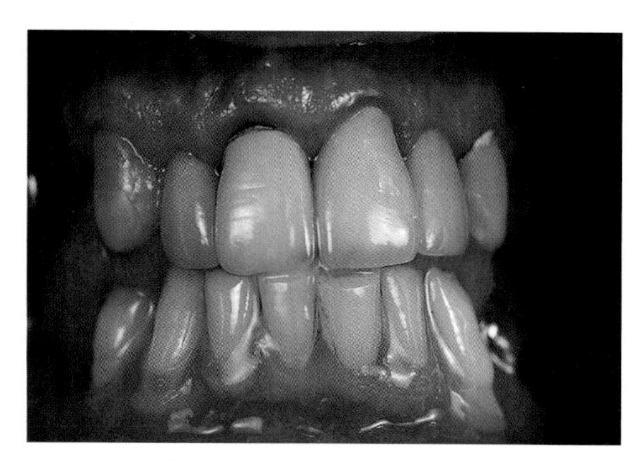

Figure 1.17 The patient was unaware of the defective anterior maxillary restorations, which are a potential site for a future disease process.

progresses, changes or alterations may be desirable or mandatory.

The presentation should encompass simple and clear verbal and written communication. Visual aids, such as radiographs, scans, study models and pictures, add credence to the written and spoken word. When starting a new aesthetic practice, it is often difficult to show treatment carried out by the clinician, and using information leaflets and dental journals is extremely helpful. However, over time, it is invaluable to build up a portfolio, especially for sceptics, who may question competence of the operator. Furthermore, showing one's own work further enhances confidence and convinces patients that what is proposed has been previously achieved by the treating dentist.

Many patients are oblivious of disease processes in their mouth, and visual aids are invaluable for raising awareness of potential or current problems (Fig. 1.17). Numerous visual aids are available, ranging from a face mirror to the latest computer software. For aesthetic treatment, intra- and extra-oral cameras are crucial at every stage of therapy, starting with pre-operative status, aesthetic analysis, shade analysis, potential complications, patient acceptance of aesthetics and post-operative results.[11] As well as a presentation tool, high-quality imagery is important for patient–dentist–specialist–ceramist communication and medico-legal documentation, especially if treatment does not proceed as anticipated. A checklist of items required, together with their diagnostic value is as follows:

- Extra- and intra-oral photographs – aesthetic and shade analysis, pathology and defective existing restorations
- Computer-generated simulations showing proposed treatment possibilities. Although useful, this form of simulation is potentially problematic since the simulation may not be clinically feasible. It is probably wiser to use a wax-up, a 'real' as opposed to a 'virtual' 3D object which can show the possibilities of a specific option
- Radiographs – infection, caries, defective margins, root fillings, bone loss, vital structures
- Scans showing bone quality and quantity if implants are considered
- Mounted study casts – occlusal assessment
- Diagnostic wax-up – intended design of the restorations (Figs. 1.18 & 1.19)
- Results of any bacteriological tests – modify periodontal therapy
- Technologically based caries and periodontal tests – verify clinical findings
- Practice internet web site – useful for showing patients the practice profile, and the type of work achievable by the treating clinician

Having gathered the visual aids, the next stage is conveying these to the patient in a logical and

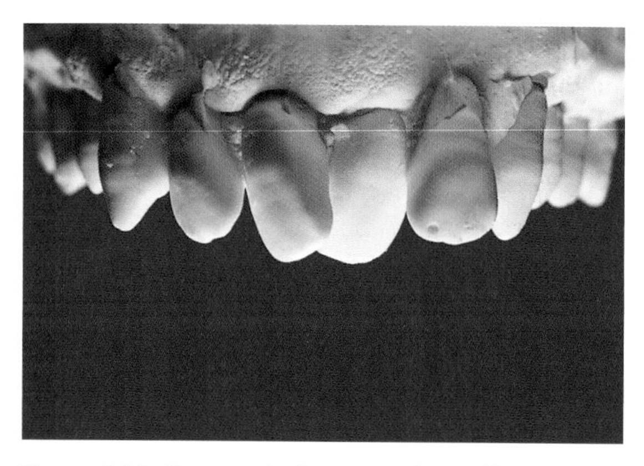

Figure 1.18 Severe misalignment of maxillary anterior sextant.

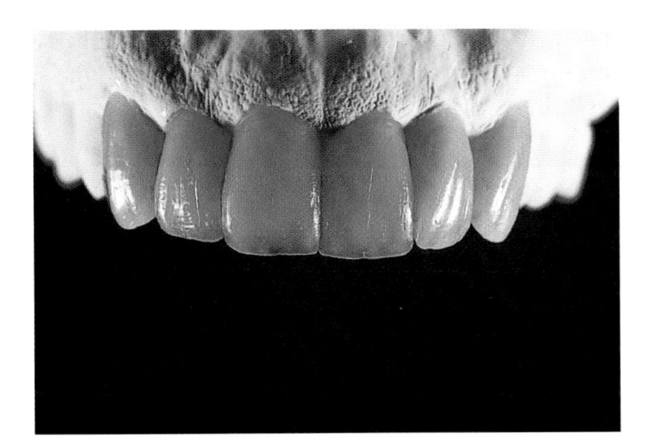

Figure 1.19 Diagnostic wax-up showing proposed appearance for maxillary incisors and canines for patient in Figure 1.18 (laboratory work by Jason Kim, New York).

organised manner. Communication is both verbal and written. Verbal communication should take place in a serene, unfettered, relaxed, unrushed ambience. The choice of words should be non-technical, non-emotive and non-phobic.[12] For example, describing intricate details of an apicectomy, including suppuration and haemorrhage details, is likely to alienate patients. Conversely, describing an apicectomy as removing bacteria, improving function and appearance is more palatable. Cautionary discretion is required regarding the current craze for cosmetic 'extreme makeovers'. These trends are predominately media propagated, often prejudicing the layman into the belief that cosmetic wonders can fulfil and enrich their lives. These views are rapidly entering dentistry, with the result that treatment is often patient driven. There is also an emerging breed of clinicians prejudging patients' desires and influencing their decisions in favour of these makeovers. Unfortunately, the motive behind this influencing is purely fiscal, where marketing takes precedence over ethics and clinical necessity. Furthermore, dentistry is not the fashion industry. It is very easy to throw away a garment once its haute couture appeal has elapsed, which is not the case for 'cosmetic restorations' created by irreversible destruction of natural teeth. The morality of this dilemma resides with the clinician.

Ultimately, the written word forms a contract between the dentist and patient. Once again, the wording should be non-technical, outlining the present clinical situation, treatment options with benefits and risks of each procedure (with scientifically based prognosis for a specific treatment option), expected time scale, costs, methods of payments and practice polices (e.g. failed appointments), and guarantees. The treatment plan should also incorporate informed consent. Informed consent, as required by most US states, has the following six elements:[13]

- Correct diagnosis of symptoms and findings
- Nature and purpose of proposed treatment
- Risks of treatment
- Likelihood of success
- Alternative options
- Prognosis

Treatment

The last part of APT is treatment. Treatment is influenced by biological, clinical, psychosocial and economic factors.[14] The biological factors include systemic and nutritional health, as well as local factors, such as periodontal biotype. Clinical aspects include knowledge, techniques and manual dexterity of the operator, while economic constraints determine the degree of sophistication of the proposed treatment. As stated above, an evidence-based approach is proactive intervention, promoting oral health, reducing tooth loss and minimising the need for future complex therapy.[15]

As well as using an evidence-based approach, aesthetic treatment also relies on the clinician's and ceramist's artistic flare. At the outset, the operator should exercise clinical self-deprecation, stepping back and asking whether he or she possesses the technical competence, experience, psychological knowledge and artistic ability to perform aesthetic treatment. One must appreciate individual limitations, professional responsibilities, effective communication and a collaborative effort when delivering quality care. Furthermore, aesthetic treatment is not the remit of every dental practice. Some practices provide routine, stereotypical, run-of-the mill treatment.

If this is the case, then referral to a specialist is prudent; the specialist should have an individual, 'more than just a restoration' approach. As a concluding comment: perfection takes time and experience, but optimal dentistry is, and should be, a tangible goal for every practice.[16]

Once a treatment plan is accepted, the stages of execution can be considered. Most aesthetic treatment plans are multiphase and multidisciplinary. The following is a summary of the chronological stages. Every stage may not be applicable for every patient, but is listed for the sake of completion. When moving from one stage to the next, it is important to remember that therapy should follow the health, function and aesthetics (HFA) triad discussed in Chapter 2.

(1) Alleviate pain and stabilise active disease
(2) Restore oral health by prophylactic measures
(3) Perform APT (assessment, planning, treatment)
(4) Ensure medical diseases are controlled or under supervision
(5) Liaise with specialist(s) for advice or treatment of skeletal, orthodontic, mucogingival or osseous anomalies
(6) Liaise with ceramist regarding shade analysis and feasibility of proposed aesthetic treatment
(7) Commence treatment

Clinical case study

The clinical case study below illustrates a systematic approach to treatment using APT.

Assessment

Initial consultation

The patient was referred by an implantologist for improvement of anterior aesthetics. The lady was 40 years old, intelligent, elegant, sophisticated and affable. She was distraught and very concerned about her dentition, recalled previous unpleasant dental experiences and failures and was sceptical about future treatment.

Histories

- Medical history – no systemic illness or medication
- Risk history – no genetic predisposition to periodontal disease, high socio-economic status, no occupational hazards, non-smoker, regular exercise, health conscious
- Nutritional history – healthy diet
- Dental history – regular attendance, visits to hygienist, poor-quality previous dental treatment, no records available from former dentist

Examination

- Chief complaint – improve anterior dental aesthetics
- Visual – no lymph swellings, low lip line (upper lip concealed maxillary incisors – Fig. 1.20)
- Intra-oral – no soft or hard tissue pathology. Retained deciduous canines, congenitally missing maxillary lateral incisors, with mesial drifting of the canines distal to the central incisors
- Triangular-shaped, chipped maxillary centrals lacking dominance due to the wide pseudo-lateral incisors. Thin scalloped periodontal biotype. Defective and chipped porcelain laminate veneers on the secondary canines (to simulate the missing laterals) and deciduous canines (to simulate secondary canines). Plaque and calculus build-up, staining and discolouration of anterior teeth. Gingival zeniths of pseudo-lateral incisors apical to central incisors (Figs. 1.21–1.23)
- Occlusion – steep anterior guidance, resulting in fractured laminates on secondary canines. Right and left group function, no eccentric working or non-working contacts, and absence of parafunctional activity
- Tactile – no muscular spasm or TMJ dysfunction
- Written – aesthetic evaluation questionnaire revealed that patient was enthusiastic about restoring her smile, but cynical due to previous poor-quality treatment

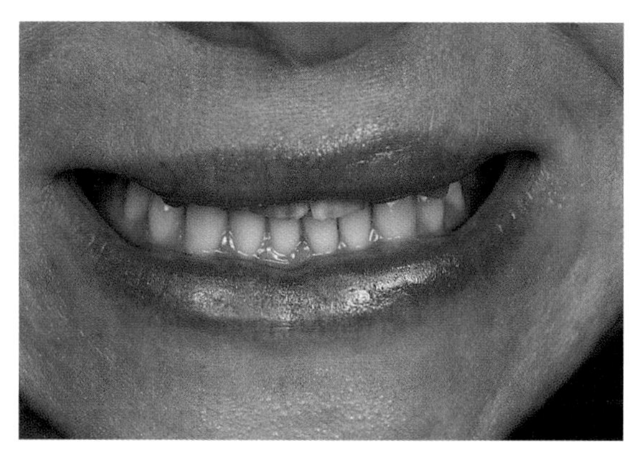

Figure 1.20 Low maxillary lip line concealing cervical margins of maxillary anterior teeth.

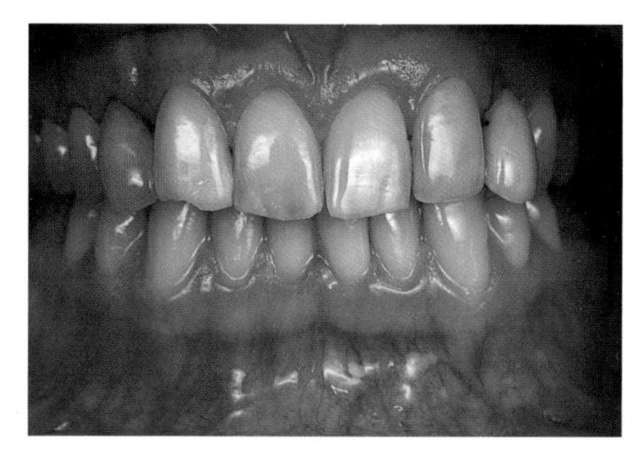

Figure 1.21 Pre-operative status in centric occlusion (see text for details).

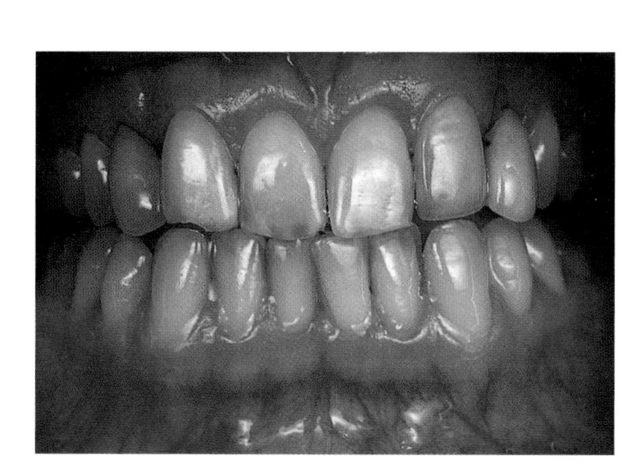

Figure 1.22 Pre-operative status in anterior protrusive excursion (see text for details).

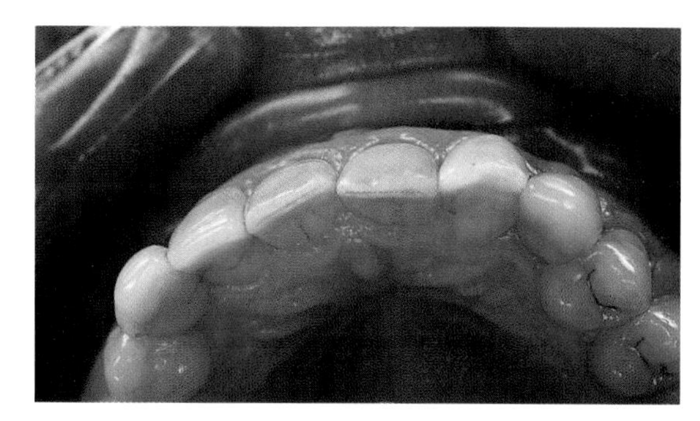

Figure 1.23 Pre-operative status: occlusal view (see text for details).

Technological

- Radiographs – periapicals showed complete root absorption of retained deciduous canine and local inflammation necessitating immediate extraction (Figs. 1.24 & 1.25).
- Upper and lower pre-operative impression with facebow and jaw registrations for mounting on semi-adjustable articulator for detailed occlusal assessment
- Diagnostic wax-up to assess feasibility of treatment options for improving anterior aesthetics (Figs. 1.26 & 1.27)
- Photographic – facial, dentofacial and detailed dental images with 35 mm camera
- Scans – none
- Shade analysis – using two shade guides, Vita Classic and Vita 3D (Figs. 1.28 & 1.29)
- Pulp vitality – all anterior teeth vital, with no periapical lesions
- Bacterial and biopsy tests – none

Planning

Diagnosis

Poor-quality dental restorations, poor anterior aesthetics, calculus and plaque deposits, staining, fractured and defective laminates on pseudo-laterals, chipped incisal edges on central incisors. Resorbed and deficient (bucco-palatal) alveolar ridge at extracted deciduous canine sites.

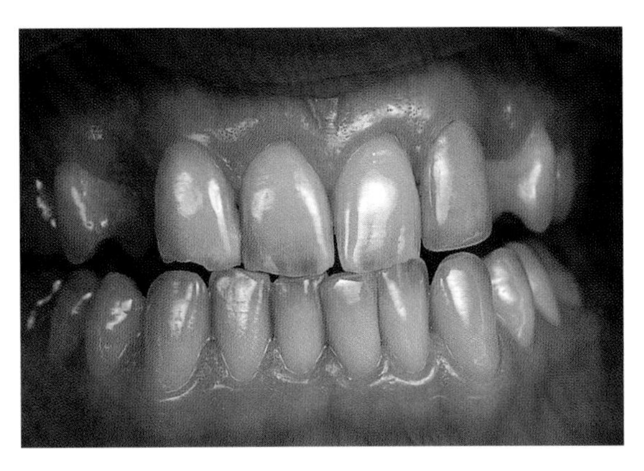

Figure 1.24 Extraction of retained deciduous canines (facial view).

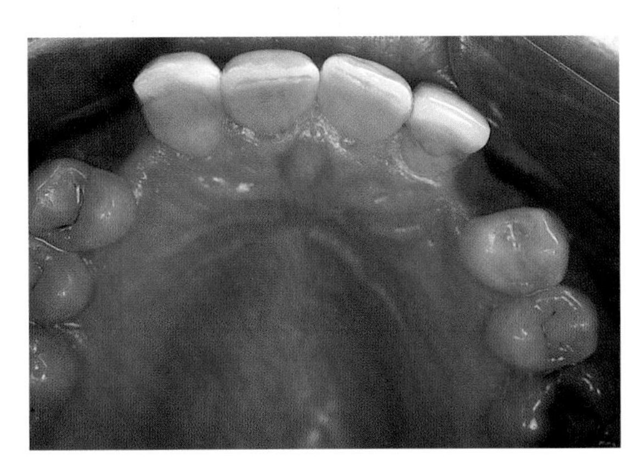

Figure 1.25 Extraction of retained deciduous canines (occlusal view).

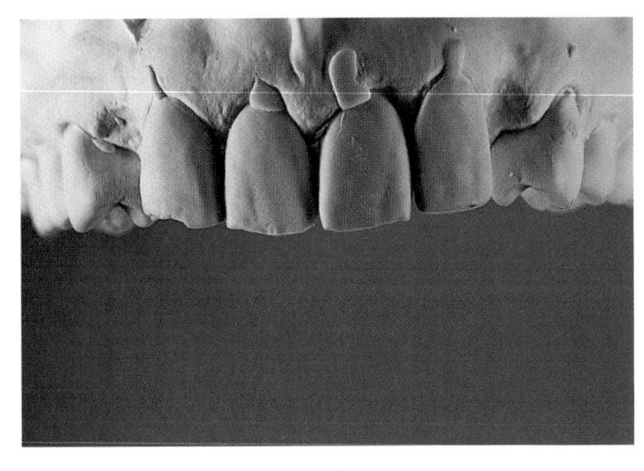

Figure 1.26 Pre-operative study cast.

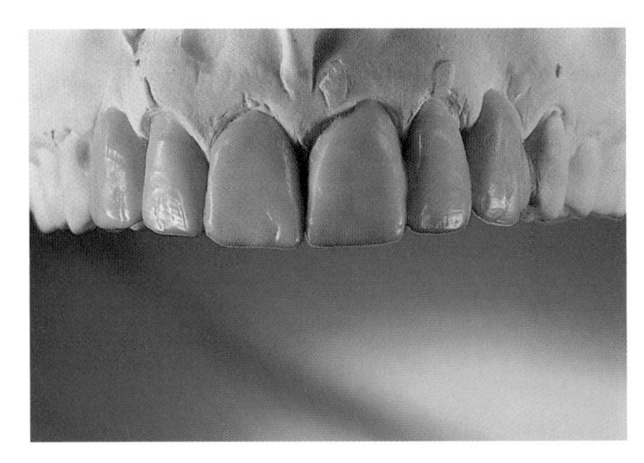

Figure 1.27 Diagnostic wax-up for anterior maxillary sextant.

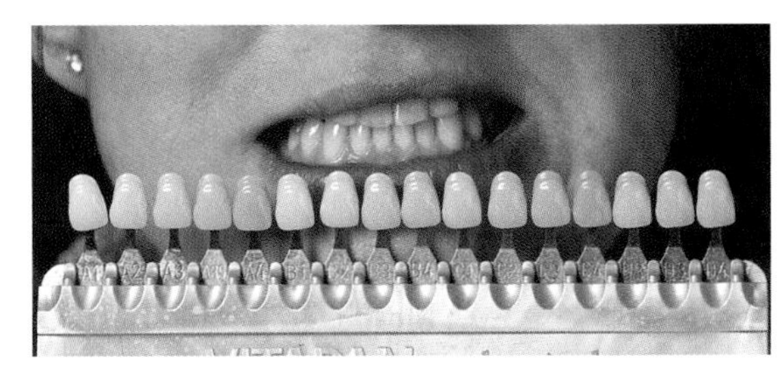

Figure 1.28 Shade analysis using the Vital Classic shade guide.

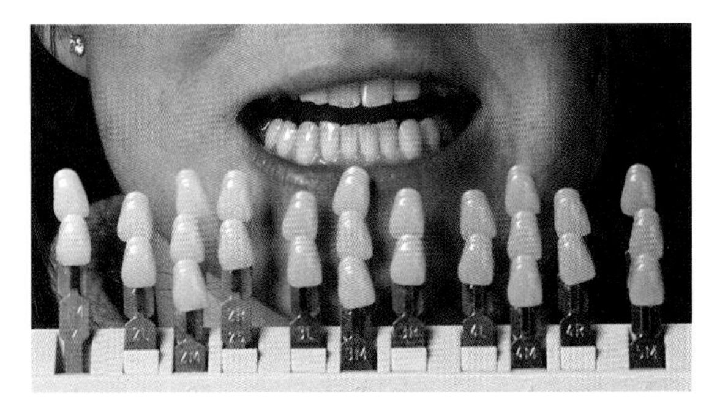

Figure 1.29 Shade analysis using the Vita 3D shade guide.

Mesial-distal space between pseudo-laterals and first premolar = 4 mm on each side of the arch, insufficient for implant placement. A minimum of 1.5 mm implant-to-tooth distance required, and even using a small platform fixture (3.5 mm), the prevailing 4 mm space is inadequate.

Treatment objectives

- Maintainance of existing occlusal scheme
- Dominance of maxillary centrals
- Narrower maxillary pseudo-laterals
- Resolving apically located gingival zeniths of pseudo-laterals
- Replacement of missing canines
- Improvement of colour of mandibular teeth

Risk assessment

Low risk of periodontal disease due to shallow pockets, no systemic illness, no genetic predisposition to periodontitis, regular dental attendance, healthy diet. However, the thin scalloped periodontal biotype necessitates care with restorative or surgical procedures to prevent gingival recession.

Evidence-based decision making and treatment

The treatment options presented to the patient were as follows:

(1) Removable upper denture
   - Benefits – expedient, non-invasive, economical
   - Risks – anti-social, onerous, food trapping, temporary solution, future replacement dentures, accelerated wear and staining of acrylic artificial teeth

(2) Bleaching mandibular teeth
   - Benefits – predictable, immediate gratification, economical
   - Risks – sensitivity, may require repeated application(s) to achieve desired result

(3) Orthodontics to increase space between pseudo-laterals and first premolar to allow endosseous fixtures (with bone grafting) and eventual implant-supported crowns. The apically located gingival zenith on the pseudo-laterals could also be rectified by orthodontic extrusion or soft tissue grafts
   - Benefits – refined, complicated, state-of-the-art treatment, minimally invasive
   - Risks – protracted, bone or root absorption due to orthodontic movement, orthodontic retainers, surgical complications, such as infection, bone loss and unpredictable soft tissue contours, costly

(4) The prosthodontic solution consisting of porcelain laminate veneers (PLVs) on the centrals, with a fixed partial denture (either two distal cantilevers from the pseudo-laterals, or two three-unit bridges from pseudo-laterals to first premolars)
   - Benefits – excellent aesthetics, expedient, predictable
   - Risks – highly invasive, technique-sensitive, possible future endodontic involvement of prepared teeth, costly

In isolation, none of the above options resolves all the treatment objectives. In order to arrive at a definitive treatment plan, more than one of the above options is necessary. After considering these four options, the patient opted for option (2) (bleaching) with option (4) (prosthodontic solution). Using an evidence-based approach, the following require consideration:

- Clinical erudition – knowledge, skill and experience. It was decided to adhere to the existing occlusal scheme, group function on both sides. Additionally, PLVs were chosen instead of full coverage crowns because of the steep anterior guidance, and a protrusive slide on natural tooth surfaces would ensure better long-term function
- Sound scientific research – bleaching is a predictable modality if judicially applied. PLVs are also predictable using an adhesive protocol for cementation. In order to maximise aesthetics, an all-ceramic alumina bridge was selected (In-Ceram, Vita), which has a reasonable short- to medium-term success rate for anterior regions of the mouth (see Chapter 3)
- Patient's needs and wants – the treatment plan was finalised once the patient expressed her wishes. The lady was totally against sur-

gical intervention and refused protracted treatment duration due to previous dental failures. Since the lip line was low, it was decided to accept the apical zeniths of the pseudo-laterals. She was also adamant about improving the tooth colour of her anterior mandibular teeth

Treatment

The treatment sequence is as follows:

(1) Achieve periodontal health and stability by prophylaxis and oral hygiene instructions
(2) Provide bleaching trays and allow 3–4 weeks for colour stabilisation before final shade determination
(3) Liaise with ceramist for detailed shade and aesthetic analysis using wax-up, photographs and discussions with patient
(4) Tooth preparations for PLVs on central incisors, and two fixed partial dentures from pseudo-laterals to first premolars. Use temporary restorations to assess health, form, occlusion, phonetics and creating ovate pontic sites for missing canines (Figs. 1.30–1.32)
(5) Verify shade after tooth preparation, especially for PLV on central incisors (Fig. 1.33)
(6) Once gingival margins are healthy and stable, make final impressions with facebow and jaw registrations (Fig. 1.34)
(7) In the dental laboratory, pour two plaster models; leave one untrimmed to confirm emergence profile and cervical contours; the second trimmed dies are mounted on an articulator for fabrication of the definitive prostheses (Figs.1.35 & 1.36)
(8) Try-in restorations, check fit, occlusion, phonetics and aesthetics (Figs. 1.37 & 1.38). In this instance the following anomalies were apparent (Fig. 1.39):
    (i) Incorrect axial inclination of the right canine pontic and left pseudo-lateral
    (ii) Marginal discrepancies on mesiobuccal and palatal aspects of abutment 14, and palatal aspects of abutments 22 and 24
    (iii) Patient requested removal of interproximal staining between pseudo-laterals and canines and a reduction in the cervical chroma stains
(9) Since the marginal discrepancies of the alumina framework cannot be corrected by adding porcelain, new bridges were fabricated. The result is shown in Fig. 1.40, correcting the aberrations listed above
(10) The restorations were cemented by using an adhesive technique with a resin luting agent
(11) The post-operative status shows impeccable periodontal health and aesthetic integration of the PLVs and fixed partial dentures (FPDs) (Figs. 1.41–1.43). The original treatment objectives are achieved as follows:
    (i) Maintenance of existing occlusal scheme
    (ii) Dominance of maxillary centrals
    (iii) Narrower maxillary pseudo-laterals
    (iv) Apically located gingival zeniths of pseudo-laterals are hidden by the low lip line
    (v) The missing canines have been replaced
    (vi) Improvement of colour of mandibular teeth

The treatment plan above has followed three sequential steps, achieving periodontal health, occlusal and phonetic function, and anterior aesthetics (the HFA triad), which is the theme of the next chapter.

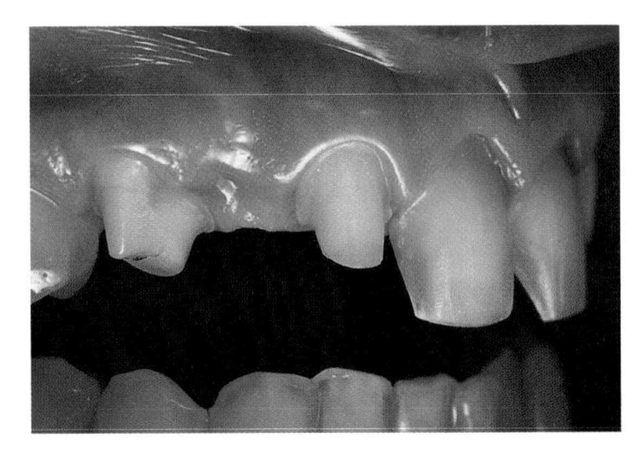

Figure 1.30 Right lateral view of tooth preparations.

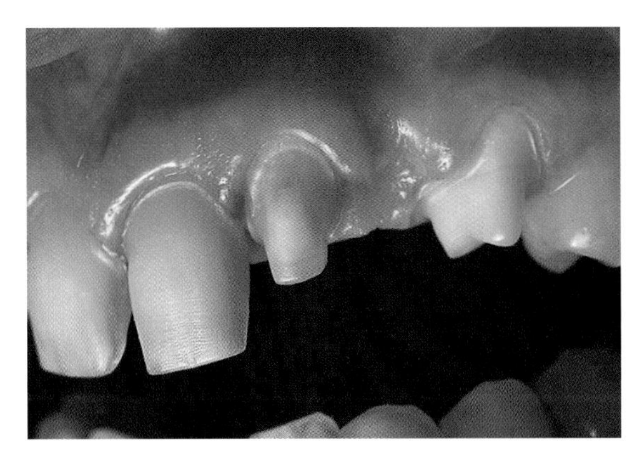

Figure 1.31 Left lateral view of tooth preparations.

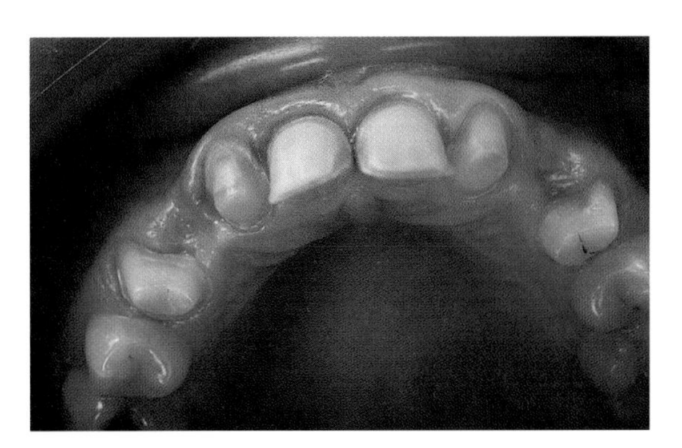

Figure 1.32 Occlusal view of tooth preparations.

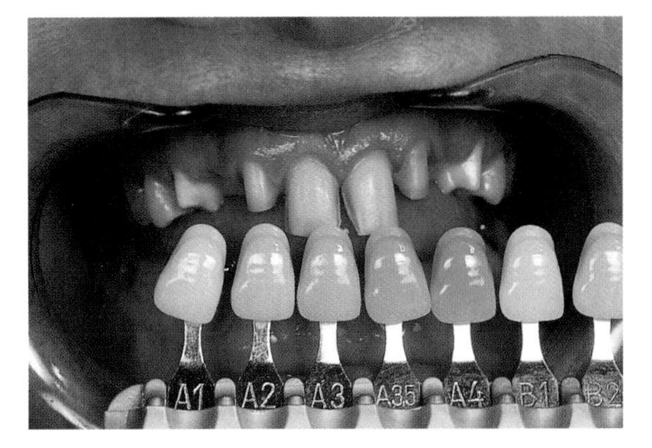

Figure 1.33 Shade analysis after tooth preparation using the Vital Classic shade guide.

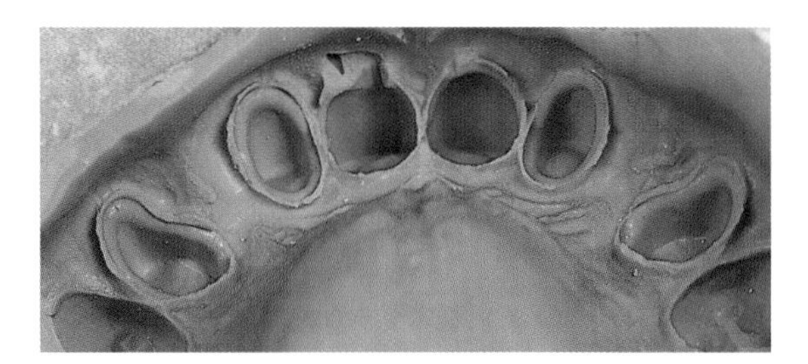

Figure 1.34 Definitive maxillary arch impression using an addition silicone material (Provil Novo, Heraeus Kulzer).

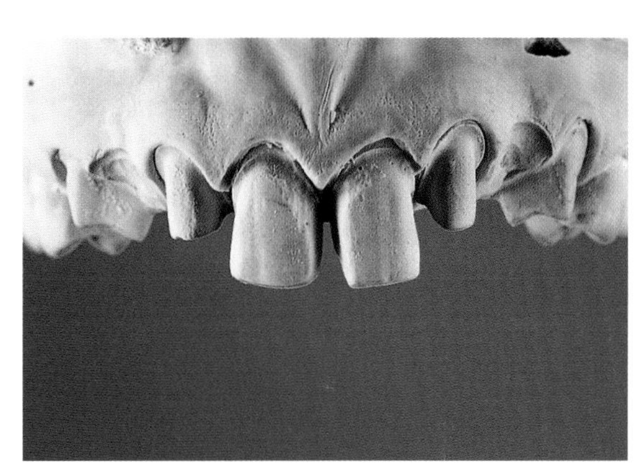

Figure 1.35 Untrimmed master cast.

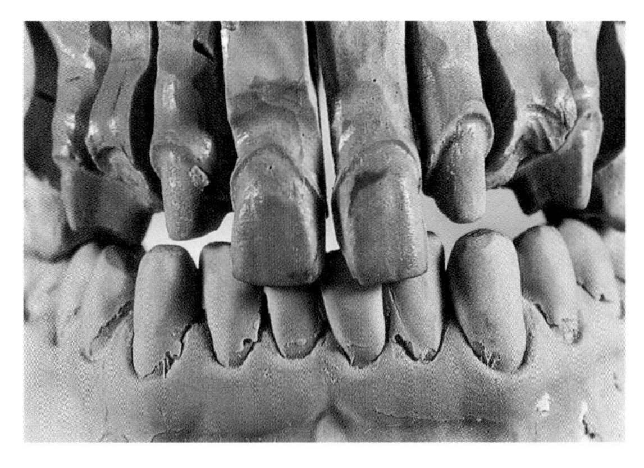

Figure 1.36 Trimmed model and dies mounted on semi-adjustable articulator.

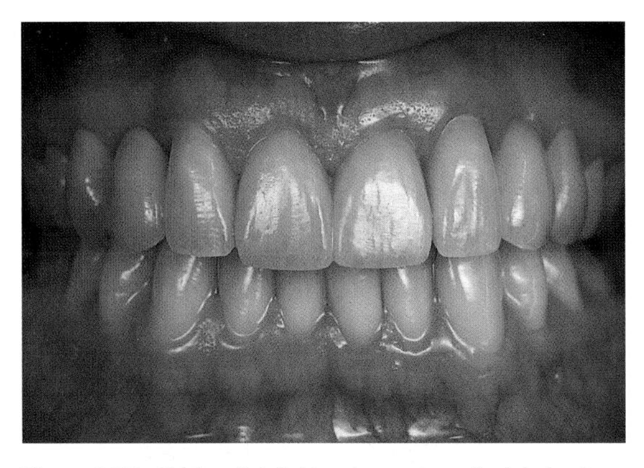

Figure 1.37 Try-in of definitive restorations (facial view).

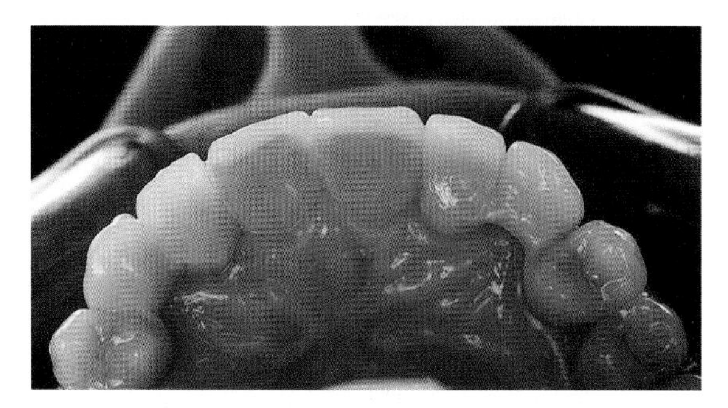

Figure 1.38 Try-in of definitive restorations (occlusal view).

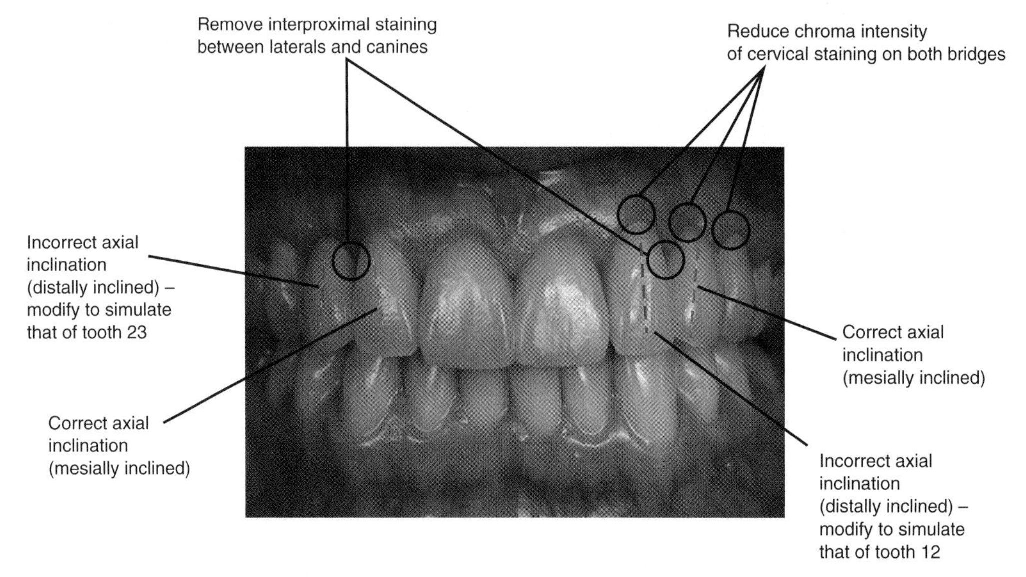

Figure 1.39 Evaluating aesthetic and technical faults at try-in stage.

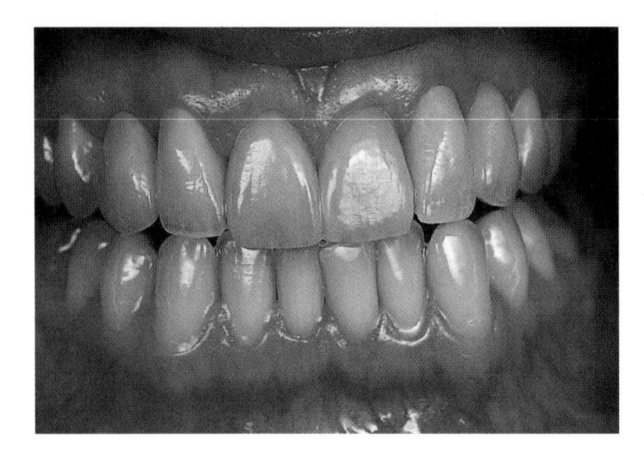

Figure 1.40 Post-operative view after correcting faults at try-in stage.

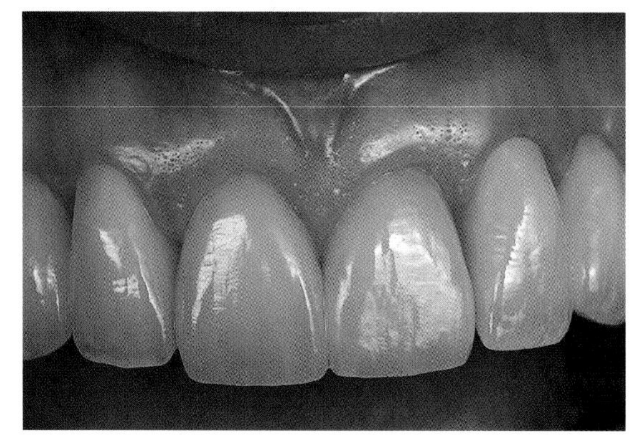

Figure 1.41 Post-operative 1:1 view showing aesthetic improvement, and immaculate integration of laminates and ceramic bridges with a healthy surrounding periodontium.

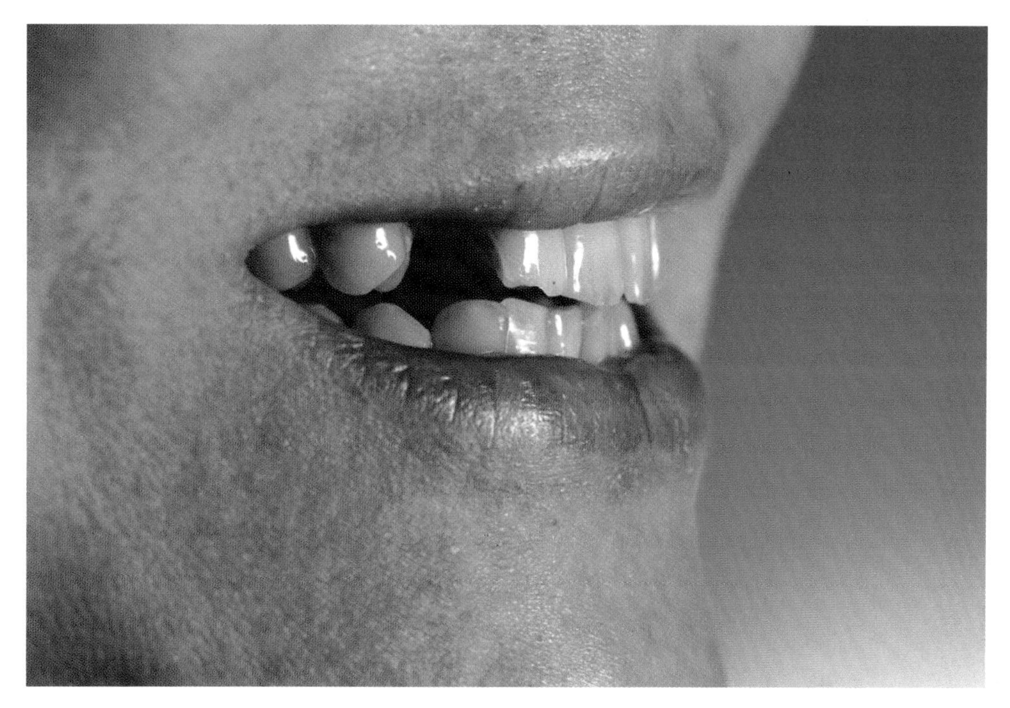

Figure 1.42 Pre-operative lateral dento-facial view.

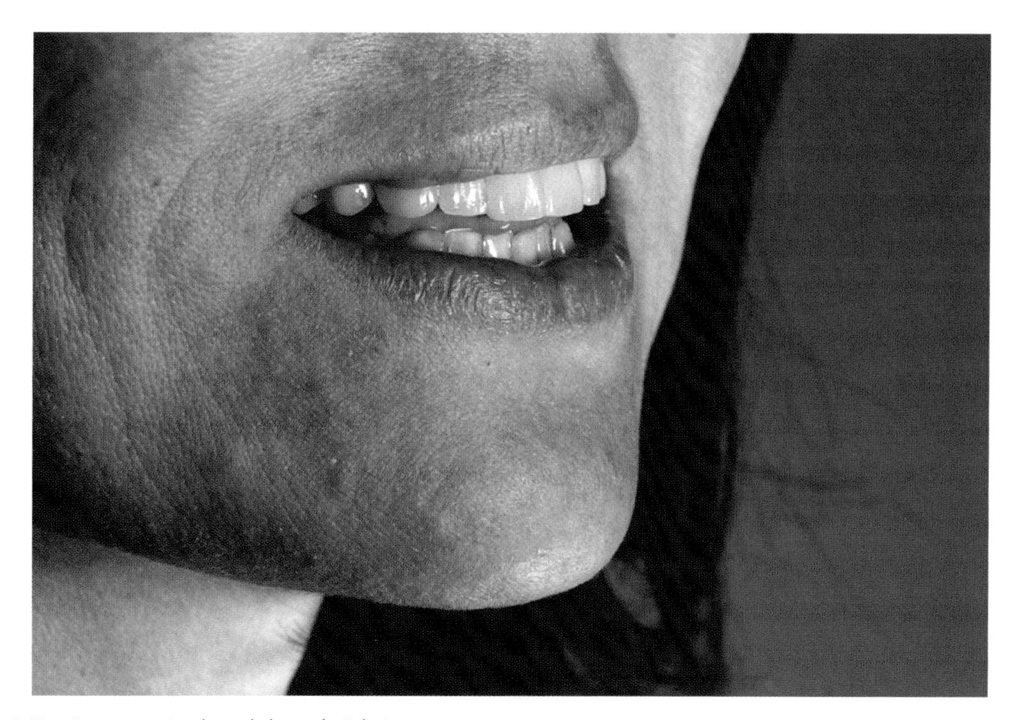

Figure 1.43 Post-operative lateral dento-facial view.

References

[1] Payne, S.H. (1968) Knowledge and skills in the practice of prosthodontics. *J Pros Dent*, **20(3)**, 255–257

[2] Misch, C.E. (1990) Division of available bone in implant dentistry. *Int J Oral Implantol*, **7**, 9–17

[3] Glick, M. (2005) Scope of practice: A matter of skills, knowledge and erudition. *JADA*, **136**, 430–431

[4] Axelsson, P., Lindhe, J. and Nystrom, B. (1991) On the prevention of caries and periodontal disease. Results of a 15-year longitudinal study in adults. *J Clin Periodontol*, **18**, 182–189

[5] Persson, G.R., Mancl, L.A., Martin, J. and Page, R.C. Assessing periodontal disease risk: a comparison of clinicians' assessment versus a computerized tool. *JADA*, **134**, 575–582

[6] Page, R.C., Martin, J.A. and Loeb, C.F. (2004) Use of risk assessment in attaining and maintaining oral health. *Compendium*, **25(9)**, 657–669

[7] Robbins, J.W. (1998) Evidence-based dentistry: What it is, and what does it have to do with practice? Anecdote vs. data – a case for evidence-based decision making. *Quintessence Int*, **29(12)**, 796–799

[8] Sackett, D.l., Rosenberg, W.M., Gray, J.A., Haynes, R.B. and Richardson, W.S. (1996) Evidence based medicine: what it is and what it isn't. *Br Med J*, **312**, 71–72

[9] McGuire, M.K. and Newman, M.G. (1995) Evidence-based periodontal treatment I. A strategy for clinical decisions. *J Periodontics Restorative Dent*, **15**, 71–83

[10] Newman, M.G. (1998) Improved clinical decision making using the evidence-based approach. *JADA*, **129**, 4–8

[11] Ahmad, I. (2004) *Digital and Conventional Dental Photography: A Practical Clinical Manual*. Quintessence Publishing Co. Inc., Chicago

[12] Bain, C. (2004) Treatment planning in general dental practice: Case presentation and communication with the patient. *Dental Update*, **March**, 72–82

[13] Mills, E.J. (2002) A clinical method for the diagnosis and treatment planning of restorative dental patients. *J Oral Implantol*, **28(3)**, 122–127

[14] Bader, J.D. and Ismail A.I. (1999) A primer on outcomes in dentistry. *J Publ Health Dent*, **59**, 131–135

[15] Axelsson, P., Paulander, J., Svardstrom, G. and Kaiser, H. (2000) Effects of population based preventive programs on oral health conditions. *J Parodontol Implantol Orale*, **19**, 255–269

[16] Drago, C.J. (1996) Clinical and laboratory parameters in fixed prosthetic treatment. *J Prosthet Dent*, **76**, 233–238

2 The health, function and aesthetic triad

Dental care can be succinctly defined by the health, function and aesthetic (HFA) triad. The primary aim of any therapy is resolution of disease, resulting in a state of well-being. It is important to realise the hierarchy of this triad, attainment of health, followed by function, followed by aesthetics. One can achieve health without function or aesthetics, and both health and function are possible without aesthetics. However, aesthetics are not possible if the first two, health and function, are absent.

To illustrate this, consider the following examples. A lateral incisor extracted following a hopeless prognosis of periapical infection achieves health, but not function or aesthetics (Fig. 2.1). Similarly, buccal amalgam fillings in the mandibular incisors achieve health and function, but are clearly unaesthetic (Fig. 2.2). Conversely, a beautifully fabricated crown for an anterior tooth without previously resolving periodontal and occlusal problems is prone to failure. The crown on the left lateral incisor is aesthetically acceptable, but due to poor periodontal health or occlusal disharmony, it is nevertheless perceived as unaesthetic (Fig. 2.3). Furthermore, because of these compromises, fracture, de-cementation or periodontal disease will ultimately cause failure. In the latter case, the treatment sequence should start by resolving periodontal and occlusal issues (health and function), before fabrication of the definitive crown.

The clinical sequence of the HFA triad is paramount for durability, longevity and success of all dental treatment. The discussion below outlines the constituents of the HFA triad (Fig. 2.4).

Health

Having treated gross soft and hard tissue pathology, the next step is achieving health of the dentition and surrounding periodontium. Attaining health of a tooth may involve decay removal, replacing defective fillings, investigating endodontic lesions or resolving occlusal dysfunction with any associated TMJ pathosis. In conjunction with the latter, a healthy periodontium is also essential for ensuring survival of a tooth. The rate of soft tissue healing depends on patient constitution, systemic disease, severity of the prevailing lesion and the degree of dental trauma during restorative procedures. This chapter focuses on general periodontal and

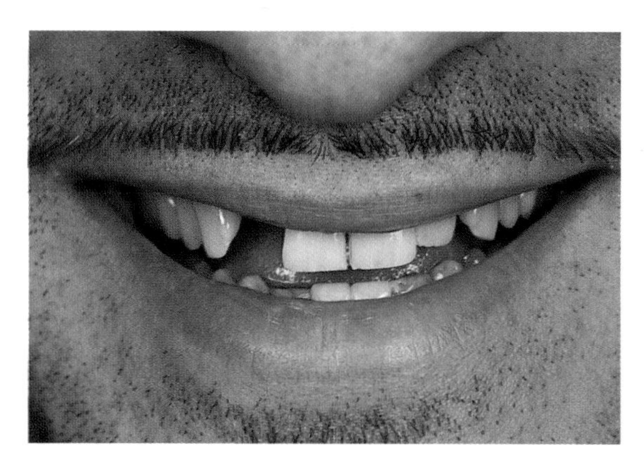

Figure 2.1 A missing right lateral incisor shows health, but lacks function and aesthetics.

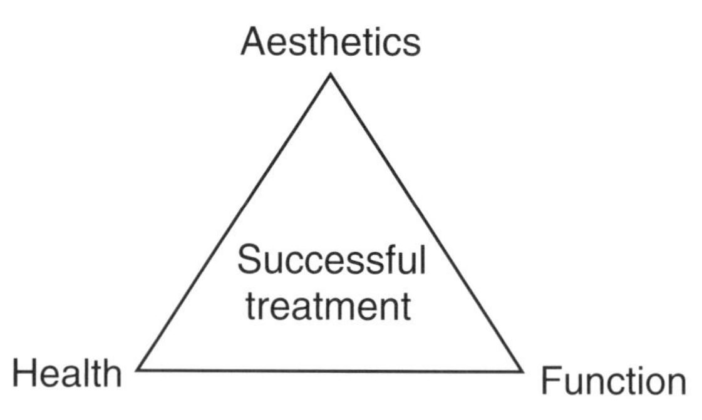

Figure 2.4 The HFA triad.

occlusal aspects, while ensuing chapters detail protocols for specific lesions.

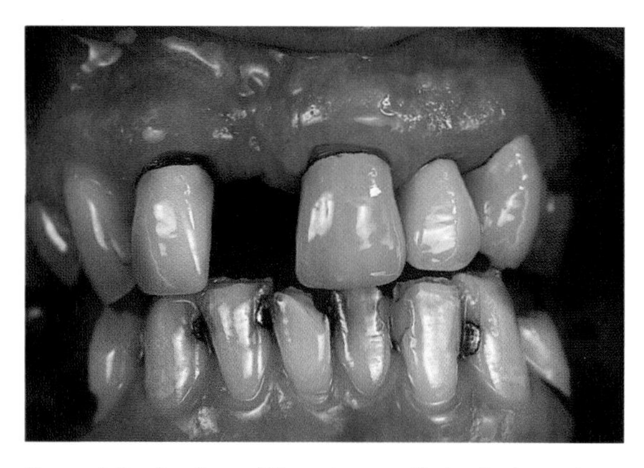

Figure 2.2 Amalgam fillings in mandibular incisors show health and function, but lack aesthetics.

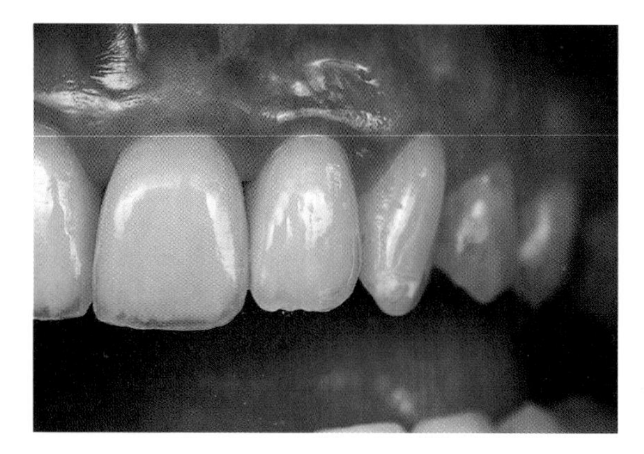

Figure 2.3 The crown on the left lateral incisor is aesthetic, but lacks periodontal health due to marginal inflammation.

The periodontium

Before commencing any reparative therapy to restore function and aesthetics, it is essential to achieve healthy tissues in the oral cavity. Only then can reconstruction of diseased and damaged tooth structure be predictably achieved and maintained.

Anatomy of the periodontium

The periodontium is a combination of hard and soft tissues. From a superficial aspect, the soft tissue covering is divided into the gingiva and alveolar mucosa. The gingiva is masticatory mucosa extending from the free gingival margin and terminating apically at the muco-gingival junction to become the alveolar mucosa (Fig. 2.5). The gingiva is keratinised and further divided into the free and attached gingiva, whose texture varies from a highly stippled to a smooth appearance. On occasions, an elevation of the free gingival margin, termed the gingival groove, is evident (Fig. 2.6). Both free and attached gingivae show huge variance in the linear dimensions (width), thickness (bucco-lingual), texture (degree of stippling) and colour (intensity of pink and/or physiological pigmentation) (Figs. 2.7–2.9). The width of the attached gingivae ranges from 0.5–8.0 mm, and its thickness from the free to attached sections decreases from

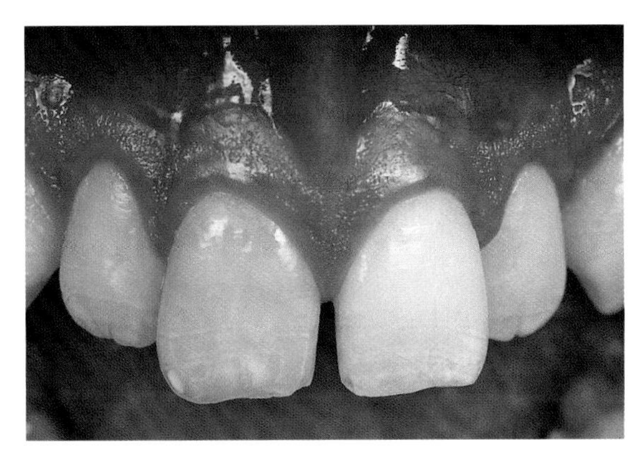

Figure 2.5 Superficial anatomy of the periodontium.

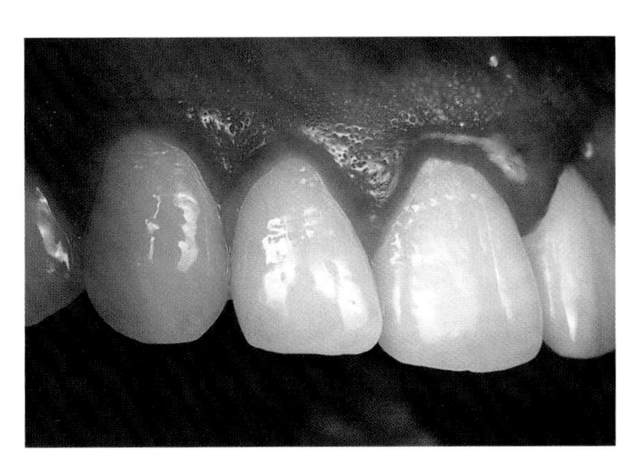

Figure 2.6 Elevation of the free gingival margin (FGM) is termed the gingival groove.

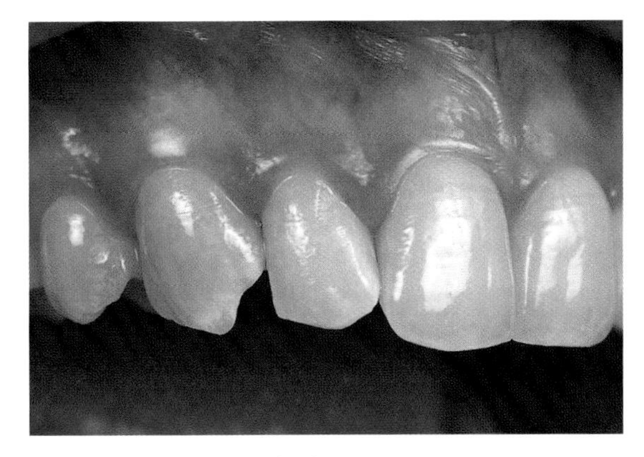

Figure 2.7 Smooth attached gingiva.

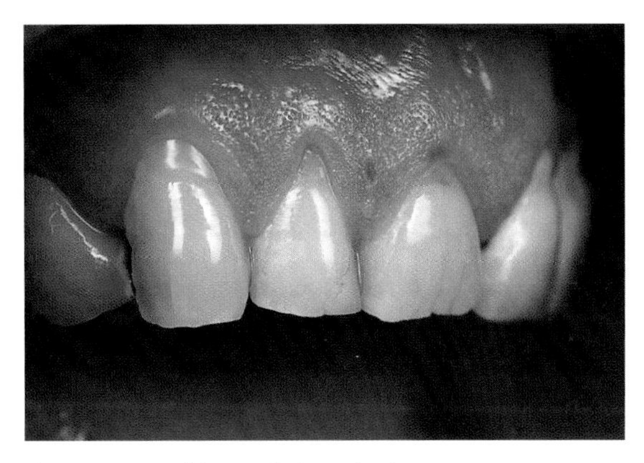

Figure 2.8 Highly stippled attached gingiva.

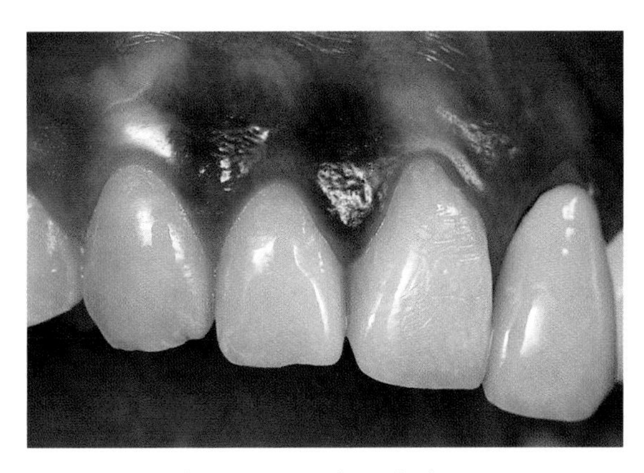

Figure 2.9 Melanin-pigmented attached gingiva.

1.56 mm to 1.25 mm, averaging at 1.41 mm. Traversing from the anterior to posterior teeth, the width decreases, while thickness increases.[1] Another correlation is that a wider and thicker attached gingiva is associated with a shallower sulcus depth.[2]

The function of the attached gingiva, which is more resilient than the non-keratinised alveolar mucosa, is to withstand normal functional masticatory trauma. When its width is diminished following surgical or implant procedures, its role is compromised. The need to have an adequate zone of attached gingiva surrounding implant-supported crowns is contentious (Fig. 2.10). Some authorities advocate that absence of an attached zone has no adverse effects on implant survival.[3] However, others stress the need for a

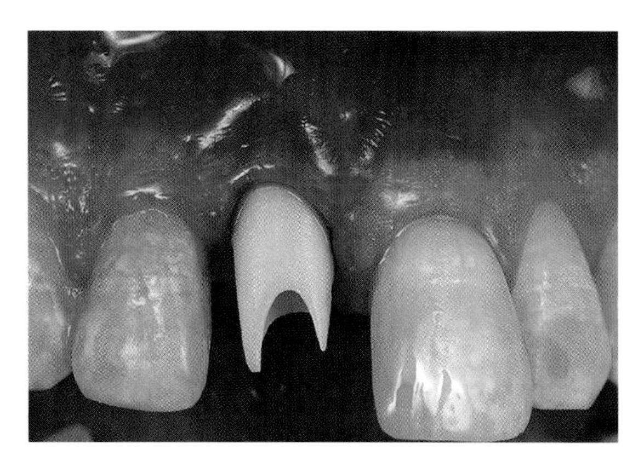

Figure 2.10 Lack of attached gingiva around a ceramic implant abutment (laboratory work by Jason Kim, New York).

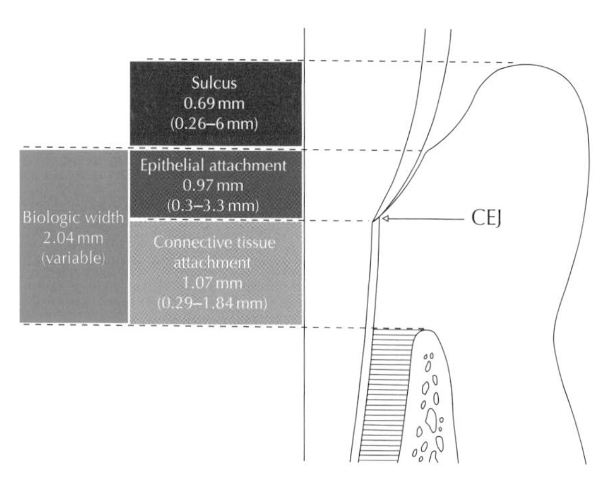

Figure 2.11 The biologic width.

soft tissue zone (minimum 1 mm around natural teeth and 2 mm around implants)[4] to prevent an inflammatory response. Indeed, it is suggested that soft tissue grafts have alleviated persistent inflammation around implants.[5] The debate continues, but is seems prudent to have a keratinised zone around implant-supported prostheses to resist trauma from food impaction and routine oral hygiene procedures, similar to that around natural teeth.

In cross-section, the periodontium is composed of three types of tissue; epithelium, connective tissue and bone. The free gingival margin forms part of the gingival crevice, which is internally lined by intact, non-keratinised or parakeratinised epithelium. This sulcus or crevice has the tooth surface on one side and the crevicular epithelium on the other. The linear dimension of the sulcus varies from 0.26–6.03 mm, depending on numerous factors, including type of tooth, site of measurement, etc. It is frequently 1 mm or less, greater at interproximal than facial sites. The epithelial attachment (EA) is located below the gingival sulcus and also exhibits variability in length from 0.32–3.27 mm.[6] A unique feature of the epithelial attachment is that if severed, by surgical or bacterial trauma, it proliferates rapidly in an apical direction in approximately 5 days.[7] The newly formed epithelial attachment is longer, limited only by the connective tissue below. However, if inflammatory response of the connective tissue is also present, this causes lysis of the connective tissue, which is then no longer capable of acting as a barrier to retard apical migration of the epithelial attachment. This process continues until the epithelial attachment encounters an intact connective tissue barrier. This is the basic sequence of periodontal pocket formation. It is important to note that the epithelial attachment can be located apical to the alveolar bone crest (ABC) on the cementum of the root surface. Another significant point is that the EA is longer around teeth with subgingival restorative margins compared with non-restored teeth.

The supracrestal fibres, emanating from the periodontal ligament, form the connective tissue attachment (CTA) below the epithelial attachment. The CTA ranges from 0.29–1.84 mm, with a mean of 0.77 mm, and is wider on posterior than anterior teeth. The connective tissue has the least variance compared with the sulcus and epithelial dimensions, and 1 mm can be safely used as a clinical guide. The EA + CTA form a soft tissue cuff termed the biologic width (Fig. 2.11).

The final component of the dentogingival complex is the alveolar bone housing the tooth, usually located apical to the epithelial and connective tissue attachments. The alveolar housing usually follows the contours of the cemento-enamel junction (CEJ), in a parabolic fashion, with peaks and troughs that are exaggerated on anterior, but diminish around posterior teeth.

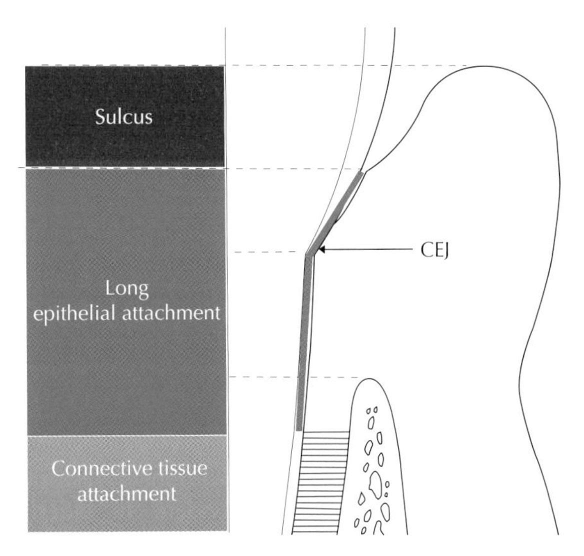

Figure 2.12 A long epithelial attachment, apical to the alveolar bone crest.

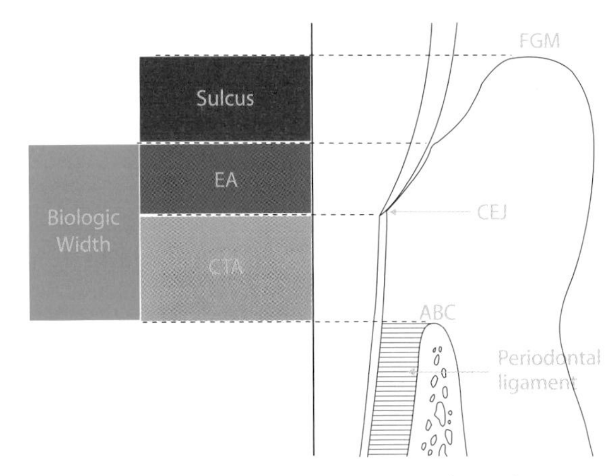

Figure 2.13 Landmarks of the dentogingival complex.

However, following periodontal disease or iatrogenic trauma, the alveolar crest may be located coronal to the epithelial attachment (Fig. 2.12).

Biologic width

The biologic width has many synonyms, including buffer zone, soft tissue cuff, soft tissue barrier, soft tissue shield or subcrevicular attachment complex. Whilst some terminology may be more descriptive than others, the most popular term is biologic width. Ingber coined the term 'biologic width' in 1977[8] based on original research by Gargiulo, Wentz and Orban in 1961.[9] The concept of the biologic width envisaged by these authors was based on autopsy and histological findings, with a mean sulcus depth of 0.69 mm, a junctional or epithelial attachment of 0.97 mm and a connective tissue attachment from the CEJ to alveolar crest of 1.07 mm. The sum of linear measurements of EA + CTA (2.04 mm) is the biologic width (Fig. 2.13). Since its introduction, the 2.04 mm measurement has been ubiquitously quoted, reported in dental journals, and indelibly ingrained in clinicians' psyche. The biologic width is nature's approach for protecting the most important part of the dentogingival complex, the periodontal ligament and alveolar crest. It is in effect a shield which endures trauma, both mechanical and bacterial, to ensure longevity of a tooth. If this soft tissue shield is inadvertently damaged or violated, its protective function is diminished, placing the survival of the tooth in jeopardy.

The main significance of the biologic width is its presence around every healthy tooth. Its integrity is indicative of gingival health, and is a guide for restorative procedures. It is obviously imperative to maintain this zone, and prevent impingement for longevity of not only the tooth, but also a reparative dental restoration. Physiologically and qualitatively, the biologic width is a valid concept, but much debate has concentrated on its quantitative values. Therefore, differential diagnosis of clinical variations of the dentogingival complex is imperative for avoiding pitfalls.

Biologic width – differential diagnosis

Ensuring the integrity of the biologic width is a shared responsibility of the patient (oral hygiene), clinician (operative trauma, margin location) and ceramist (precision restorations). The quoted dimension of 2.04 mm is an average ideal, not applicable for each site or every tooth. Furthermore, even if violated, a biologic width re-establishes, although with a reduced dimension. This suggests that the ideal 2 mm is not essential for gingival health, and the minimum dimension required for health is still unknown.[10] It is also relevant to note the relationship of various landmarks: EA, CEJ and ABC. Usually, the EA and CEJ are both coronal to the ABC.

Type of tooth and restored teeth variations

The biologic width (EA + CTA) dimensions vary according to the type of tooth. There is a progressive increase of the biologic width from anterior to posterior teeth. The mean dimensions are:

- Anterior teeth 1.75 mm
- Premolars 1.97 mm
- Molars 2.08 mm (almost the same as the ubiquitously quoted width of 2.04 mm)

All these measurements are average values, indicating that a viable biologic width as small as 0.59 mm can exist around healthy teeth. Another variation is that restored, compared with non-restored teeth, have a wider biologic width. As stated above, the increase in the biologic width around restored teeth is usually due to a longer EA, while the CTA and sulcus seems fairly constant for both restored and non-restored teeth. This clinical observation is irrespective of the type of restoration.[11]

Population variations

In 85% of invididuals, the ABC position is in a normal relationship to the CEJ, with a sulcus depth of 1 mm. However, in 13% of the population, both ABC and EA are more apical, in a relative normal relationship, but with a long epithelial attachment (and if violated, results in gingival recession and forming of the so-called 'black triangles'). Finally in 2% of the population, both ABC and EA are more coronal, in a relative normal relationship, but with a smaller EA and a minimal or non-existent crevice. In these circumstances, subgingival crown margin location should be avoided, as it will almost certainly violate the biologic width.

Apical location of epithelial attachment

Another situation is when the EA is located apical to the ABC. This is a sequela of either periodic intervals of periodontitis or surgical intervention. After episodes of periodontitis and subsequent pseudo-healing, the apical proliferation of a long healthy EA occurs before connective tissue formation. Similarly, following surgical curettage, without bone grafting or membrane barriers, the epithelium may migrate apically before the connective tissue or bone has had a chance to regenerate.

Passive and altered passive eruption

Other factors to consider are passive and altered passive eruptions, both of which can be deceptive when deciding margin location of restorations. Passive eruption is evident in elderly patients where the dentogingival complex migrates apically, resulting in recession, but maintaining a normal relationship of the CEJ to the ABC. Much debate has concentrated on whether this phenomenon is a physiological or pathological process. The physiological explanation is that recession is an ageing process, and the migration of the dentogingival complex is a normal occurrence. On the other hand, the pathological explanation is that during a lifetime, an individual will be inflicted with episodes of acute and chronic gingival inflammation with apical migration of the crestal bone. Which opinion is correct is irrelevant, but the result is gingival recession.

Altered passive (or delayed) eruption is evident when the epithelial attachment fails to migrate apically, resulting in a long junctional epithelium with short clinical crowns, but with a normal relationship between the CEJ and ABC. The latter usually occurs during permanent tooth eruption, and, over a period, the EA establishes a normal relationship with the ABC (Fig. 2.14). Failure to diagnose this condition, with inappropriate crown margin location, may cause gingival recession leading to exposure of crown margins.

Periodontal bioform and biotypes

Besides biologic width, the other factor to consider before considering dental restoration is the patient's periodontal bioform and biotype. These

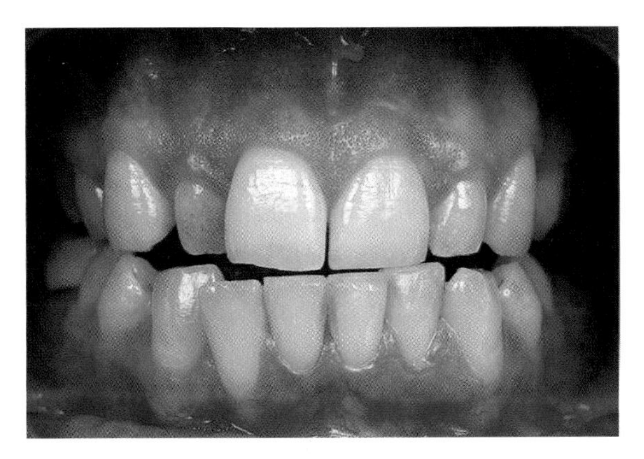

Figure 2.14 Alternated passive eruption on right maxillary lateral.

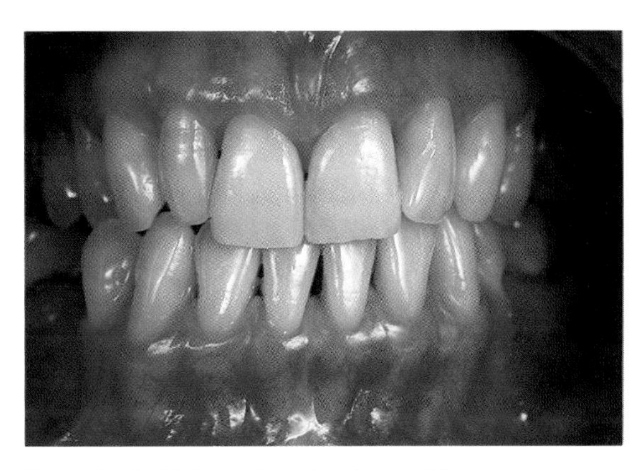

Figure 2.16 Thin, scalloped periodontal biotype.

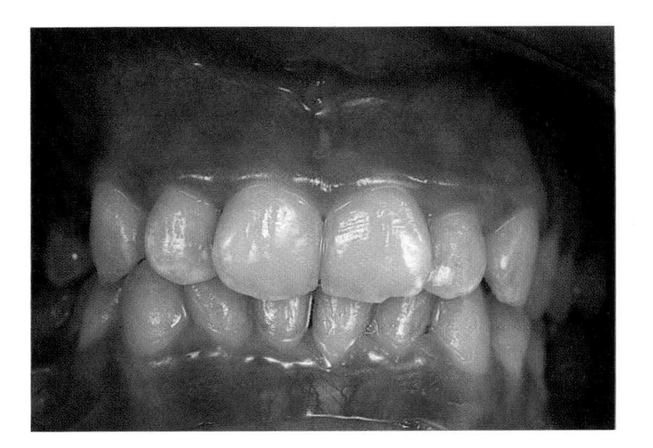

Figure 2.15 Thick, flat periodontal biotype.

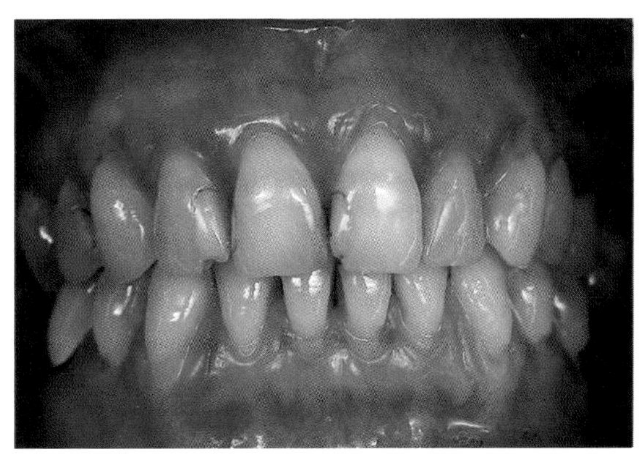

Figure 2.17 Pronounced, scalloped periodontal biotype.

two elements influence treatment modalities, and the anticipated type of healing response.

The shape of the gingival scallop envelope is determined by the position and morphology of the teeth. Teeth are categorised into three basic shapes: square, oval and triangular. These three basic shapes determine the gingival topography into thick flat, thin scalloped and pronounced scallop (Figs. 2.15–2.17).[12] The underlying alveolar bone architecture (distance from interproximal crestal peak to mid-facial crestal peak) of the three different periodontal bioforms is shown in Table 2.1 below.

The flat type scallop is prevalent in 85% of the population, and the thin type in 15% of cases.

Table 2.1 Periodontal forms.

Periodontal form	Mean distance from interproximal crestal peak to mid-facial crestal peak (mm)
Flat	2.1
Scalloped	2.8
Pronounced scallop	4.1

The flat, thick type is associated with a dense fibrotic appearance, and if manipulated or violated by surgical procedures reacts by forming periodontal pockets. On the other hand, a thin scalloped type has a smooth appearance, with less attached masticatory mucosa, predisposing to dehiscences and fenestrations. Trauma to this type of periodontium usually results in recession.

The clinical significance of the type of periodontium is that violation of the biologic width in thick types causes pocketing, while in thin types gingival recession is expected (Figs. 2.18 & 2.19). If subgingival crown margins with a thin type violate the biologic width, gingival recession will expose the crown–tooth interface and compromise aesthetics for patients with high lip lines. This is particularly significant interproximally when the distance from the crestal bone to contact point is 5 mm or less, causing incomplete papilla fill of the gingival embrasures (black triangles).[13] Tooth shape also determines the degree of interproximal bone between teeth. In a thin scalloped type, the teeth are triangular with narrower conical roots, and the interproximal bone volume is greater (Figs. 2.20 & 2.21). Conversely, in a thick, flat type, the squarer teeth have wider cylindrical roots, reducing the space available for the interproximal bone volume. For this reason, bone loss in thin, scalloped types is greater and wider causing pronounced gingival recession, compared with the thick, flat types, in which bone loss results in pocket formation.

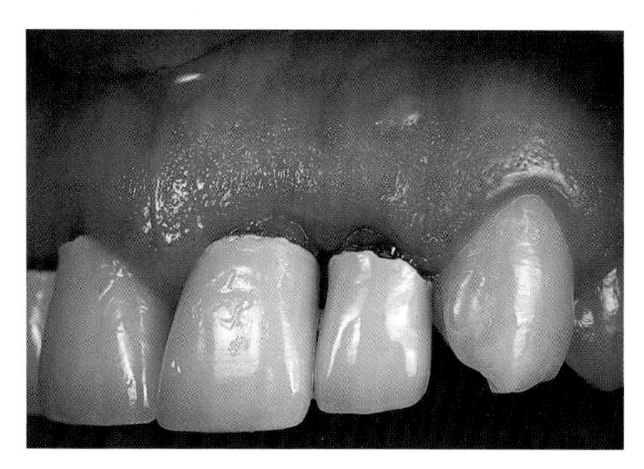

Figure 2.18 Pocket formation with a thick biotype due to defective crowns (note abscess associated with left lateral incisor).

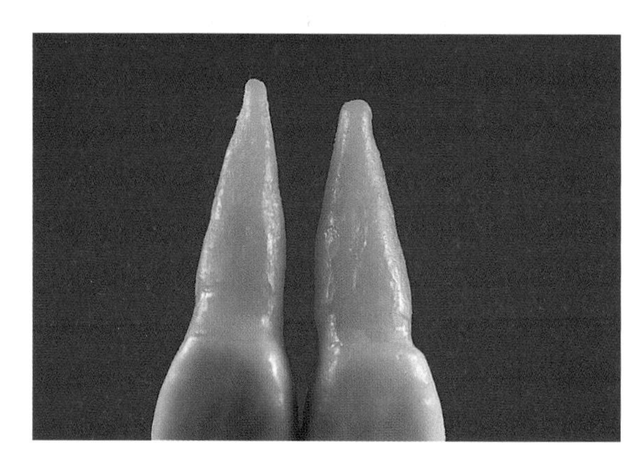

Figure 2.20 Triangular teeth have conical roots with greater interproximal bone volume.

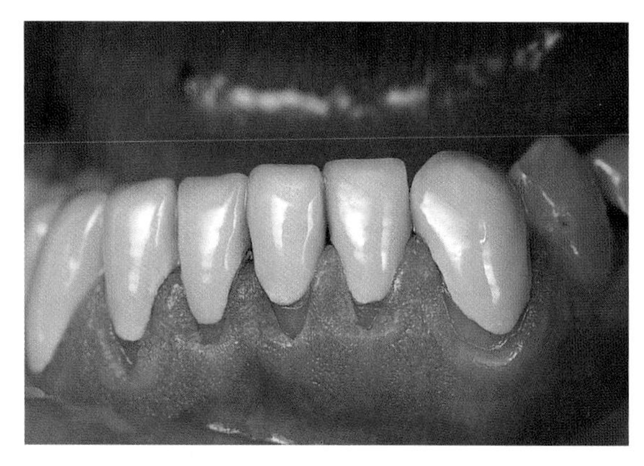

Figure 2.19 Gingival recession around defective crowns with a thin biotype.

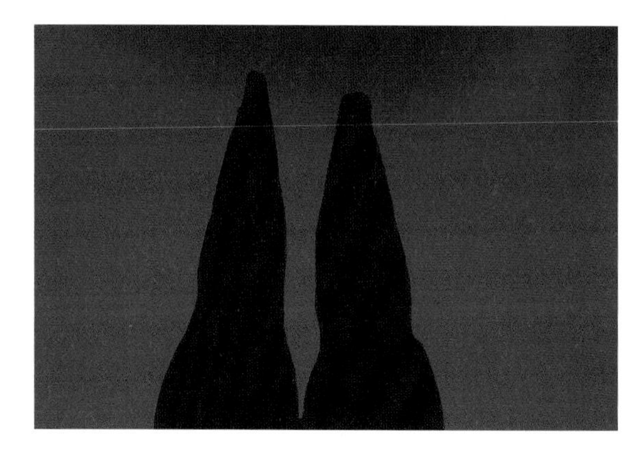

Figure 2.21 Silhouette of triangular teeth and conical roots, emphasising the increased interproximal bone volume.

Restorative implications

For dental therapy, evaluation of the biologic width and periodontal biotype are necessary for the following treatment modalities:

- Restorative procedures
- Surgical crown lengthening
- Implants

Restorative procedures

Restorative procedures include fillings and intra- and extra-coronal restorations (direct or indirect), which either approach or encroach the dentogingival complex. The biologic width is not clinically visible, and numerous guidelines are proposed to speculate its location and dimensions.[14] Basically, there are two schools of thought focusing on definite anatomical references. The two proposed landmarks are either the ABC, or a healthy and stable free gingival margin (FGM).

The rationale for using the ABC is that the average dimension of the biologic width is 2 mm, verified histologically; this fails to account for clinical variations, however. Many authors and clinicians recommend that restorative margins and procedures be 2–3 mm coronal to the ABC ensuring integrity of the biologic width.[15] If this method is used, differential diagnosis, and individual variations assessments are essential to avoid entering the EA, or worse, the CTA.

An alternative reference point is a healthy FGM, placing margins 0.5 mm apical into the sulcus.[16] The rationale for this method is a tangible landmark, as opposed to a physiological or histological reference point of the biologic width. This method obviously avoids encroachment of the biologic width, since the margins will undoubtedly be coronal to the EA. However, this approach also has disadvantages. In patients with a thin biotype or altered passive eruption, gingival recession following restorative procedures may expose the crown margin/tooth interface, which is significant if the crown cement line is stained and there is a high lip line. In conclusion, both methods offer benefits and limitations, but the key to success is assessing each patient individually, before choosing the ABC or FGM as a reference point.

Surgical crown lengthening

When therapy involves crown lengthening or implant placement, assessment of both the biologic width and periodontal biotypes is essential. For crown lengthening procedures, a supracrestal tissue barrier is vital for stability of the FGM and periodontal health.[17] For crown lengthening procedures, using the FGM as a reference point is difficult following flap elevation and surgical trauma, which distort the pliable soft tissues. Although the average dimension of the biologic width of 2 mm is not applicable to clinical findings around every tooth, it is however, a useful guide for practical purposes. The variations discussed above can obviously be incorporated into treatment planning, but for crown lengthening, a minimum distance of 2–3 mm is recommended between ABC and the proposed location of the FGM.

Implants

Similar to natural teeth, healthy peri-implant tissues also possess a biologic width. This soft tissue cuff is prerequisite for a stable periodontal architecture around implant-supported prostheses.[18] For dental implants, both thick, flat or thin, scalloped periodontal biotypes offer advantages and disadvantages.

With a thin, scalloped periodontal biotype the interproximal volume of bone is greater, due to the narrower conical shape of the roots. This is advantageous for ensuring the minimum necessary implant-to-tooth or implant-to-implant distance, 1.5 mm and 3 mm, respectively (Fig. 2.22). However, because the gingival tissue is thin and delicate, inadvertent trauma or incorrect fixture placement predisposes to gingival recession (exposing implant–abutment interface), or formation of unsightly 'black triangles'.

For thick, flat biotypes, the roots are broader and conical, with reduced interproximal bone volume, leaving less space between adjacent teeth or proposed implants. If implants are considered

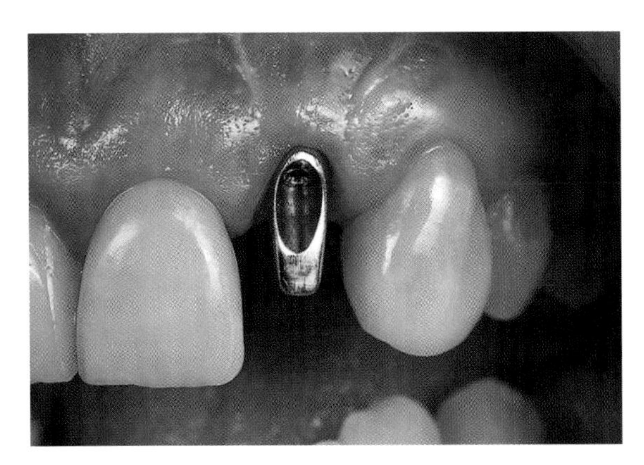

Figure 2.22 Implant (Replace Select, Nobel Biocare) replacing missing left lateral showing 2 mm mesial and distal space between adjacent teeth.

in these circumstances, the situation can be resolved either by using narrower fixtures with concurrent mesial-distal bone grafting, or grafting on the buccal aspect to compensate for the reduced mesial-distal implant spacing.[19] The advantage of a thick periodontal biotype is that due to the bulky fibrotic attached gingiva, recession is less likely than with a thin, scalloped form.

Finally, margins of any extra-coronal restoration (on natural teeth or implant fixtures) should mimic the undulations of the CEJ and ACB, with coronal peaks in the interproximal regions, and apical peaks on facial and lingual aspects. The introduction of scalloped (Nobel Perfect, Nobel Biocare) and parabolic implants is an endeavour to mimic these natural contours of the CEJ and alveolar crest, with the aim of minimising bone loss in the interproximal regions that often occurs with conventional flat implant platforms.[20] Using these novel implant designs, the implantogingival junction simulates a natural dentogingival junction.

Function

The following discussion about function assumes that periodontal health is reinstated and maintained. The basic premise of function is ensuring comfort and free range of movement. Function is divided into two categories: phonetics and occlusion. The former has reasonable concord in the dental literature, but the latter has an aura of mystique and confusion amongst dental professionals.

Occlusion

Occlusion is bewildering for clinicians because of the following reasons:

- The thinking about occlusion has undergone drastic changes in the last century
- Many theories abound, and depending on which literature or lecture one cares to follow, the research is conflicting with varied conclusions
- There is a tendency to overstate and complicate this subject, leading to alienation, and speculation by the recipient audience

In reality, no ideal occlusion exists that is applicable to every individual. Occlusion, like other physical features, is genetically determined. Therefore, prescribing a theoretically ideal scheme is at best futile, and at worst detrimental. Most dental restorations are carried out with a superficial knowledge of occlusion, but nevertheless integrate without due concern with the patient's dentition. However, occlusal interference should not be flippantly introduced, nor should occlusion be regarded as superfluous. On the contrary, many failures are avoidable by correctly and carefully addressing occlusal factors.

Ultimately, the practitioner craves for practical guidance, applicable to the clinical scenario. The purpose of this discussion is not to present academic nuances for a scholarly dissertation, but to clarify basic concepts of occlusion that are relevant to daily practice.

The first ambiguity is terminology, since many synonyms are employed.[21] For the sake of simplicity and clinical relevance, widely accepted nomenclature and definitions are used. These are centric occlusion (CO), centric relation (CR), working and non-working (contacts and interferences), guidance (lateral and anterior) and occlusal vertical dimension (OVD).[22]

Centric occlusion

CO is defined as maximum intercuspation of the maxillary and mandibular teeth. This is probably the most significant occlusal position, for the following reasons:

- CO is readily reproducible when a patient is asked to close on to the back teeth (Fig. 2.23)
- CO is the ideal position for dissipation of occlusal forces by the periodontal ligament, since the load is axially directly through the teeth
- CO is a neuromuscular learned behaviour representing the end of the chewing cycle with maximum force excursion

Consequently, an artificial restoration should be shaped to integrate with CO, which is the case for the majority of restorations routinely supplied by dentists. Assuming that the existing occlusion is asymptomatic, and a limited number of units are restored (one or two) which do not violate the existing occlusal equilibrium, CO is probably the only occlusal position that requires attention. Specifically, a restoration fabricated in CO, should not create interferences, especially in CR.

Centric relation

CR is the position of mandibular closure when the condyles are maximally seated in their respective fossae and initial contact is observed between maxillary and mandibular teeth (Fig. 2.24). From this position, there is mandibular protrusive or lateral excursion into CO. In 90% of the population, CO does not coincide with CR without deleterious effect.[23] Hence, pretreatment occlusal adjustments to achieve harmony with CR and CO are unwarranted and unjustifiable. However, it is necessary to identify CR, together with the initial antagonist tooth-to-tooth contact, because in certain situations it may become relevant. This is particularly significant when extensive restorative treatment is envisaged, for example altering the OVD, or a profound slide is evident on to anterior teeth that are being restored, or in the presence of a slide between CR and CO with the aim to distalise the mandible for creating lingual space for anterior crowns. In these cases, the CR is an ideal and reproducible starting point. Finally, when a restoration involves teeth that make the initial contact in CR, pre-operative identification and occlusal adjustment is beneficial, thus avoiding grinding the definitive prostheses into occlusion.[24]

Working and non-working contacts and interferences

Lateral movement of the mandible distinguishes two sides, termed working side (direction of movement) and the contralateral side (away from the movement) or the non-working side.

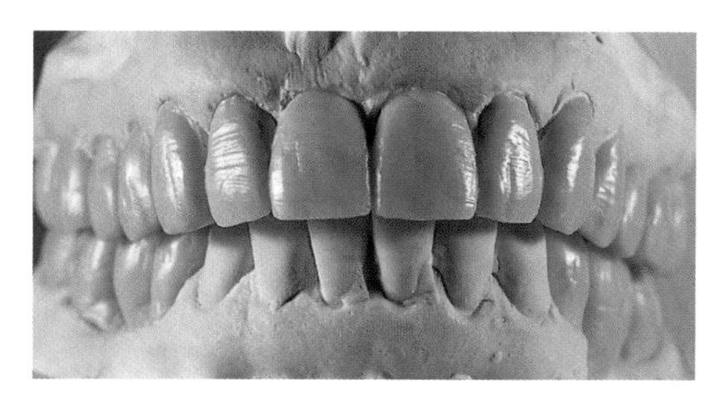

Figure 2.23 Diagnostic wax-up in centric occlusion (CO).

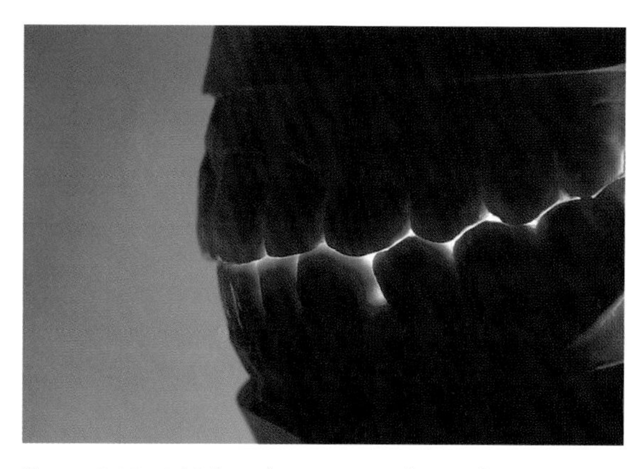

Figure 2.24 Initial tooth contact on first molars in centric relation (CR).

Contacts can occur on either side guiding mandibular movement, as is the case of balanced articulation for complete upper and lower dentures. For dentate patients, balanced articulation is a rarity, since the laterally generated forces, unlike axially directed forces in CO, place undue stress on the teeth. These eccentric occlusal forces, if repeatedly applied for long durations are detrimental to the stomatognathic system, involving teeth, periodontium, muscles of mastication and the TMJ. However, neuromuscular adaptation makes these interferences insignificant, and restores physiological function. A potential problem only emerges when restorations are planned which involve these interferences. This applies equally to single as well as multiple units. When contemplating dental prostheses that necessitate tooth preparation, interferences are often eliminated, but with resultant reduced inter-occlusal clearance for the proposed restorative materials. This results in a grossly overbuilt prosthesis, preventing mandibular closure and freedom of movement in lateral excursions. In these instances, it is prudent to identify all interferences, and to perform pre-operative judicial adjustments, stabilise the occlusion, and then proceed to the definitive restoration(s), ensuring that the prepared abutments have adequate clearance in CO and lateral excursions. It is also imperative to avoid introducing new interferences during prosthetic rehabilitation.

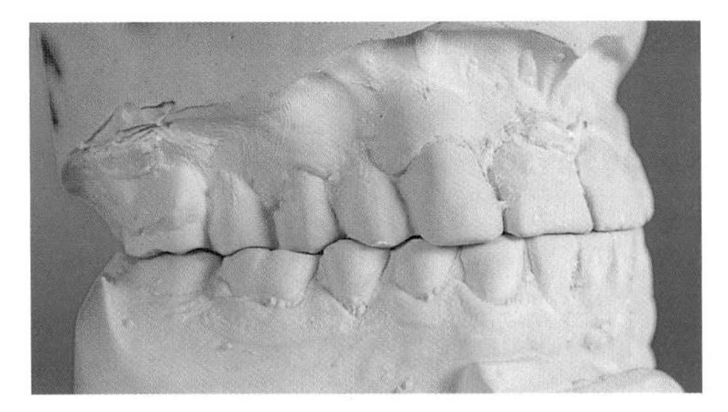

Figure 2.25 Study casts showing group function.

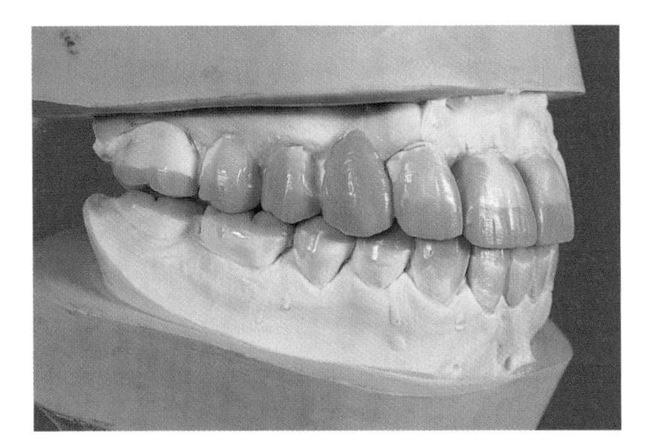

Figure 2.26 Diagnostic wax-up of case study in Figure 2.25, restored to canine guidance.

Lateral excursions

Mandibular excursions are complicated, but for simplicity are divided into lateral and anterior. Lateral translation results in guidance of the mandible by one or more teeth. In a healthy dentition, this movement can be canine guided or group function (involving more than one tooth, e.g. the premolars), but can also involve incisors and molars (Figs. 2.25–2.27). Once again, the biological adaptive capacity allows harmony and clinical intervention is unnecessary. When prostheses are planned involving guidance teeth, care is crucial. The reason is that the forces placed on the guidance teeth are lateral, and therefore potentially more harmful; they may result in

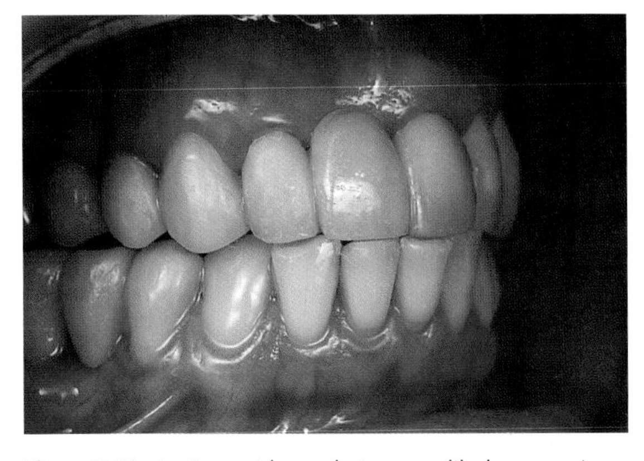

Figure 2.27 Incisor guidance during mandibular excursions.

fracture or dislodgement of the prostheses or damage to the stomatognathic system, including TMJ dysfunction, increased wear, mobility or drifting of the opposing dentition. Therefore, the proposed prosthesis should emulate this guidance, and be sufficiently resilient, if no change to the occlusal scheme is envisaged. Furthermore, the prepared teeth should be checked for sufficient occlusal clearance in all excursions to accommodate the proposed metal and/or ceramic material.

Another aspect to consider is whether the patient predominantly masticates in a vertical or horizontal direction. Vertical biting is preferred since forces are axial, compared to horizontal chewing patterns with non-axial forces that are detrimental. In the latter, bruxism is evident with loss of occlusal anatomy. Providing artificial, especially ceramic, restorations should be approached with caution until diagnosis is confirmed and grinding stabilised.

If, however, the occlusion requires drastic change by extensive restorations, a new scheme is planned before treatment commences. Ideally, canine guidance is recommended because it elicits a 30–40% lower muscular activity compared to group function.[25] However, when a canine is compromised (by periodontal or endodontic involvement), and in order to spread the load during lateral movements, changing to group function may be advisable. This protocol is also prudent if a missing canine is replaced by an implant-supported prosthesis. Because implants lack a periodontal ligament and proprioception, it may be prudent to adopt group function, in order to dissipate forces via natural teeth during lateral excursions.

Anterior guidance

Anterior guidance is the protrusive movement of the mandible. When aesthetic restorations are planned for the anterior mandibular and maxillary teeth, anterior guidance is of paramount concern. Conforming to the existing guidance is relatively simple, but when the occlusion is reorganised, anterior guidance requires re-establishment. A steep guidance causes elevated muscular activity, while the opposite is true for a flatter guidance (Figs. 2.28–2.31).[26] Consequently, a steep angle may cause cement failure, fracturing of all-ceramic units, tooth mobility and TMJ pain. A reduced or absent anterior guidance (incomplete anterior overbite) facilitates anterior restorations, but complicates posterior prostheses since the posterior teeth remain in contact during excursions. The opposite is true for a steep anterior guidance, which facilitates posterior prostheses due to canine disclusion, but hampers anterior crowns due to limited space between the maxillary and mandibular anterior teeth.[27]

The angle of anterior guidance and direction of the forces also impact on the design of anterior restorations. In the natural dentition, even if the mandibular teeth contact the palatal aspect of the maxillary teeth at a steep angle, the

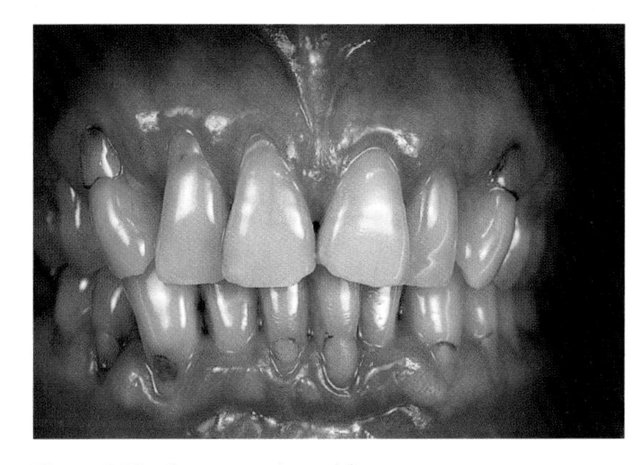

Figure 2.28 Steep anterior guidance.

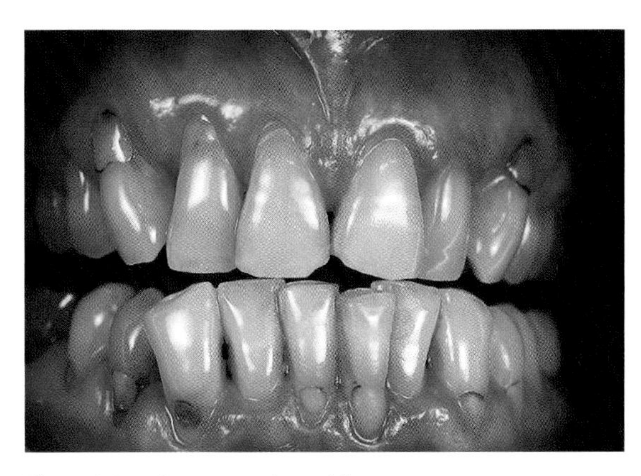

Figure 2.29 Steep anterior guidance.

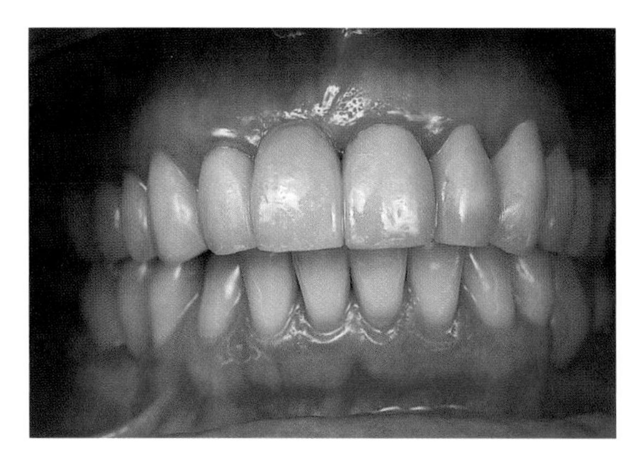

Figure 2.30 Shallow anterior guidance.

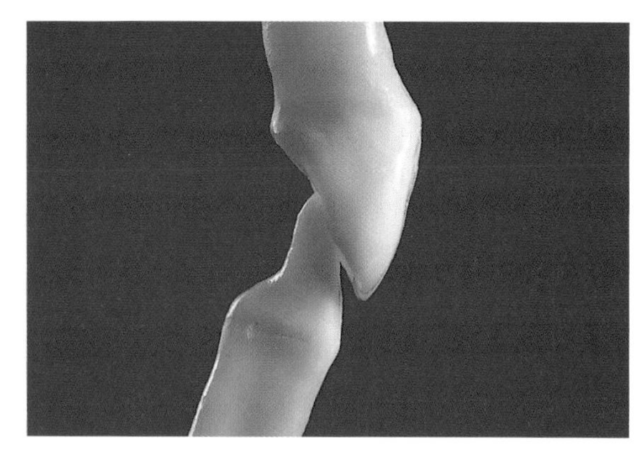

Figure 2.32 Mandibular incisor contacting palatal surface of maxillary incisor in a non-axial direction.

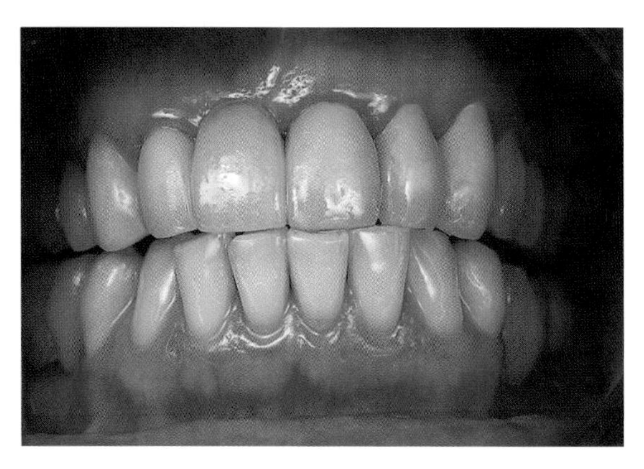

Figure 2.31 Shallow anterior guidance.

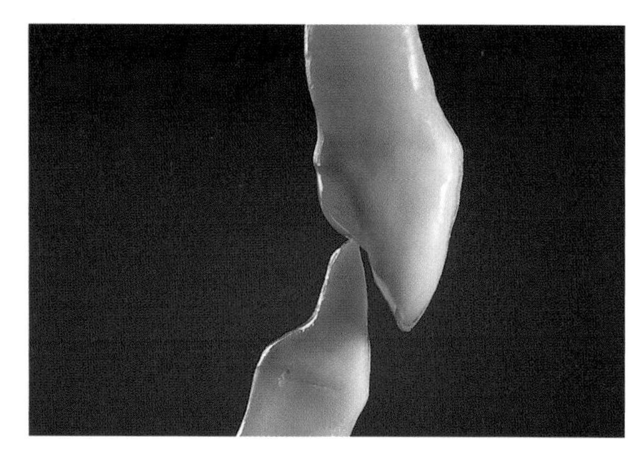

Figure 2.33 Addition of restorative material to palatal surface of maxillary incisor to flatten cingulum, and direct forces from mandibular incisor in an axial direction.

dentine and enamel dissipate the forces to the periodontal ligament (Fig. 2.32). However, artificial restorative materials do not possess similar biomechanical properties to natural dentine and enamel. These inferior substitutes are often incapable of performing as well in the oral environment. Ultimately, the weak link yields; this can be the restorative material (fracture, dislodgement), opposing natural teeth (fractures, wear) or soft or hard tissues (periodontal or TMJ pathosis). As mentioned above, if an occlusal change is envisaged (e.g. altering occlusal schemes or increasing the OVD), it is wiser to shape the palatal cingulum of the maxillary teeth so that it is flatter and makes perpendicular contact with the mandibular teeth to direct forces axially, placing less stress on the restorative material (Fig. 2.33). This procedure of reducing the anterior guidance from steep to shallow also reduces muscular stress.

The protocol to adopt is determining the start and end points of the anterior slide, and ensuring freedom of movement with a shallow angle for reduced muscular activity.

Occlusal vertical dimension

In order to improve dental aesthetics, the OVD may need to be increased in certain circumstances, and therefore warrants special attention. Two aspects require elaboration, the determination and alteration of the OVD.[28]

Proposed methods for determining the existing OVD include nocturnal acrylic splints, neuromuscular activity, freeway space, positions of FGMs or CEJs of anterior teeth, facial landmarks, cephalometric analysis and masticatory muscle lengths. Nearly all these methods are limited in their conclusions with questionable results.

Wearing an acrylic splint for ascertaining whether the proposed increase in vertical height can be tolerated is flawed, since any transient pain experienced by the patient usually disappears after 1 or 2 weeks, irrespective of the degree of proposed increase. Due to neuromuscular reprogramming, any increase in OVD is compensated for by an adaptive response; therefore measuring the level of muscle activity or the freeway space becomes irrelevant.[29] Another method is measuring the distance between the FGMs or CEJs of maxillary and mandibular anterior teeth (Fig. 2.34). The important point to realise is that the existing OVD is not determined by the anterior but posterior teeth. This is clearly illustrated with bulimic erosion of anterior teeth. In this scenario, the anterior teeth lose incisal height, but due to over-eruption, anterior centric contact is re-established. However, the posterior teeth are intact without showing signs of wear. In these circumstances, the anterior teeth require either orthodontic intrusion or surgical crown lengthening. Carrying out extensive restorations on the posterior teeth for increasing OVD is unjustified.

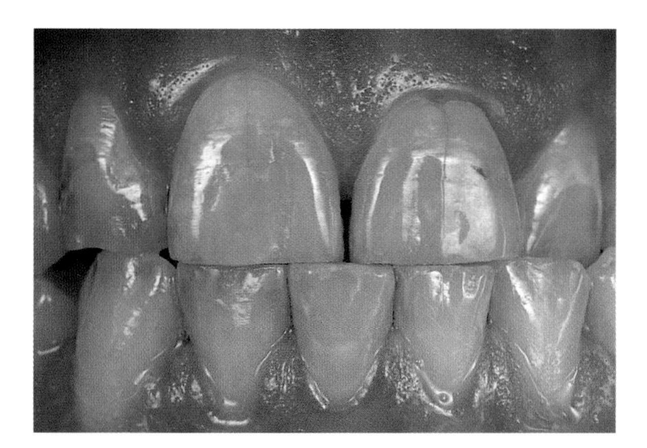

Figure 2.34 Disparity of gingival zeniths of the maxillary centrals.

Facial dimensions are another spurious method for OVD determination.[30] For ideal facial dimensions, the middle-face (from eyebrows to base of the nose) should equal the lower-face (base of nose to tip of chin). The latter is genetically determined, and if a patient has a short chin, should the OVD be increased to compensate for this anatomical anomaly? Cephalometric analysis is invaluable for orthodontic tooth movement, when both soft tissues and the alveolus are altered for restorative dentistry; when only the teeth are affected, however, its use is limited. Finally, lengths of the masseter and medial pterygoid muscles are yet another suggested method. The latter is simply calculated by geometric analysis of the condylar position relative to the muscles and anterior teeth. For every 3 mm anterior opening, the masseter length increases by 1 mm, but due to the 1 mm posterior seating of the condyles, the apparent increase in muscle length is nullified. Therefore, altering the OVD anteriorly by up to 3 mm has no effect on muscle length; muscle length is therefore not an accurate determinant of OVD.

Having outlined methods for OVD determination, the next step is altering the OVD. This is primarily carried out for improving anterior aesthetics, gaining space for dental prostheses or altering the occlusion. The first myth to dispel about altering OVD is that there is no such thing as an ideal vertical dimension. Consequently, performing extensive dentistry for attaining this erroneous goal is not only futile, but also grossly unethical.

As a general guideline, an anterior opening of 3 mm produces posterior space of 1 mm. As stated previously, with this amount of increase in OVD the masseter is lengthened by 1 mm, but because the condyles seat 1 mm posteriorly the increased muscle length is negated (Figs. 2.35 & 2.36). Put another way, an anterior increase of 3 mm is tolerable without any muscular adaptation or pain.[31] However, if the increase is greater than 3 mm, certain concerns need to be addressed:

- Pain associated with an increase in OVD is ephemeral, usually subsiding within 2 weeks

- In certain patients there is a degree of relapse when the OVD is increased, by remodelling of the alveolar bone and muscular adaptation, stabilising in 6 months. Therefore, if the precise increase in OVD is crucial, it is wise to place temporaries and wait 6 months before progressing to the definitive restorations
- Increased bite forces could potentially be detrimental to new prostheses. Initially there is an increase in bite force, which normalises within 3 months, and is of no clinical significance
- Violation of the freeway space may cause concern. When fabricating dentures for an edentulous patient, the freeway space of 2–4 mm is essential for preventing the upper and lower dentures clicking during speech or mastication.[32] However, in the dentate patient, the proprioceptive response of the periodontal ligament ensures that if the freeway space is encroached, neuromuscular adaptation recreates the freeway space within 2–4 weeks

Phonetics

The second part of function is unimpeded phonetics, verified by speaking certain words or letters such as the 'M', 'S', 'F' or 'V'. The 'M' sound, erroneously referred to as the rest position, is when the teeth are separated with a freeway space (Fig. 2.37). In fact, this position is not one of rest, but a habitual muscular position of the mandible.[33] A true rest position is observed when the elevator muscles are completely relaxed, such as during sleep. This 'M' position assesses the amount of maxillary incisal display and confirms that the freeway space has 'returned', following an increase in the OVD. The 'F' sound determines the sagittal inclination of the maxillary incisors. If correct, the buccal aspects of incisal third of the maxillary incisors should contact the mucosal, not the cutaneous, part of the lower lip (Fig. 2.38). If contact is absent, the incisors may be either too short or protruded.[34]

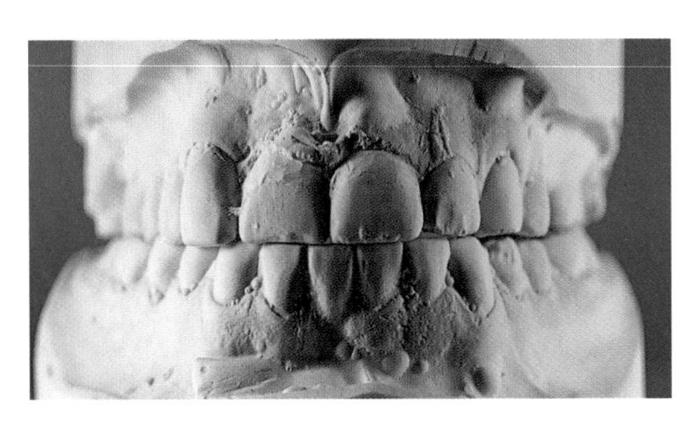

Figure 2.35 Proposed increase in OVD to enhance function and aesthetics (laboratory work by Gerald Ubassy, France).

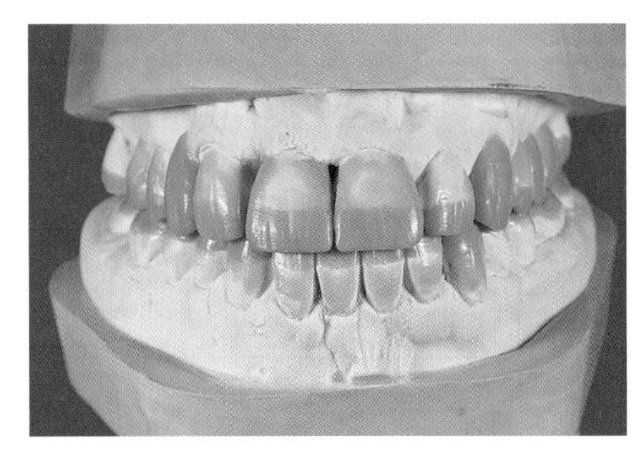

Figure 2.36 Proposed increase in OVD to enhance function and aesthetics (laboratory work by Gerald Ubassy, France).

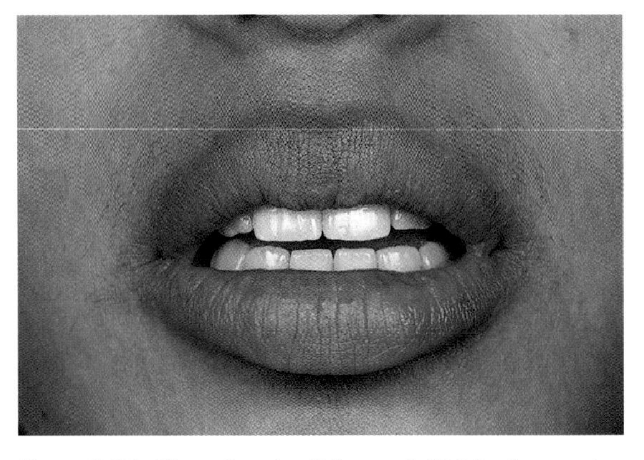

Figure 2.37 Phonetics: the 'M' sound. Habitual muscular position for determining amount of maxillary incisor display.

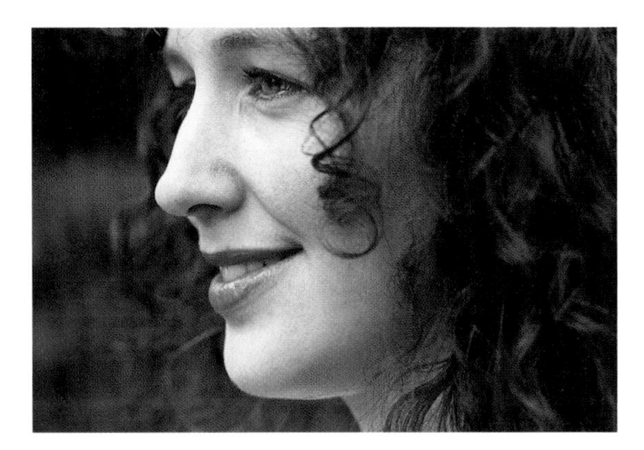

Figure 2.38 Phonetics: the 'F' and 'V' sounds. Maxillary incisors touching mucosal part of mandibular lip.

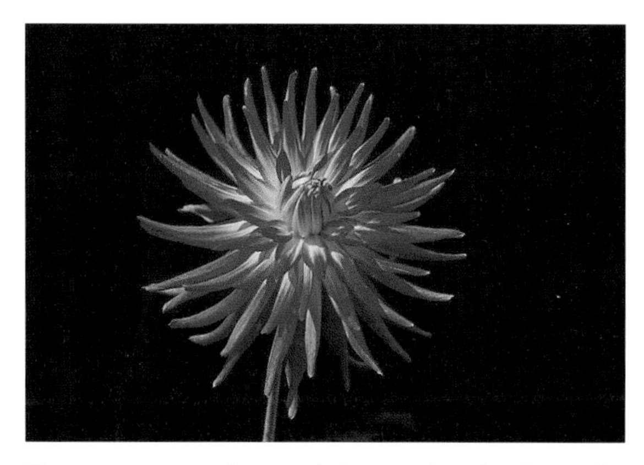

Figure 2.40 Innate beauty of plants can be related to mathematical concepts of beauty.

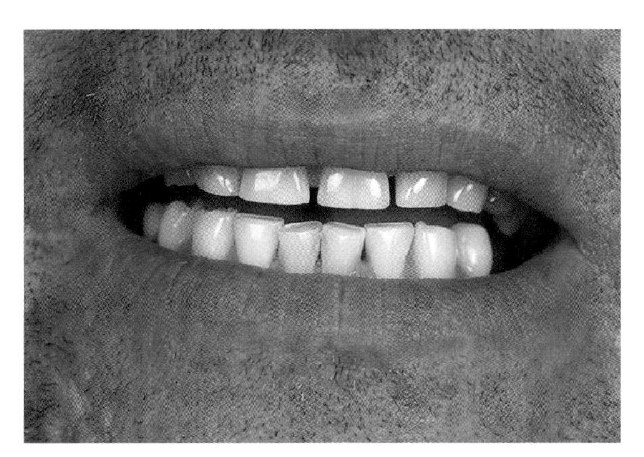

Figure 2.39 Phonetics: the 'S' sound. Vertical dimension of speech.

Finally, the 'S' sound assesses the vertical dimension of speech (Fig. 2.39). In order to avoid lisping, a 1 mm separation between the maxillary and mandibular incisors is necessary. Two scenarios are evident:

- The patient postures the mandibular incisors forward to make the 'S' sound, i.e. the postural position of the mandible is NOT coincident with CO. In this situation, adjusting the incisors (usually shortening the mandibular incisors) re-creates the requisite 1 mm separation. However, when the patient now occludes in CO, there is lack of contact between the anterior teeth. The latter is easily corrected by addition of the relevant restorative material(s) to the palatal aspect of the maxillary incisors
- The mandible coincides with CO during the 'S' sound, evident in some Class II and III occlusions. Adjusting the incisors to obtain 1 mm separation to prevent lisping will obviously create an unwanted anterior space. In these cases, the only option is to close the OVD posteriorly to obtain centric contact between maxillary and mandibular incisors

Aesthetics

Dental aesthetics is a vast topic, encompassing many scientific and artistic principles. The section below on aesthetics is not exhaustive, but furnishes the reader with basic outlines and practical guidelines for providing aesthetic restorations. For a detailed analysis, further reading is essential to grasp the theoretical concepts pertaining to dental aesthetics.[35]

Aesthetics is an art, not a science.[36] But like so many works of art, scientific principles are used for creating aesthetics. The morphology of animals and plants is based on fundamental geometric principles, with modifications, to create beings that are unique (Figs. 2.40 & 2.41). Dental aesthetics are also governed by mathematical concepts to create unique artificial pros-

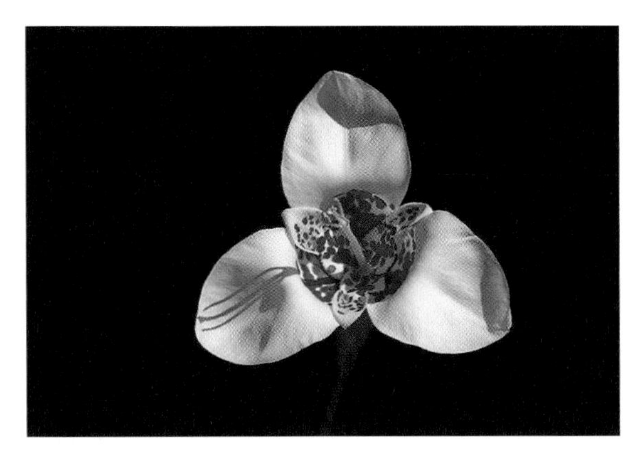

Figure 2.41 Innate beauty of plants can be related to mathematical concepts of beauty.

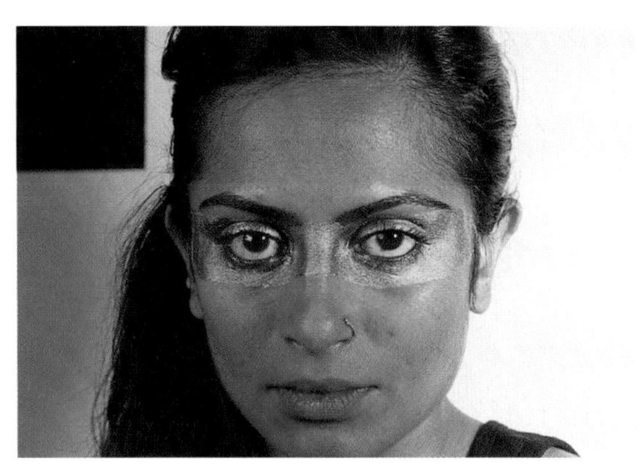

Figure 2.42 Facial composition.

theses. Nature, however, goes one step further by using its 'imagination', and avoids generating clones of a particular species. Geometric laws are not 'carved in stone', but are invaluable as a starting point for inspiration as opposed to emulation. The ensuing discussion outlines basic geometric rules for the anterior maxillary six teeth, which the clinician can readily incorporate into daily practice for an aesthetic prescription.

The starting point of an aesthetic appraisal is listening to the desires and wishes of the patient. Patients have an image of themselves, which they project and preserve. This image is constantly fluctuating by the id, peer and media pressure. Whilst these opinions are highly subjective, the only objective method of aesthetic analysis is mathematical. Indeed, mathematical language has been considered the only reference by which nature can be comprehended.[37] The clinician should therefore be familiar with geometric concepts governing anterior dental aesthetics. For elucidation, dental aesthetics can be arbitrarily divided into four compositions; facial, dentofacial, dental and gingival (Figs. 2.42–2.45).

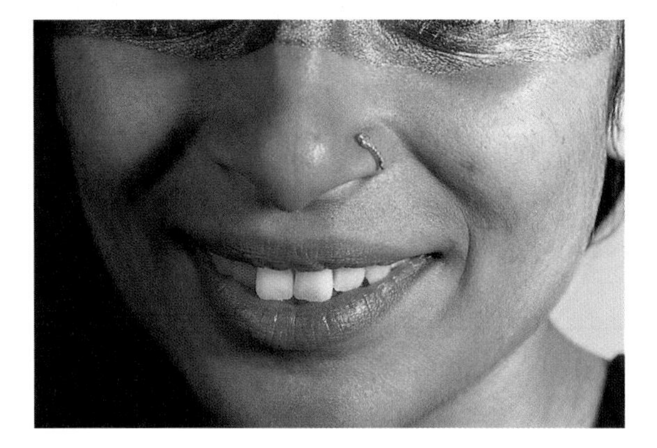

Figure 2.43 Dentofacial composition.

Facial composition

The facial composition is the one most important to the patient. This composition influences most patients' preconceived ideas of a 'perfect smile'.

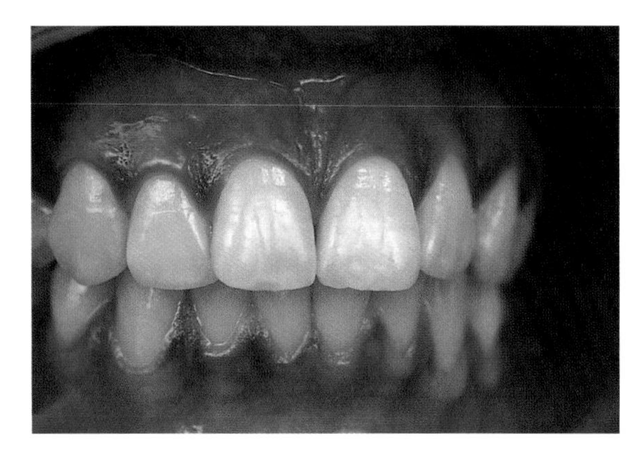

Figure 2.44 Dental composition.

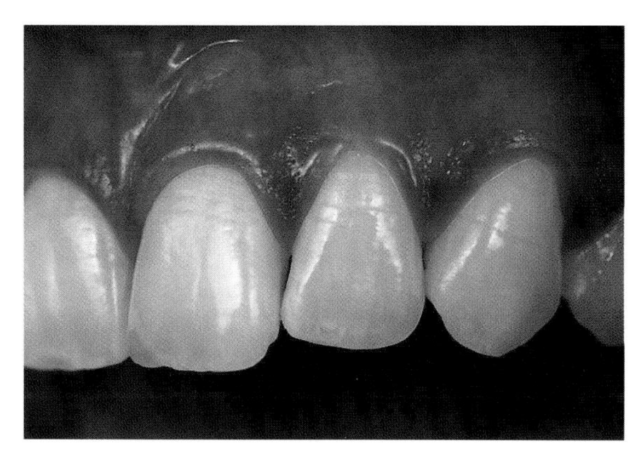

Figure 2.45 Gingival composition.

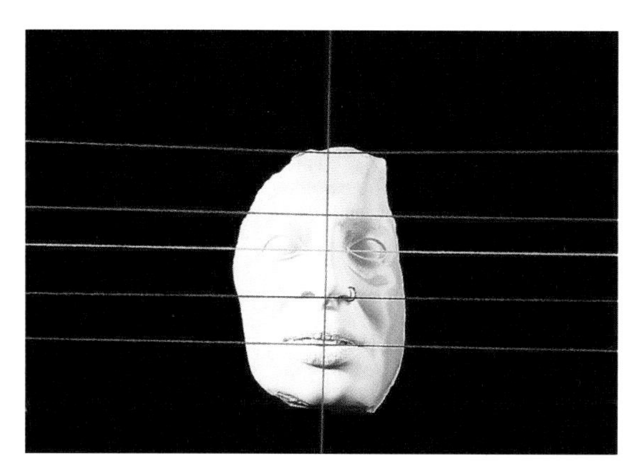

Figure 2.46 Parallelism of facial lines results in horizontal symmetry.

The reason for this is that most media images of beauty are concentrated around the face. The public is rarely accustomed to viewing a smile at a close distance that is routine in dentistry. At the facial distance of focus, the teeth appear white and straight. At a closer field of view, for example the dentofacial composition, the teeth rarely exhibit exact regularity, but have distinct proportions and embrasures. It is important to convey this to the layman, so that he or she appreciates that the media image is only one aspect of a smile.

Two aspects are significant when analysing the face: the frontal and sagittal. From the frontal aspect, numerous landmarks are used as guides for aesthetic appraisal. Horizontally, several imaginary reference lines are discernible, commencing from the upper to lower part of the face including the hair, ophriac, interpupillary, interalar and commissural lines. These parallel lines create horizontal symmetry, acting as cohesive forces to unify the facial composition. The facial midline is perpendicular to the horizontal lines and opposes their cohesiveness. These are termed segregative forces and are essential in a composition to add interest and harmony (Fig. 2.46). The cohesive forces are paramount for achieving pleasing aesthetics; the deviation of the facial midline is secondary, varying in many individuals without a deleterious effect. It is the general parallelism of the horizontal lines which is important, rather than orientation of a specific line.[38]

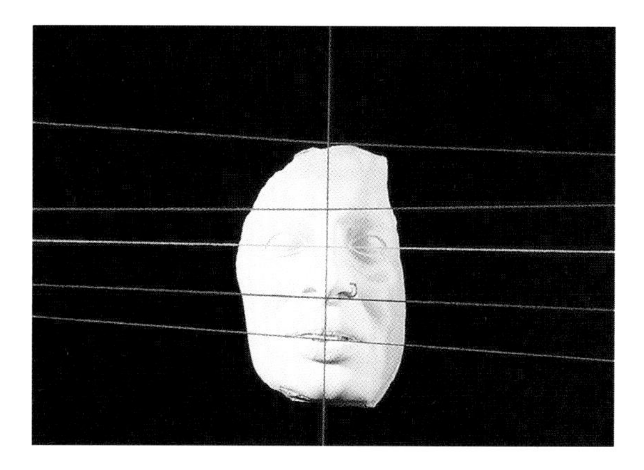

Figure 2.47 Frequently, the secondary facial lines are eschewed, and absolute parallelism is not a prerequisite for aesthetic appraisal.

The interpupillary line is used as a reference for the occlusal and incisal plane orientations. The other horizontal lines can be eschewed and therefore do not act as definite references; but they are useful accessory makers (Fig. 2.47). The incisal edges of the anterior teeth should be parallel to the interpupillary line and perpendicular to the midline (Fig. 2.48). Canting of the incisal plane is attributed to either dental or skeletal factors. The dental factors include wear (attrition, erosion, abrasion), altered patterns of eruption or periodontal disease. If the dental factors are eliminated, the tilting could be due to a slanted maxilla. It is crucial to ascertain causes

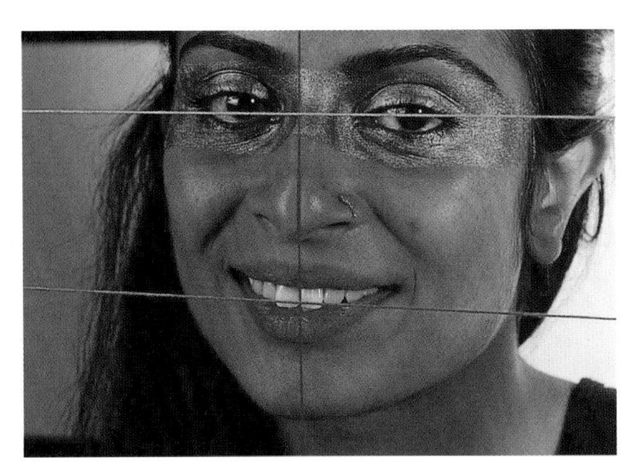

Figure 2.48 Coincidence of the interpupillary and incisal plane lines is used as a guide for dental aesthetics.

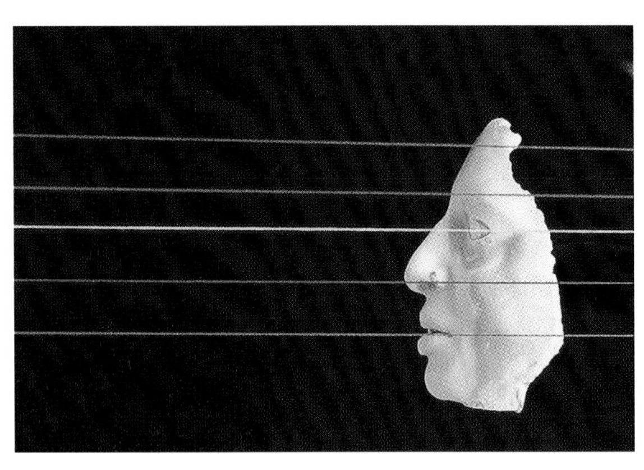

Figure 2.50 Sagittal view showing parallelism of the facial lines.

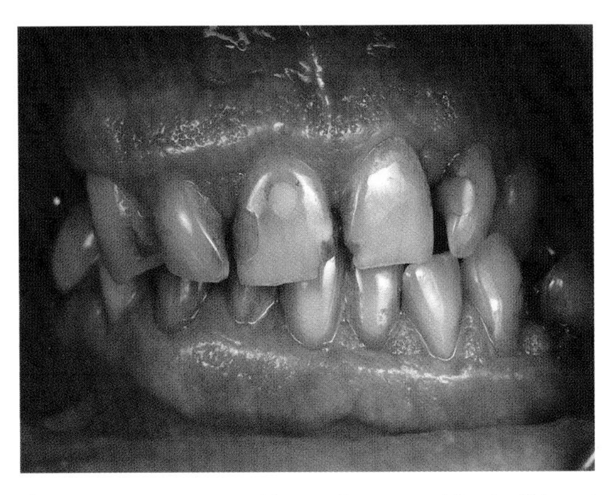

Figure 2.49 Uneven attrition and wear resulting in tilting of the incisal plane.

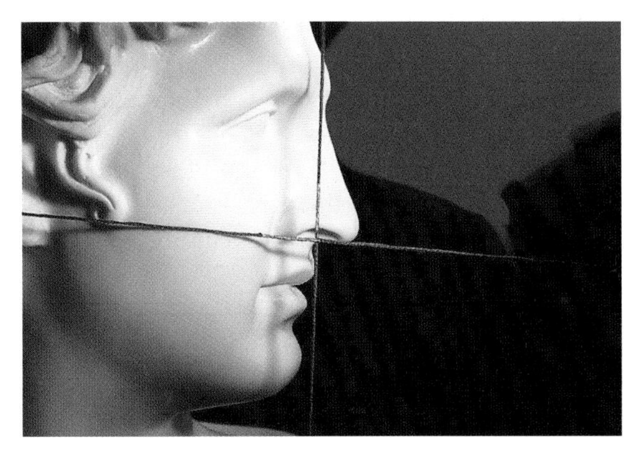

Figure 2.51 Nasolabial angle (golden highlight).

of misalignment of the incisal plane, since these impact on the proposed treatment plan (Fig. 2.49).

From the sagittal aspect, the horizontal lines also reinforce the cohesiveness of the profile (Fig. 2.50). In this aspect two additional reference lines require consideration: the nasolabial angle (Fig. 2.51) and the Rickett's E-plane (Fig. 2.52).[39] The nasolabial angle is formed by the intersection of two lines using the nose and lips as reference points. For males this angle ranges from 90–95° and for females from 100–105°. The Rickett's E-plane is a line drawn from the tip of the nose to the chin prominence. Accepted norms for the distance from the upper lip to this imaginary line is 4 mm, while that for lower lip is

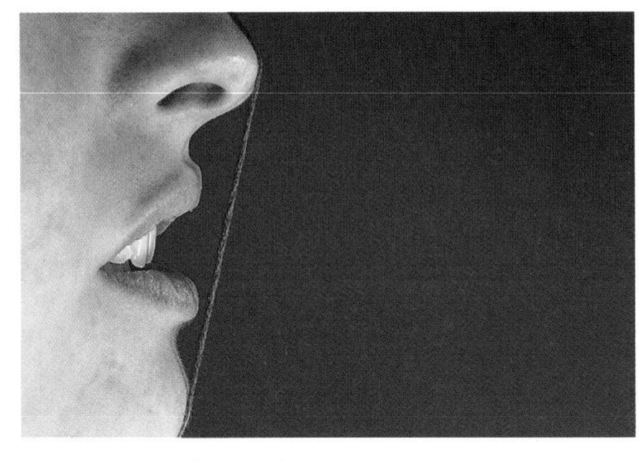

Figure 2.52 Rickett's E-plane.

2 mm. Using the nasolabial angle and Rickett's E-plane, the protrusion or retrusion of the maxilla can be assessed. Assuming 90° as the normal, if the nasolabial angle is <90°, and the distance of the upper lip to the E-plane is greater than 4 mm, the maxilla is prominent and the facial profile is convex. In these cases, less dominant maxillary anterior restorations should be considered. If the reverse, a concave profile is evident, i.e. nasolabial angle is >90°, and the distance of the upper lip to the E-plane is <4 mm, a prominent maxillary anterior dental sextant is desirable. Spear[40] has termed this concept of facial profile to determine the position and degree of dominance of the maxillary anterior teeth as 'facially generated treatment planning'.

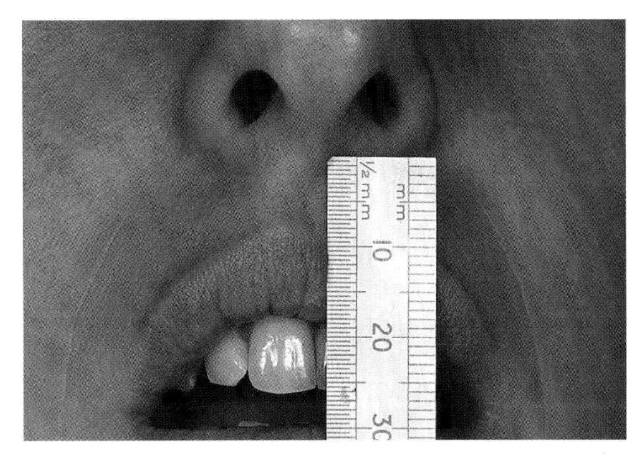

Figure 2.53 Maxillary lip length determines the degree of maxillary incisor display.

Dentofacial composition

The second constituent of anterior dental aesthetics is the orofacial view known as the dentofacial composition, consisting of the teeth surrounded by the highly vascularised lips. The red colour of the lips and the lighter teeth create a colour contrast, adding interest to this composition. The aesthetic appraisal of this view is determined by two muscular positions, the static and dynamic.

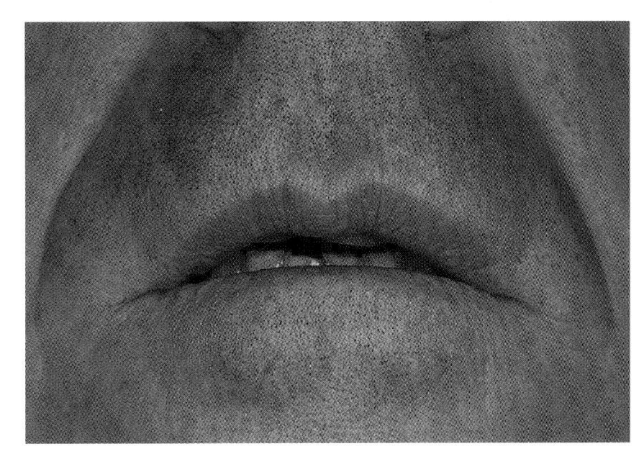

Figure 2.54 Elderly males have long maxillary lips, with reduced maxillary incisor display.

Static

In the static position, the lips are slightly parted, the teeth out of occlusion. This is a habitual muscular position, often incorrectly referred to as the 'rest position'. In this position four features influence tooth exposure: lip length, age, race and sex, known as the LARS factor (Figs. 2.53–2.56).[41] Table 2.2 displays the amount of maxillary and mandibular central incisor teeth visible in relation to the length of the maxillary lip. The length of the upper lip varies from 10–36 mm, and individuals with a long maxillary lip show more mandibular than maxillary incisors.

Age is the second part of the LARS factor which, in a similar manner to lip length, influences the amount of tooth visibility. The amount of maxillary incisor tooth display is inversely proportional to increasing age, while degree of

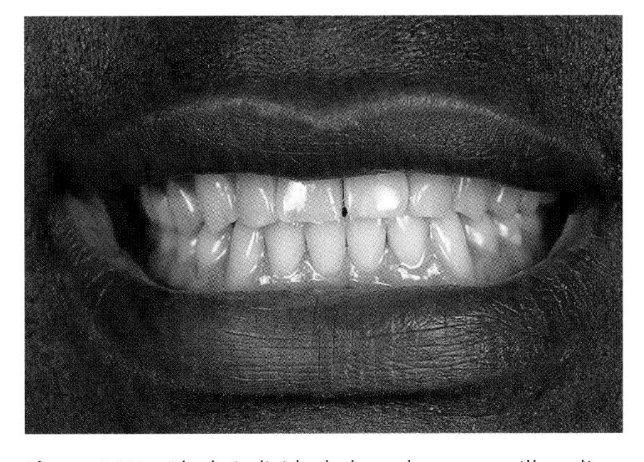

Figure 2.55 Black individuals have longer maxillary lips, with reduced maxillary incisor display.

Table 2.2 Maxillary lip length in relation to anterior tooth exposure.

Maxillary lip	Maxillary lip length (mm)	Exposure of maxillary central incisors (mm)	Exposure of mandibular central incisors (mm)
Short	10–15	3.92	0.64
Medium	16–20	3.44	0.77
Medium	21–25	2.18	0.98
Long	26–30	0.93	1.95
Long	31–36	0.25	2.25

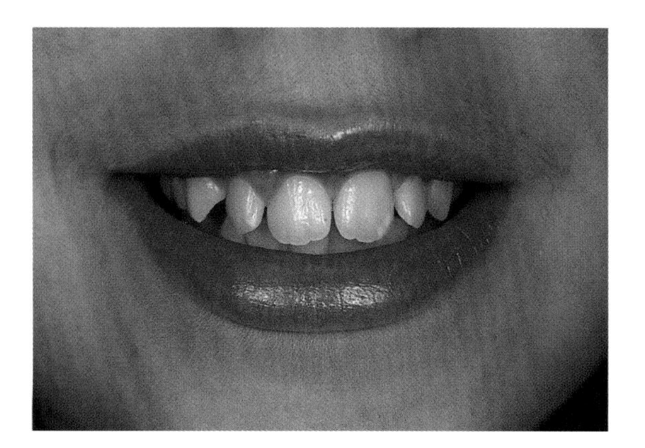

Figure 2.56 Females have short maxillary lips, with increased maxillary incisor display.

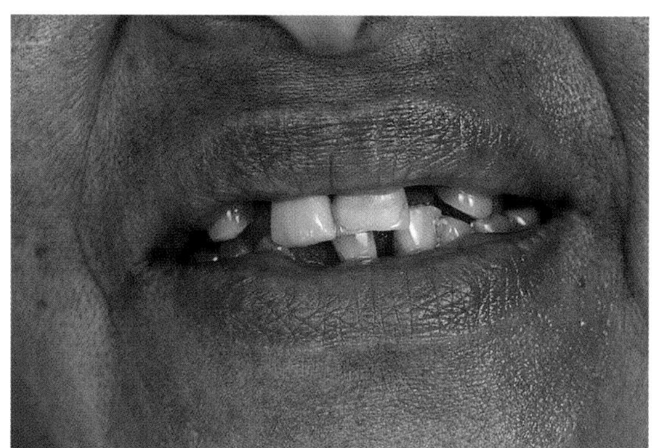

Figure 2.57 Early tooth loss due to periodontitis results in accelerated formation of nasolabial grooves.

mandibular incisor display is directly proportional to increasing age.

People age at different rates, because ageing is a multifactorial phenomenon described by the three Ps:

- Programmed ageing
- Pathological ageing
- Psychological ageing

In youth, the process of destruction and formation of cells is in a state of equilibrium. With advancing years the balance shifts in favour of increased destruction and reduced replacement. This change is triggered by an internal 'biological clock', the reason for which is unknown. Pathological ageing is due to diseases of the oral cavity and surrounding structures leading to an accelerated degradation of tissues. For example, if anterior teeth are lost due to refractory periodontitis, there is premature development of nasolabial grooves (Fig. 2.57). Psychological ageing is the result of psychosomatic changes due to emotional and personal traumas. Irrespective of cause, the three Ps of ageing cause reduced tonicity of the orofacial muscles and laxness of tegumental relief in the lower third of the face. This leads to formation of the labial, nasolabial and mental grooves and ridges. The loss of elasticity and tooth support (gingival two-thirds of upper incisor) of the upper lip accounts for less maxillary and more mandibular incisors display at rest. Attrition is another factor in the aged, contributing to further reduced amount of tooth display.

The last two determinants of the LARS factor are race and sex. A decreasing amount of maxillary and increasing amount of mandibular tooth visibility is evident from Caucasians, Asians to Blacks. Finally, gender considerations reveal that females display nearly twice the amount of tooth as compared to men, 3.40 mm and 1.91 mm, respectively.

In conclusion, each patient should be assessed according to the LARS factor before finalising the final amount of tooth exposure in the static position, e.g. an increased maxillary tooth display is indicated for young females, while the opposite is true for elderly men.

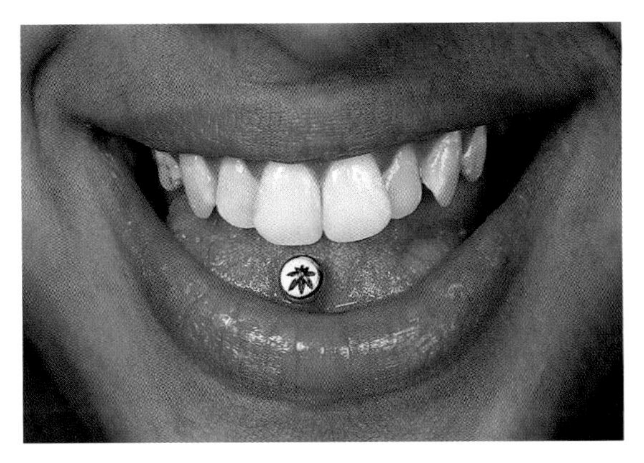

Figure 2.58 Balance: perfect alignment of the anterior maxillary sextant is less important than balance on contralateral sides.

Dynamic

The dynamic position of the dentofacial composition is characterised by a smile. The extent of tooth exposure during a smile varies, depending on the degree of contraction of the facial muscles, the shape and thickness of the lips, the skeletal make-up, and the shape and size of the dental elements. Whereas in the facial composition horizontal symmetry was the most important factor, in the dentofacial view it is radiating symmetry that takes precedence. Radiating symmetry is the central point of an object from which the right and left sides are mirror images.[42] In the dental context, the maxillary dental midline is the fulcrum or central point, and the right and left upper anterior teeth are balanced mirror images. This is relatively uncommon due to erratic patterns of wear and attrition of the incisal and canine edges. Lack of radiating symmetry is not crucial, so long as there is balance on the right and left sides of the anterior dental sextant (Fig. 2.58). The incisal plane and commissural lines should coincide to act as cohesive forces, and the dental midline as the segregative force, adding interest to the composition (Fig. 2.59).

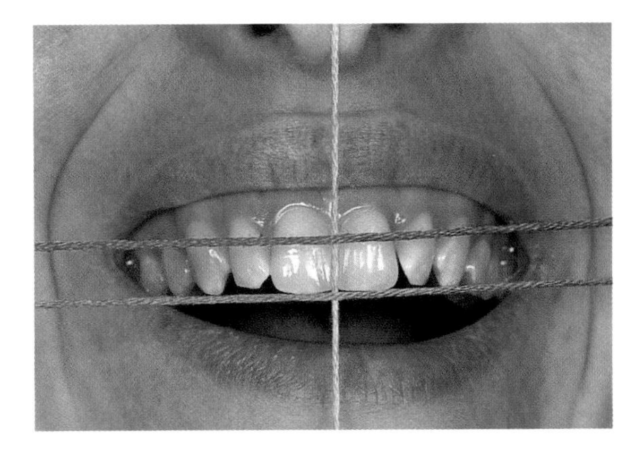

Figure 2.59 Ideally, the commissural plane (blue) should coincide with the incisal plane (lime green) and be perpendicular to the dental midline (yellow).

Placement of the dental midline has evoked considerable controversy in the dental literature. One school of thought states that the maxillary dental midline should coincide exactly with the labial frenum and the facial midline[43] as it does in 70% of the population. The opposing view states that placing the midline exactly in the centre contributes to a sense of artificiality.[44] Where to place this midline should be determined after an aesthetic appraisal. If a dominant central point of focus exists, e.g. a maxillary median diastema, then the midline should be placed with this focal point as the fulcrum. Another reason for placing a vertically aligned midline precisely in the centre is to detract attention from asymmetries and disharmonies of the face. The concept of guiding the eye to a particular point of focus on the face is extensively used by opticians and the cosmetic industry with great effect. On the other hand, a slightly off-centre placement of the dental midline, in relation to the facial midline, is not detrimental to aesthetic approval (Figs. 2.60 & 2.61). The mandibular

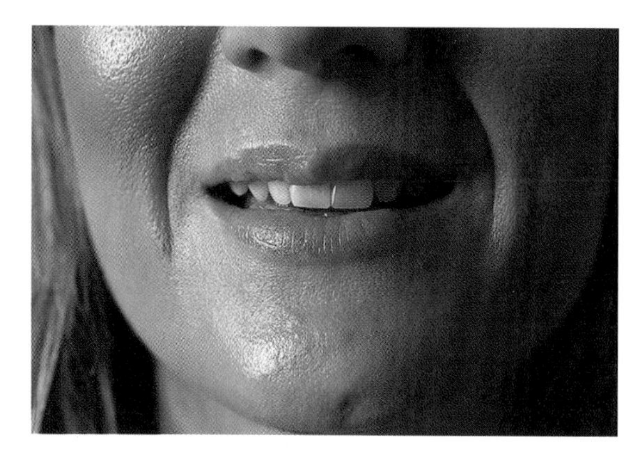

Figure 2.60 For a pleasing appearance, coincidence of the facial and dental midlines is not mandatory.

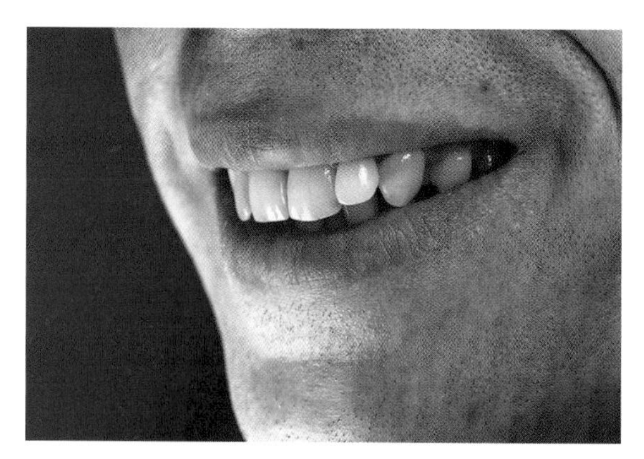

Figure 2.62 Parallelism of the incisal plane with the curvature of the mandibular lip.

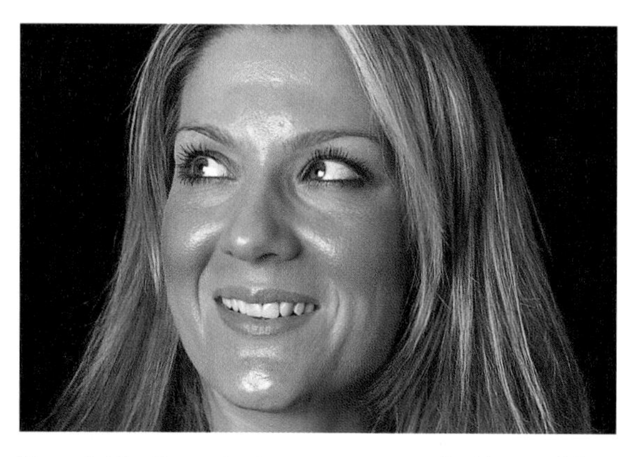

Figure 2.61 For a pleasing appearance, coincidence of the facial and dental midlines is not mandatory.

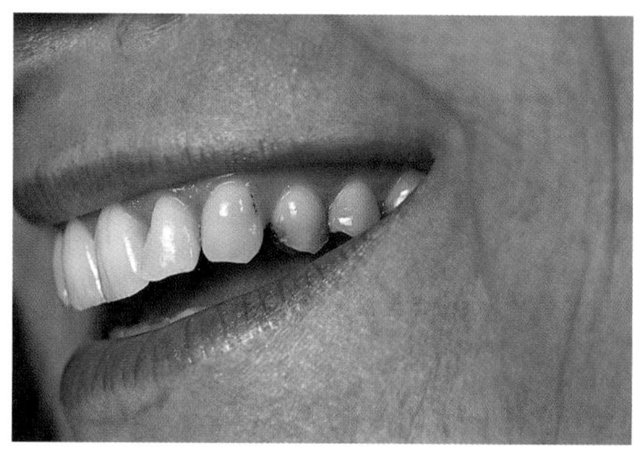

Figure 2.63 Anterior negative space during laughter.

midline should not be used as a reference point, because in 75% of cases this does not coincide with the maxillary midline.[45]

The smile line is an imaginary line of the tips of the maxillary teeth, parallel to the curvature of the mandibular lip (Fig. 2.62). The coincidence between the incisal table and the lower lip is often lost because of wear, and, if possible, should be restored by restorative procedures. The anterior and lateral negative spaces act as a border to the dental elements, similar to the border around a painting, while the lips represent a frame. Anterior negative space is evident during speech and laughter (Fig. 2.63), while the bilateral negative spaces are seen during a smile (Fig. 2.64). These negative spaces provide cohe-

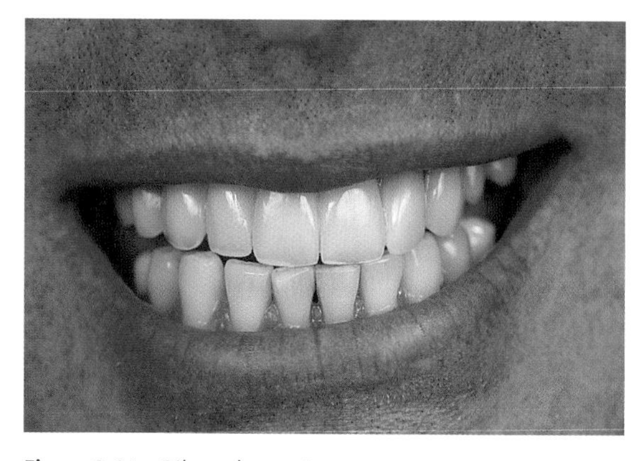

Figure 2.64 Bilateral negative space.

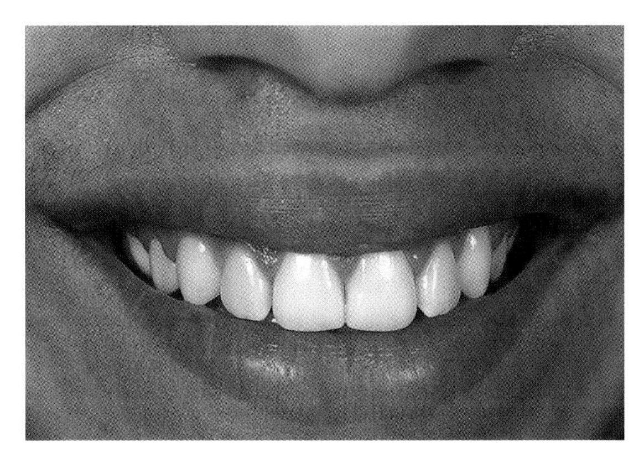

Figure 2.65 The 'perfect' smile.

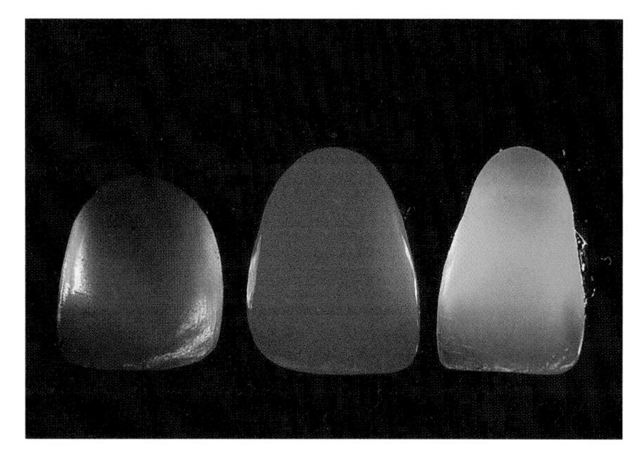

Figure 2.66 Width/length ratio. Blue tooth – wide (0.8); red tooth – 'ideal' (0.75); green tooth – narrow (0.6).

siveness and a frame to the dentofacial composition.[46] Some authorities advocate elimination of bilateral negative spaces, during a so-called 'complete aesthetics makeover'. This results in excessive tooth display during a smile conveying artificiality, and is unwarranted because of irreversible destructive prosthetic procedures.

To summarise, the perfect smile is when the upper anterior teeth are in line with the curvature of the lower lip, the corners of the lips are elevated to the same height on both sides (smile symmetry), with bilateral negative space separating the teeth from the corners of the lips (Fig. 2.65).

Dental composition

The dental composition consists of the teeth (size and shape), and their intra- and inter-arch relationships. Tooth size is determined by measuring the inciso-gingival length and dividing by the mesio-distal width to obtain the width/length ratio:

$$\text{width/length (w/l) ratio of a tooth} = \frac{\textit{width}}{\textit{length}}$$

Clinicians and authors have subjective opinions, as no definitive value exists for the w/l ratio. The mesio-distal width is more important than the inciso-gingival length[47], and it is the former measurement that has attracted much debate. Research has focused on measurements of extracted orthodontic teeth, racial and gender differences, and facial landmarks such as the bizygomatic width. The latter was described by House and Loop[48] who stated that the mesio-distal measurement of the central incisor was 1/16 of the bizygomatic width. Other studies have assigned geometric values to the mesio-distal width of the centrals to the size of the face, while Rufenacht[49] has proposed morphopsychological determination of the ideal proportion and suggested that the width of the central incisor should be considered constant throughout life. Which theory a clinician chooses is open to discussion as none of the research is conclusive. Nevertheless, general guidelines are necessary to create pleasing dimensions:

- The w/l ratio of the central incisor should range from 0.75–0.8, less than this value creates a long narrow tooth, while a larger w/l ratio results in a short wide tooth (Fig. 2.66)
- The central incisor is dominant in the anterior dental composition (Fig. 2.67)
- The vertical overbite in relation to speech requires attention (discussed above).

Besides these fundamental principles, subtle variations can be introduced, accounting for sex, race, morphopsychological and facial factors.

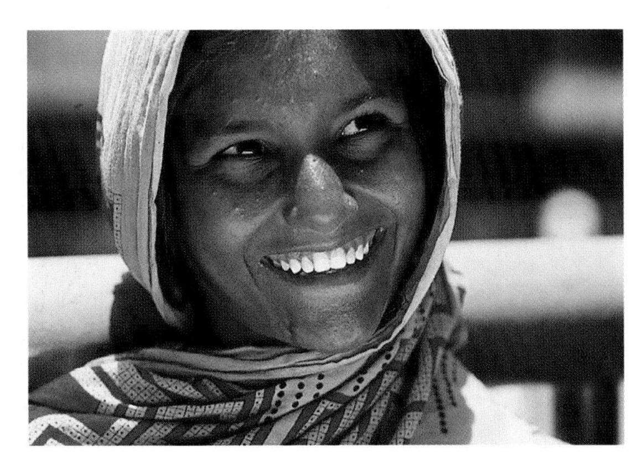

Figure 2.67 The dominance of the maxillary central is essential for a pleasing smile.

The shape of the upper anterior teeth is also widely debated. The two prominent studies are by Williams[50] and Frush and Fisher.[51,52,53] Williams established a relationship between the shape of the central incisor and the face, while Frush and Fisher related sex, age and personality (SAP) to the contour of the anterior dental segment. The Williams theory was invalidated by subsequent studies. The Frush and Fisher concept is concerned with the dominance of the central incisor and its wear in advancing years. Other theories have proposed a correlation of tooth shape to skeletal and soft tissue landmarks, but have proved inconclusive. The shape of teeth is inherited, and if possible, the prosthodontist should obtain pictures of patients' relatives before determining the final shape of anterior teeth. If this is not possible, the items to consider are age, sex, race and personality. For example, youthful teeth have sharp, unworn incisal edges; the centrals dominate the composition, and are in harmony with the laterals and canines.

The next factor to consider is tooth-to-tooth progression. Ancient Greeks endeavoured to formulate beauty as an exact mathematical principle. They believed that beauty could be quantified and represented in a mathematical formula. This lead Pythagoras to conceive the Golden proportion (1/1.618 = 0.618), and Plato the Beautiful proportion (1/1.733 = 0.577). Both ideas stipulate that an object with specific proportions is perceived as having innate beauty. The most widely used concept in dentistry is the Golden proportion, whose formula is as follows:

$$\frac{S}{L} = \frac{L}{S+L} = \frac{2}{1+\sqrt{5}} = 0.618$$

where S is the smaller and L the larger part. The uniqueness of this ratio is that when applied by three different methods of calculations, linear, geometric and arithmetic, the proportional progression from the smaller to the larger to the whole part always produces the same results. This concept has been described by Lombardi[54] and Levin[55] (Fig. 2.68). However, researchers have indicated that a Golden proportion is not always evident, and variations are often apparent in the natural dentition.[56] It is imperative to mention that many healthy dentitions do not conform to this 'ideal' ratio, but are still perceived as aesthetically pleasing (Fig. 2.69). To create an aesthetically pleasing result, the most important aspect is repeating proportions, rather than a specific ratio. Therefore, providing 'cosmetic dentistry' for healthy teeth not in the ideal ratio 0.618 is grossly unnecessary and highly unethical.

The axial inclination of the maxillary anterior teeth is ideally aligned so that the incisal edges converge mesially (Fig. 2.70). The contact points are also coincident with the incisal edges and the curvature of the lower lip, enhancing the cohesiveness of the dentofacial composition.

Incisal embrasures have a distinct appearance depending on age and sex. For virgin teeth, an increase of the embrasure angle from the maxillary central incisor to the canine is apparent (Fig. 2.71). Pronounced embrasures are a feature of youth or femininity, while shortened, worn edges convey advancing age or masculinity (Fig. 2.72). Discussion with the patient is essential to incorporate their wishes and desires, before deciding on the angle of the incisal embrasures.

The buccolingual thickness of teeth varies, e.g. the upper central incisor has a range between 2.5 and 3.3 mm.[57] This is measured with a width gauge at the junction of the middle third and incisal third of the tooth (Fig. 2.73). If the buccolingual thickness of a prosthesis is more than 3.5 mm, over-contouring should be suspected.

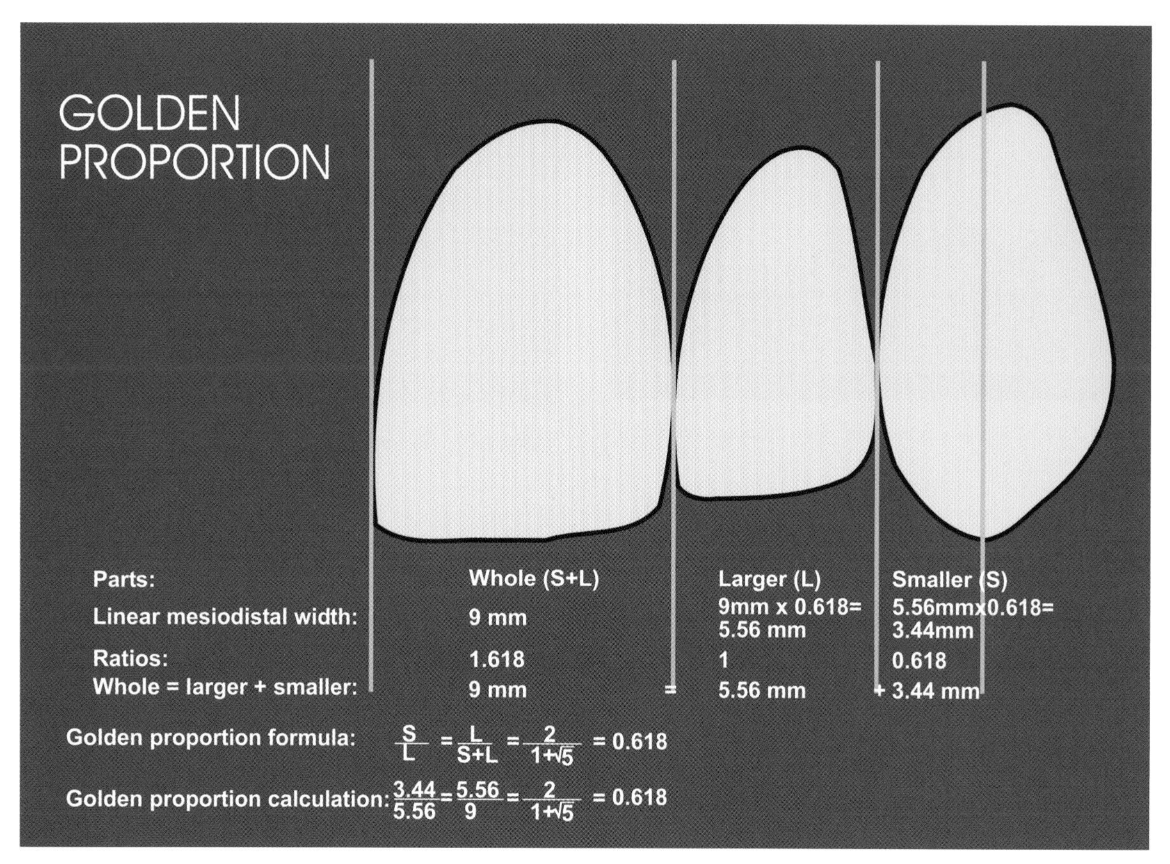

Figure 2.68 The Golden proportion.

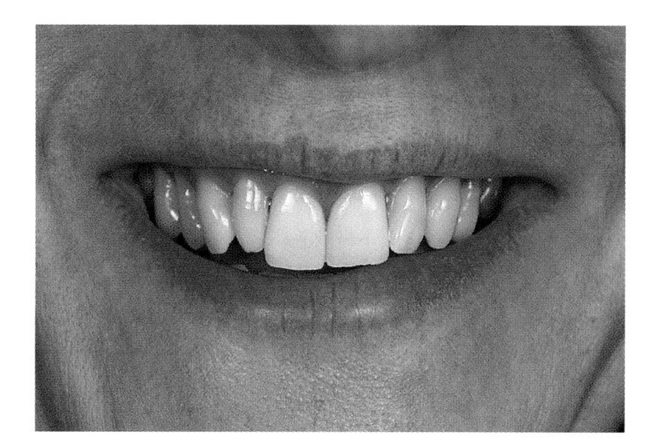

Figure 2.69 Although not in the Golden proportion, this natural dentition is nevertheless aesthetically pleasing.

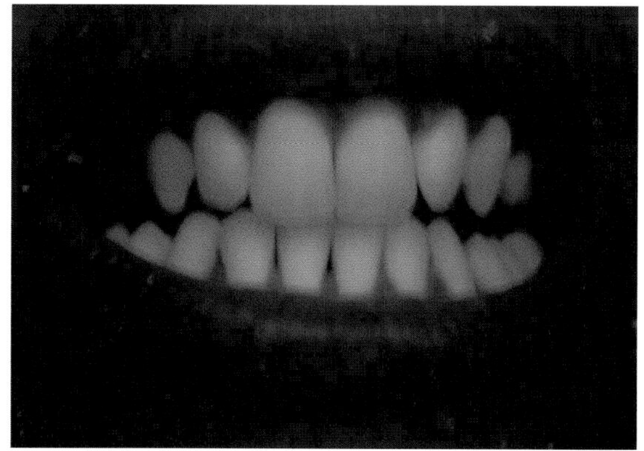

Figure 2.70 Mesial axial inclination of maxillary anterior teeth.

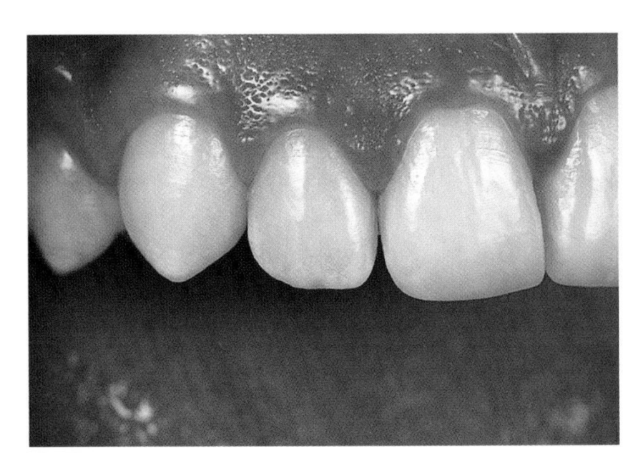

Figure 2.71 Pristine virgin teeth with pronounced incisal embrasures.

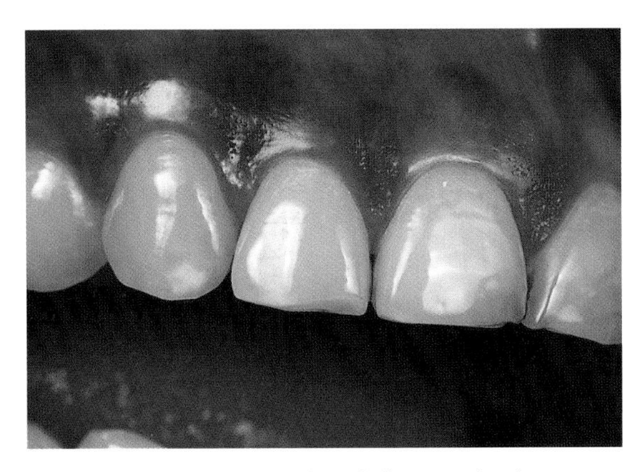

Figure 2.72 Worn aged teeth with flat incisal embrasures.

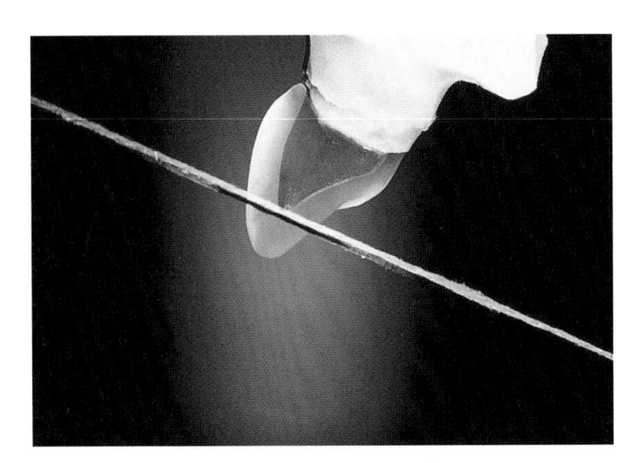

Figure 2.73 Bucco-lingual thickness.

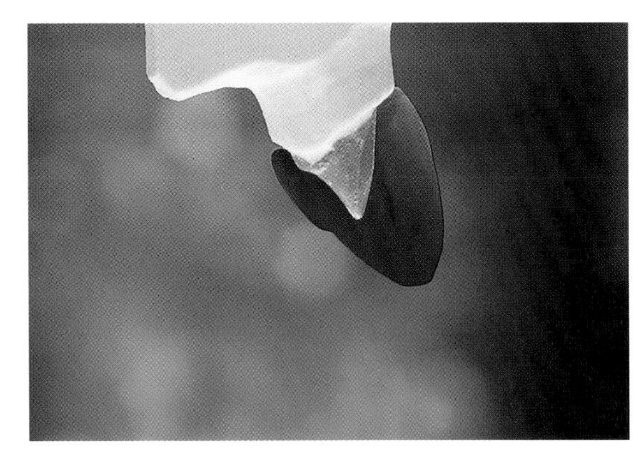

Figure 2.74 Over-contoured, bulbous crown.

This is usually caused by insufficient tooth preparation, leaving inadequate space for the restorative materials, resulting in a bulbous restoration (Fig. 2.74). If the buccolingual thickness is less than 2.5 mm, elective endodontic therapy may be necessary to achieve the desired aesthetic result.

Gingival composition

The gingival apparatus is the last constitutent of aesthetic appraisal. Gingival contour mimics the underlying bone architecture. The gingival zenith is the most apical part of the FGM and is located distally for the maxillary central and canine, and in line for the lateral, to the long axis of the tooth. This zenith disappears due to poor dentistry, but can be regained by replacing defective restorations (Figs. 2.75 & 2.76).

Extension of the FGM apically from the contact point to the attached gingiva forms the interdental papilla. Following recession, periodontal or iatrogenic insult, the gingival embrasures become visible and form so-called 'black triangles' (Fig. 2.77). Numerous techniques for preserving[58] and restoring[59] the interdental papilla have been described, and the prosthodontist should strive to fill these open gingival embrasures for optimal aesthetics.

During a relaxed 'ideal smile', the upper lip exposes the cervical aspects of the upper anterior

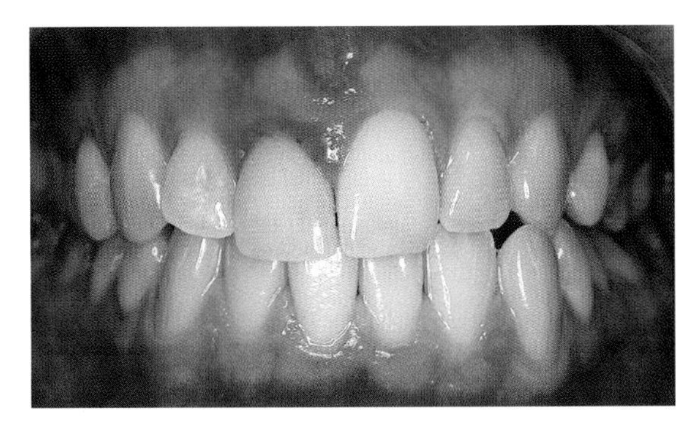

Figure 2.75 Amorphous free gingival margin associated with defective crown on maxillary right central incisor.

teeth. The gingival margins of the maxillary central should be at the same height, and symmetrical. Up to 3 mm exposure above the cervical margins of the teeth is aesthetically acceptable (Fig. 2.78).[60] More than 3 mm exposure leads to a 'gummy' smile, requiring correction in order to avoid visual tension (Fig. 2.79). Treatment modalities depend on the type of pathosis, e.g. hyperplastic gingivae require gingivectomy or crown lengthening; recession can be corrected by cosmetic periodontal plastic surgery using tissue grafts or guided tissue regenerative membranes; over-eruption by orthodontic intrusion; deficient pontic sites by ridge

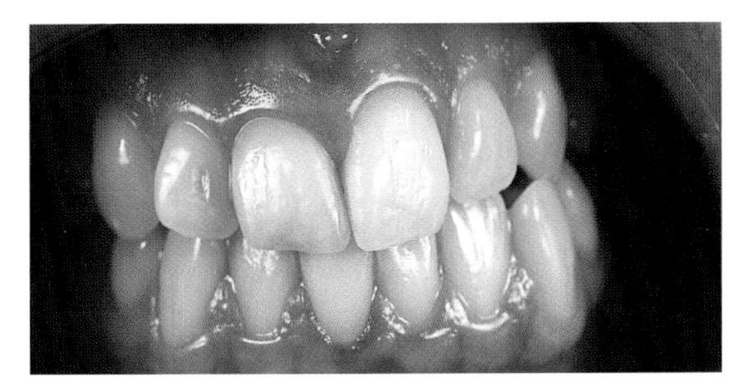

Figure 2.76 Replacement crown for patient in Figure 2.75, and following gingival health the gingival zenith peaks distal to long axis of tooth.

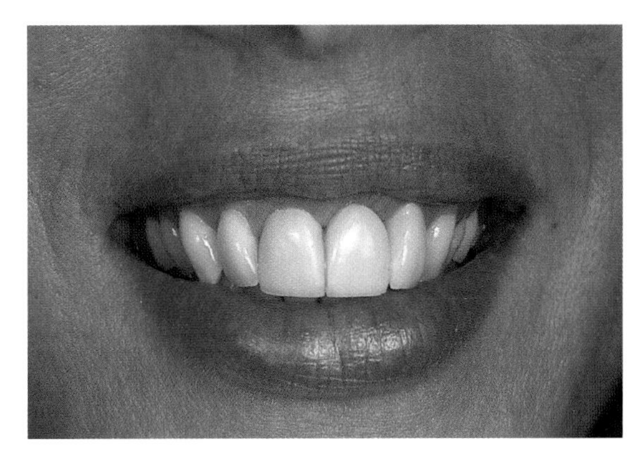

Figure 2.78 Up to 3 mm of gingival exposure during a relaxed smile is acceptable for a pleasing smile.

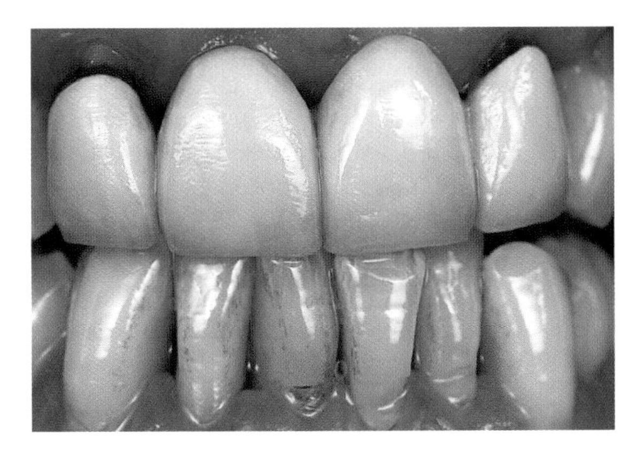

Figure 2.77 Gingival embrasures causing 'black triangles' between defective metal–ceramic crowns.

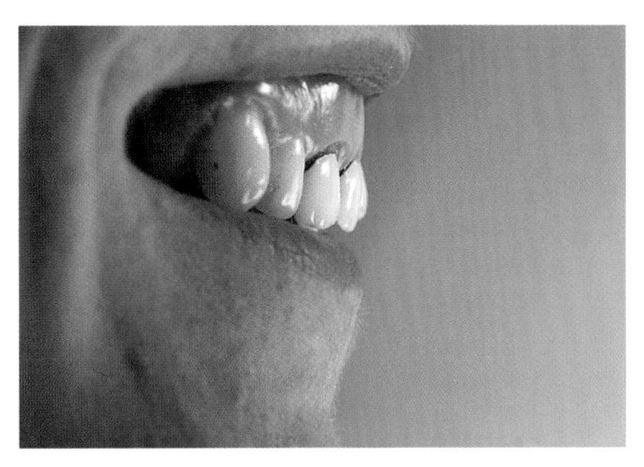

Figure 2.79 Greater than 3 mm of gingival exposure is aesthetically unacceptable.

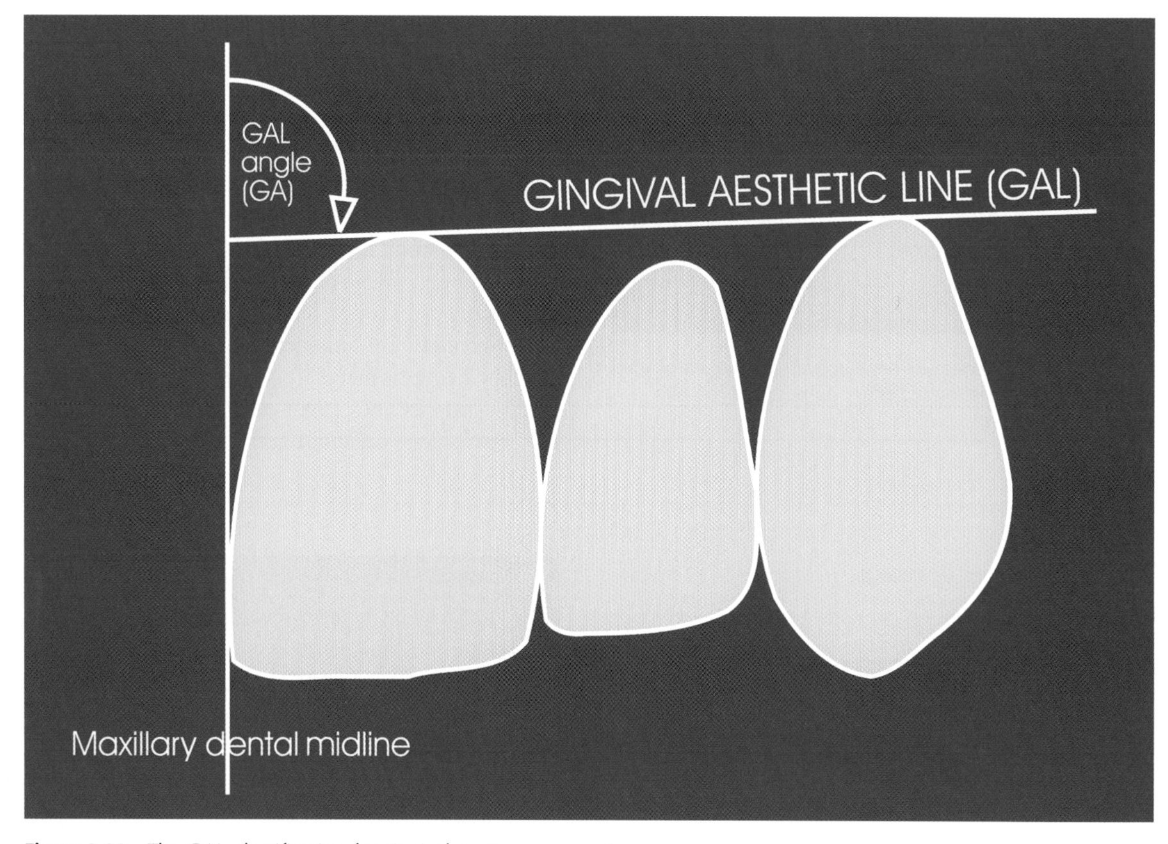

Figure 2.80 The GAL classification for gingival contour progression.

augmentation procedures; and skeletal abnormalities by orthognathic surgery.

One of the most significant features of gingival aesthetics is its contour progression from the incisors to canine. The gingival aesthetic line (GAL) can be defined as a line joining the tangents of the zeniths of the gingival margins of the central incisor and canine. The GAL angle (GA) is the intersection of the GAL line with the maxillary dental midline (Fig. 2.80). Assuming a normal w/l ratio, anatomy, position and alignment of the anterior dental segment, four classes of GAL are described, as follows:

- Class I – the GAL angle is between 45° and 90° and the lateral incisor is touching or below (1–2 mm) the GAL (Fig. 2.81)
- Class II – the GAL angle is between 45° and 90° but the lateral incisor is above (1–2 mm) the GAL and its mesial part overlaps the distal aspect of the central incisor. This situation often occurs in Angle's class II or pseudo-class II conditions, adding variety to the dental composition (Fig. 2.82)
- Class III – the GAL angle is 90°, and the canine, lateral and central all lie below the GAL (Fig. 2.83)
- Class IV – the gingival contour can not be assigned to any of the above three classes. The GAL angle can be acute or obtuse. A myriad of gingival conditions present as gingival asymmetries, including recession, altered patterns of eruption, loss of interdental papillae, clefts and high frenal insertions (Fig. 2.84)

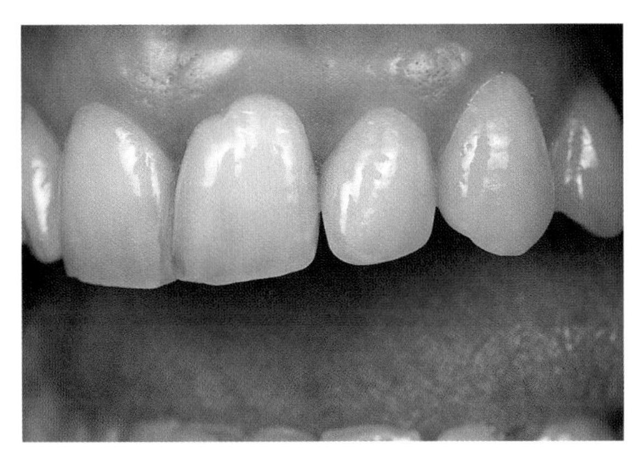

Figure 2.81 GAL class I.

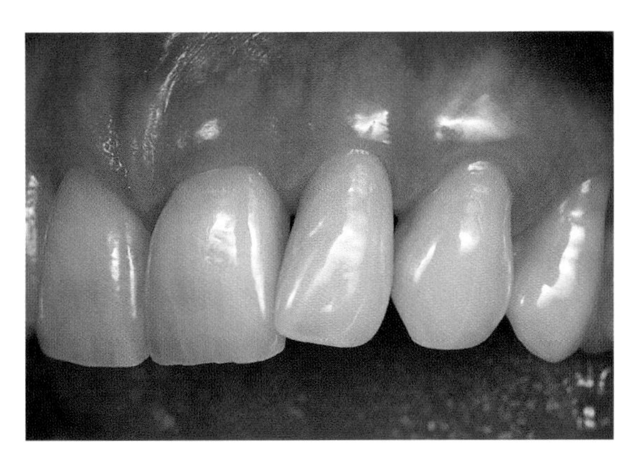

Figure 2.82 GAL class II.

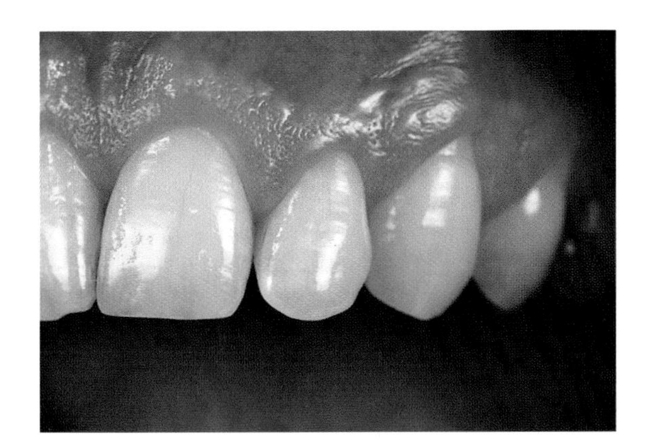

Figure 2.83 GAL class III.

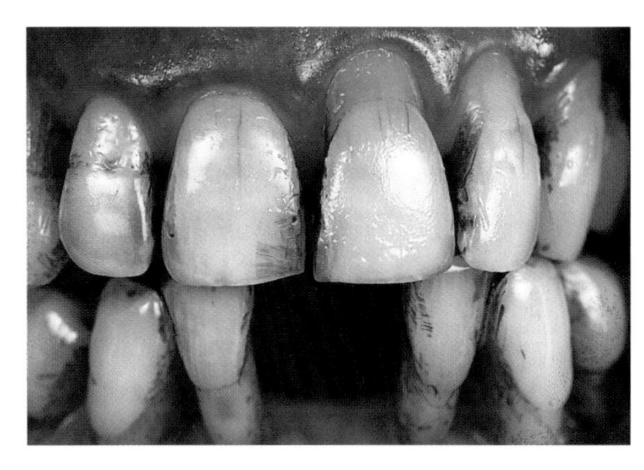

Figure 2.84 GAL class IV.

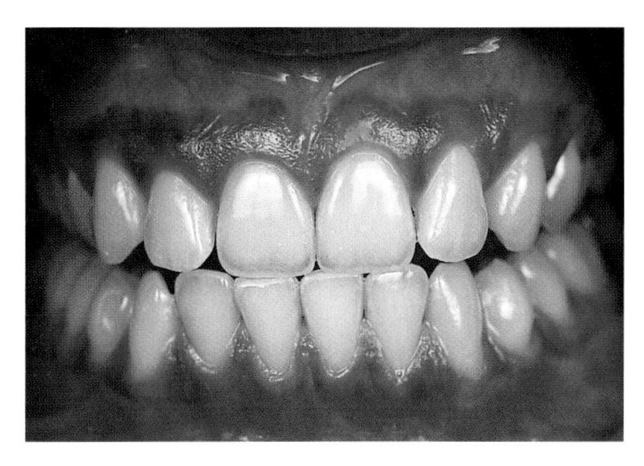

Figure 2.85 GAL class I on right maxillary sextant and GAL class III on left maxillary sextant.

In a single mouth, the right and left sides can display different GAL classes (Fig. 2.85). The aim is to restore the gingival contour to a GAL class I, II or III in order to achieve aesthetic approval and favourable 'pink aesthetics'.

Table 2.3 summarises the salient items to consider during an aesthetic appraisal.

Table 2.3 Aesthetic appraisal.

Composition	Evaluate	Determine by . . .
Facial	Cohesive forces (horizontal symmetry)	Horizontal facial lines
	Segregative forces	Facial midline
	Incisal plane	Relation to interpupillary line
	Protrusion/retrusion of maxilla	Rickett's E-plane and nasolabial angle
Dentofacial	Tooth exposure in static position	LARS factor
	Tooth exposure during a smile	Radiating symmetry
	Fulcrum of smile	Dental midline
	Smile line	Relation of maxillary teeth to lower lip during a smile
Dental	Tooth dimensions	Width/length ratio
	Tooth morphology	Genetics (hereditary)
	Tooth-to-tooth relationship	Modified Golden proportion, repeated proportion more significant than a specific ratio
	Axial inclination	Mesially inclined maxillary anterior dental segment
	Incisal embrasures	Age, sex and personality
	Buccolingual thickness	Normal range = 2.5–3.3 mm
	Phonetics	M, F, V and S sounds
Gingival	Contour around individual tooth	Underlying bone architecture and tooth morphology
	Exposure during smile	Acceptable range is less than or equal to 3 mm
	Contour progression from central incisor to canine	GAL and GA

References

1. Goaslind, G.D., Robertson, P.B., Mahan, C.J., Morrison, W.W. and Olson, J.V. (1977) Thickness of facial gingiva. *J Periodontol*, **48(12)**, 768–771
2. Alpiste-Illueca, F. (2004) Dimensions of the dentogingival unit in maxillary anterior teeth: A new exploration technique (Parallel Profile Radiography). *Int J Periodontics Restorative Dent*, **24**, 386–396
3. Wennstrom, J.L., Bengazi, F. and Lekholm, U. (1994) The influence of the masticatory mucosa on the peri-implant soft tissue condition. *Clin Oral Implant Res*, **5**, 1–8
4. Meffert, R.M. (1988) The soft tissue interface in dental implantology. *J Dent Educ*, **52**, 810–811
5. Silverstein, L.H., Lefkove, M.D. and Garnick, J.J. (1994) The use of free gingival soft tissue to improve the implant/soft tissue interface. *J Oral Implantol*, **20**, 36–40
6. Stanley, H.R. The cyclic phenomenon of periodontitis. *Oral Surg*, **8**, 598–610
7. Frank, R., Fiore-Donno, G., Cimasoni, G. and Matter, J. (1974) Ultrastructural study of epithelial and connective gingival reattachment in man. *J Periodontol*, **45**, 626–635
8. Ingber, J.S., Rose, L.F. and Caslet, J.G. (1977) The biological width – a concept in periodontics and restorative dentistry. *Alpha Omegan*, **70**, 62–65
9. Garguilo, A.W., Wentz, F.M. and Orban, B. (1961) Dimensions and relations of the dentogingival junction in humans. *J Periodontol*, **32**, 321
10. Tal, H., Soldinger, M., Dreiangel, A. and Pitarus, S. Periodontal response to long-term abuse of the gingival attachment by supracrestal amalgam restorations. *J Clin Periodont*, **16**, 654–689
11. Vacek, J.S., Gher, M.E., Assad, D.A., Richardson, A.C. and Giambarresi, L.I. (1994) The dimensions of the human dentogingival junc-

tion. *Int J Periodontics Restorative Dent*, **14(2)**, 155–165

[12] Becker, W., Ochsenbein, C., Tibbets, L. and Becker, B. (1997) Alveolar bone anatomic profiles as measured from dry skulls. *J Clin Periodontal*, **24**, 727–731

[13] Tarnow, D., Mager, A. and Fletcher, P. (1992) The effect of the distance from the contact point to the crest of bone on the presence or absence of the interproximal dental papilla. *J Periodontol*, **63**, 995–996

[14] Kois, J.C. (1998) New paradigms for anterior tooth preparation: Rationale and technique. *Oral Heath*, **April**, 19–30

[15] Nevins, M. and Skurow, H.M. (1984) The intracrevicular restorative margin, the biologic width, and the maintenance of gingival margin. *Int J Periodontics Restorative Dent*, **4**, 30–49

[16] Block, P.L. (1987) Restorative margins and periodontal health: A new look at an old perspective. *J Prosthet Dent*, **57(6)**, 683–689

[17] deWaal, H. and Castelucci G. The importance of restorative margin placement to the biologic width and periodontal health: part 1. *Int J Periodontics Restorative Dent*, **13**, 461–471

[18] American Academy of Periodontology (2000) Dental implants in periodontal therapy. *J Periodontol*, **71**, 1934–1942

[19] Grundler, U., Gracis, S. and Capelli, M. (2005) Influence of the 3-D bone-to-implant relationship on esthetics. *Int J Periodontics Restorative Dent*, **25**, 113–119

[20] Holt, R.L., Rosenberg, M.M., Zinser, P.J. and Ganeles, J. (2002) A concept for a biologically derived parabolic implant design. *Int J Periodontics Restorative Dent*, **22**, 473–481

[21] (1999) The glossary of prosthodontic terms. *J Prosthet Dent*, **81(1)**, 39–110

[22] Dawson, P. (1989) *Evaluation, Diagnosis and Treatment of Occlusal Problems*, 2nd edn. Mosby, St Louis

[23] Posselt, U. (1952) Studies in the mobility of the human mandible. *Acta Odontol Scand*, **10**, 109

[24] Steele, J.G., Nohl, F.S.A. and Wassell, R.W. (2002) Crowns and other extra-coronal restorations: Occlusal considerations and articulator selection. *Br Dent J*, **192(7)**, 377–387

[25] Manns, A., Chan, C. and Miralles, R. (1987) Influence of group function and canine guidance on electromyographic activity of elevator muscles. *J Prosthet Dent*, **57(4)**: 494–501

[26] Williamson, E.H. and Lundquist, D.O. (1983) Anterior guidance: its effect on electromyographic activity of the temporal and masseter muscles. *J Prosthet Dent*, **49(6)**, 816–823

[27] Bartlett, D.W. and Fisher, N.L. (1995) Factors influencing treatment planning of restorative dentistry in general practice: Part 2. *Dental Update*, **October**, 334–337

[28] Speak, F. (2004) Occlusion in the new millennium: The controversy continues – Part 2. *Spear Perspective*, **3(2)**

[29] Rugh, J.D. and Johnson, R.W. (1984) Vertical dimension discrepancies and masticatory pain/dysfunction. In: *Abnormal Jaw Mechanics*. Ed. Solberg, W.K. and Clark, G. Quintessence, Chicago

[30] McGee, G.F. (1947) Use of facial measurements in determining vertical dimension. *J Am Dent Assoc*, **35**, 342–350

[31] Rivera-Morales, W.C. and Mohl, N. (1991) Relationship of occlusal vertical dimension to the health of the masticatory system. *J Prosthet Dent*, **65**, 547–553

[32] Gattozzi, J.G., Nichols, B.R., Somes, G.W. and Ellinger, C.W. (1976) Variations in mandibular rest positions with and without dentures in place. *J Prosthet Dent*, **36**, 159

[33] Rugh, J.D. and Drago, C.J. (1981) Vertical dimension: A study of clinical rest position and jaw muscle activity. *J Prosthet Dent*, **45**, 677–675

[34] Chiche, G.J. and Pinault, A. (1994) *Esthetics of Anterior Fixed Prosthodontics*. Quintessence Publishing Co. Inc., Chicago

[35] Ahmad, I. (2005) *Clinical Guide to Anterior Dental Aesthetics*. Nature Publishing, London

[36] HeGAL, G.W.F. (1944) Montaigne, ed. *Vorlesungen über die Ästhetik*. Paris

[37] Rufenacht, C.R. (1990) *Fundamental of Esthetics*. p. 20. Quintessence Publishing Co. Inc., Chicago

[38] Chiche, G.J. and Pinault, A. (1994) *Esthetics of Anterior Fixed Prosthodontics*. Quintessence Publishing Co. Inc., Chicago
[39] Levin, J.B. (1995) Esthetic diagnosis. *Current Opinion in Cosmetic Dentistry, Current Science*, 9–17
[40] Spear, F. (1995) Creating Esthetic Excellence Part I, A Complete Approach. Presented at the ADA Meeting, Las Vegas
[41] Vig, R.G. and Brundo, G.C. (1972) The kinetics of anterior tooth display. *J Prosthet Dent*, **39**, 502
[42] Rufenacht, C.R. (1990) *Fundamental of Esthetics*. Quintessence Publishing Co. Inc., Chicago
[43] Heartwell, C.M. (1968) *Syllabus of Complete Dentures*. Lea and Febiger, Philadelphia
[44] Swissedent Foundation (1990) *Dental Office Procedures*. Swissedent Foundation, California
[45] Miller, E.C., Bodden, E.R. and Jamison, H.C. (1979) A study of the relationship of the dental midline to the facial median line. *J Prosthet Dent*, **41**, 657–660
[46] Levin, E.I. (1978) Dental esthetics and the golden proportion. *J Prosthet Dent*, **40**, 244–252
[47] MacArthur, D.R. (1987) Are anterior replacement teeth too small? *J Prosthet Dent*, **57**, 462–465
[48] House, M.M. and Loop, J.L. (1939) *Forum and Colour Harmony in the Dental Art*. Whittier, Calf, MM House
[49] Rufenacht, C.R. (1990) *Fundamental of Esthetics*. p. 114. Quintessence Publishing Co. Inc., Chicago
[50] Williams, J.L. (1914) A new classification of human tooth forms with a special reference to a new system of artificial teeth. *Dent Cosmos*, **56**, 627
[51] Frush, J.P. and Fisher R.D. (1956) How dentinogenics integrate the sex factor. *J Prosthet Dent*, **6**, 160–172
[52] Frush, J.P. and Fisher, R.D. (1956) How dentogenics integrate the personality factor. *J Prosthet Dent*, **6**, 441–449
[53] Frush, J.P. and Fisher, R.D. (1957) The age factor in dentogenics. *J Prosthet Dent*, **7**, 5
[54] Lombardi, R.E. (1973) The principles of visual perception and their clinical application to dental esthetics. *J Prosthet Dent*, **29**, 358–381
[55] Levin, E.I. (1978) Dental aesthetics and the golden proportion. *J Prosthet Dent*, **40**, 244–252
[56] Woelfel, J.B. (1990) *Dental Anatomy: Its relevance to Dentistry*. 4th edn. Lea and Febiger, Philadelphia
[57] Chiche, G.J. and Pinault, A. *Esthetics of Anterior Fixed Prosthodontics*. p. 59. Quintessence Publishing Co. Inc., Chicago
[58] Beagle, J.R. (1992) Surgical reconstruction of the interdental papilla: case report. *Int J Periodont Rest Dent*, **12**, 145–151
[59] Lie, T. (1992) Periodontal surgery for the maxillary anterior area. *Int J Periodont Rest Dent*, **12**, 73–82
[60] Allen, P. (1988) Use of mucogingival surgical procedures to enhance esthetics. *Dent Clin North Am*, **32**, 307

3 Choice of all-ceramic systems

Having established an ideal treatment modality using APT and the HFA triad in the previous two chapters, the clinician, ceramist and patient are now confronted with choosing the type of restoration which will achieve these objectives. The dental market is awash with crown systems, with wide-ranging claims. However, it should be emphasised that no system offers everything, and, very often, a compromise is inevitable. The discussion below concentrates on all-ceramic systems, allowing the operator to select the most appropriate material for a given clinical situation. The clinical performance of all-ceramic restorations is influenced by many factors, which are discussed in other chapters of this book, including material properties, tooth preparation design, fabrication, luting, occlusion and fatigue. This chapter is limited to material properties of various ceramics.

SCIENTIFIC RATIONALE

Rationale for all-ceramic restorations

The first question to ask is 'Why?' Why choose an all-ceramic, rather than a metal–ceramic restoration? It is a fait accompli that metal–ceramic restorations have exhibited remarkable durability since their introduction over four decades ago. The major reason for this success is attributed to the relatively forgiving and established clinical and laboratory techniques. While mechanical endurance of metal–ceramic restorations is undisputed, their major disadvantage is poor appearance in aesthetically challenging areas of the mouth. In these circumstances, the familiar shadowing or metal shine-through at the cervical margins severely compromises aesthetics. Additionally, corrosion by-products and allergic responses to casting alloy constituents are also a concern. These disadvantages have fuelled the introduction of all-ceramic systems, with superior aesthetics and biocompatibility, and elimination of unwanted corrosion or allergic responses. The rationale for improved aesthetics with ceramic prostheses is as follows.

A tooth appears 'natural' due to the interaction of light with dental tissues. The process by which light interacts with dentine and enamel is complex, consisting of reflection, transmission, diffusion, fluorescence, opalescence and iridescence, which are elaborated further in Chapter 4 (Colour and Shade Analysis). Nevertheless, for the present discussion, the following simplified explanation is sufficient. Light enters a tooth by two pathways, via the root through the periodontium, and the crown, the part that is visible in the oral cavity (Figs. 3.1 & 3.2). The vitality and authenticity of natural dentition is due to the unimpeded mingling of light rays through these two routes. Ideally, an artificial restoration should endeavour to emulate this free flow of light within the entire tooth structure (Fig. 3.3).

This phenomenon is illustrated by models of a natural tooth, a metal–ceramic crown and an all-ceramic crown (Figs. 3.4–3.6). In a natural tooth, blue light (representing light entering the root) and red light (representing light entering from the crown) is free to mingle, and utilise 100% of the optical capacity of enamel and dentine (Fig. 3.7). When a metal–ceramic crown is placed on

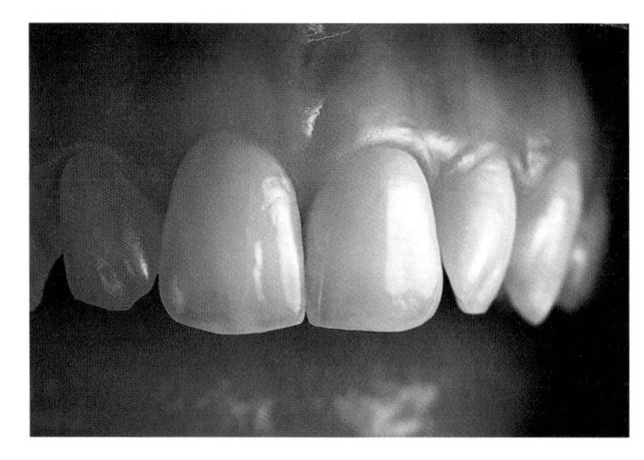

Figure 3.3 The vitality of natural dentition is attributed to unimpeded light flow through the root and crown of a tooth.

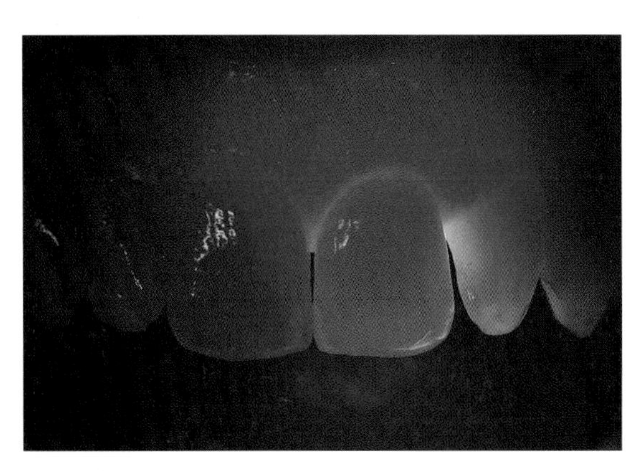

Figure 3.1 Light entering a tooth by the root via the periodontium.

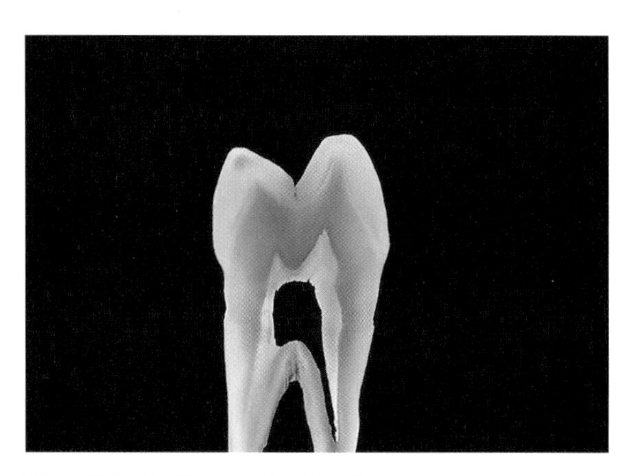

Figure 3.4 Sectioned natural tooth.

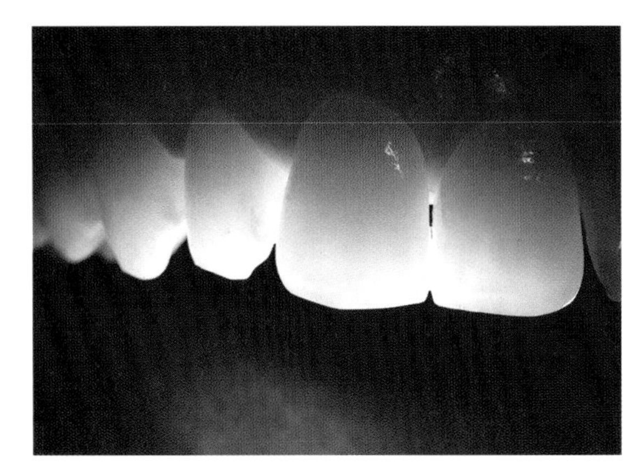

Figure 3.2 Light entering a tooth by the crown.

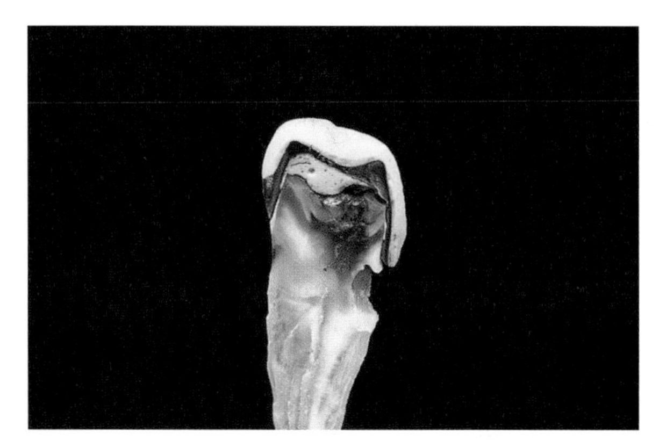

Figure 3.5 Section tooth with metal–ceramic crown.

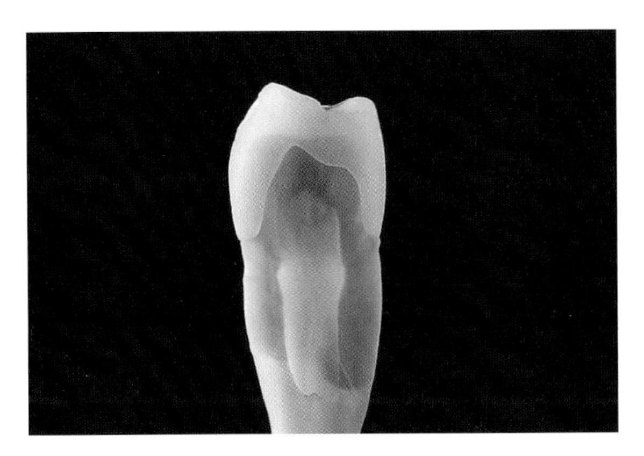

Figure 3.6 Sectioned tooth with all-ceramic crown.

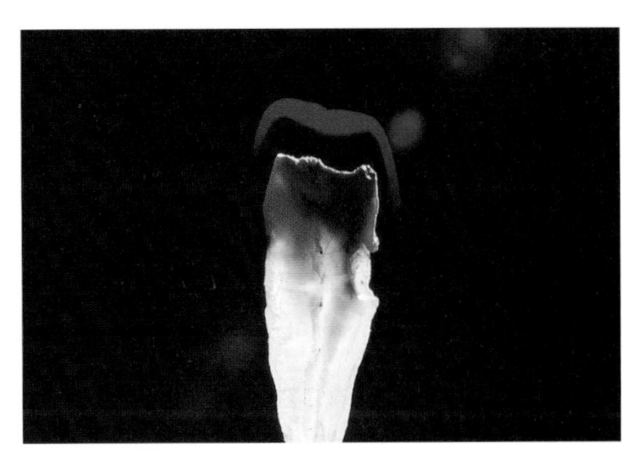

Figure 3.8 Metal–ceramic crown: the metal substructure blocks all light via the root (blue), and aesthetics or appearance of the crown is limited to the veneering porcelain (red).

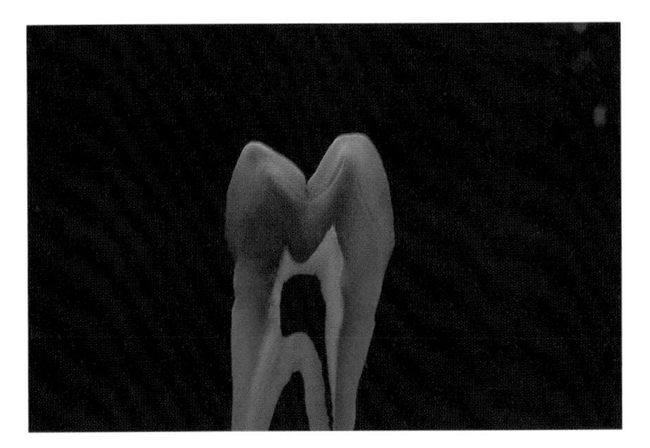

Figure 3.7 Natural tooth: light entering through the root (blue) is free to mingle with light entering from the crown (red).

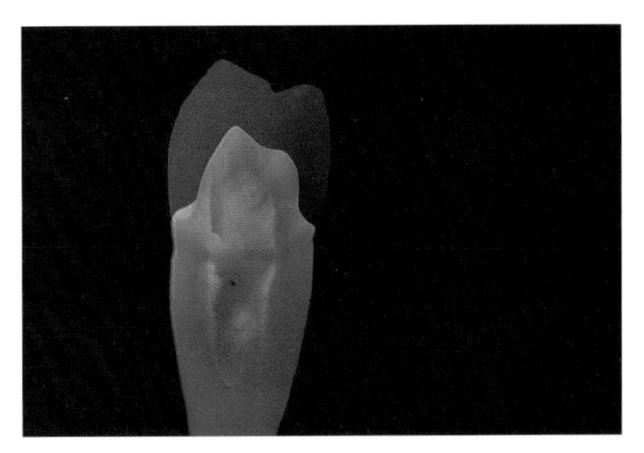

Figure 3.9 All-ceramic crown: light via the root (blue) and crown (red) is free to mingle (red), similar to in a natural tooth, especially at the crucial cervical area.

to a tooth, the metal substructure blocks 90% (by surface area) of the optical capacity of a tooth. In effect, aesthetics, or appearance, of the metal–ceramic crown is limited to the veneering porcelain, less than 10% of the surface area (Fig. 3.8). Although not impossible, it is extremely difficult to simulate the entire optics of a tooth within only 10% of its surface area. The ceramist is faced with mimicking light flow of the entire tooth in the veneering porcelain, which requires skill and a high degree of aptitude. If not achieved, the resultant metal–ceramic crown appears artificial and dull, often with greying or shadowing at the cervical margin.

With an all-ceramic crown, similar to a natural tooth, light is able to flow freely, utilising 100% of the optical capacity of enamel and dentine (Fig. 3.9). Hence, all-ceramic restorations display vitality, vibrancy, and are often indistinguishable from the surrounding natural dentition. The optical advantage of all-ceramic units helps the ceramist to create life-like restorations, without the constraints of working within the limited surface area of the veneering porcelain. This is also relevant when using posts for non-vital teeth that require intra-radicular support, since metallic posts hinder light transmission into the root.

Physical and mechanical properties of ceramic

Generally, a high-glass content yields superior optical properties, but inferior mechanical strength (e.g. feldspathic and leucite-reinforced glass ceramics). The opposite is true for low-glass content, which has better mechanical strength but reduced translucency (e.g. pure densely sintered alumina and zirconia). Of course, optical properties alone are insufficient for a ceramic to perform adequately in the oral cavity. Additionally, a ceramic should possess sufficient strength (flexural strength, fracture toughness), longevity (resistance to fracture), reduced wear of opposing teeth and biocompatibility. Finally, simple, expedient and precise laboratory protocols are desirable for ease of manipulation for facilitating fabrication of the restoration, e.g. possessing a linear coefficient of thermal expansion.

The following properties are applicable for most ceramics, while specific differences of a given class of ceramic are discussed later. Ceramics are highly biocompatible with dental tissues, producing few allergic reactions or corrosion by-products that plague certain dental restorations.[1] They are also chromatically stable and plaque repellent, with insignificant colour change over time, and diminished staining, respectively.[2] Another concern with older feldspathic porcelains is pronounced hardness, leading to unwanted opposing tooth wear; this can be as much as 230 µm per annum,[3] in comparison to natural enamel-to-enamel wear of only 60 µm per annum. The smallest amount of wear is with gold restoration (9 µm per annum). However, newer low-fusing porcelains have an annual wear comparable to natural teeth at approximately 60 µm per annum.

Uni-layer and bi-layer all-ceramic systems

All porcelains, from the early feldspathic to the latest zirconia ceramics, are beleaguered with inherent brittleness and low fracture toughness; these compromise mechanical resilience and, ultimately, longevity. In order for a ceramic to endure the oral environment, it must be adequately supported. Unsupported porcelain, because of its inherent high modulus of elasticity (MOE) (brittleness), is prone to fracture under masticatory loads. There are two solutions to this predicament. The first is to gain support from the underlying tooth to dissipate occlusal forces. The second is to support the weaker veneering porcelain by a stronger substructure. Both methods are used for different all-ceramic systems.

To gain support from natural tooth involves adhesive bonding to form a unified structure. To achieve this, the ceramic must be amenable to etching with hydrofluoric acid. This is followed by silane application of the intaglio surface and bonding the restoration to dentine using dentine bonding agents (DBAs) and appropriate resin luting cements. The ceramics conducive to etching with hydrofluoric acid are the silica-based varieties, e.g. feldspathic, or pressed ceramics. Before the advent of silane coupling agents, most porcelain laminate veneer (PLV) failures were attributed to lack of adhesion to the underlying tooth. Silane resolved this issue by forming a chemical link between etched feldspathic porcelain and the underlying tooth, creating a hermetic seal between two disparate materials, with the natural tooth acting as the support for the brittle porcelain. This type of all-ceramic system, in which the support of the porcelain is gained from the natural tooth, is termed a uni-layer all-ceramic system (Fig. 3.10).

Instead of using the natural tooth for a support, the alternative is a resilient infrastructure to support the fragile veneering porcelain. The initial substructures were casting alloys for metal–ceramic restorations. To circumvent poor aesthetics of the latter, high-strength ceramics, such as alumina or zirconia, can be a substitute for the metallic substructure, which also obviates the necessity to gain support from the underlying tooth. This is termed a bi-layer all-ceramic system, and is employed by most of the currently available ceramic systems (Fig. 3.11). Furthermore, the intaglio surfaces of restorations fabricated from alumina and zirconia are not etchable

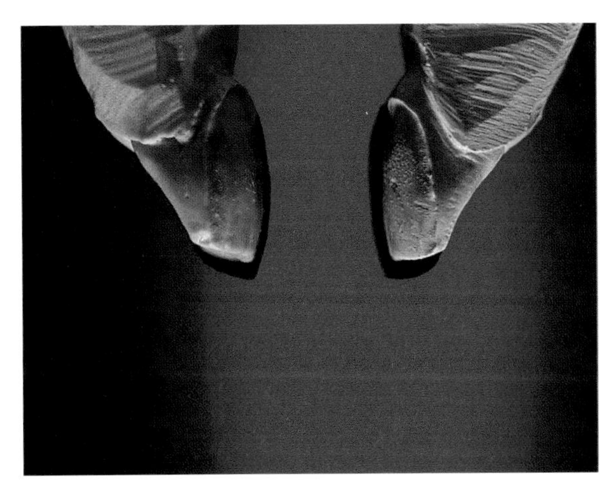

Figure 3.10 Uni-layer ceramic restorations: silhouette of cross-sections of porcelain laminate veneers.

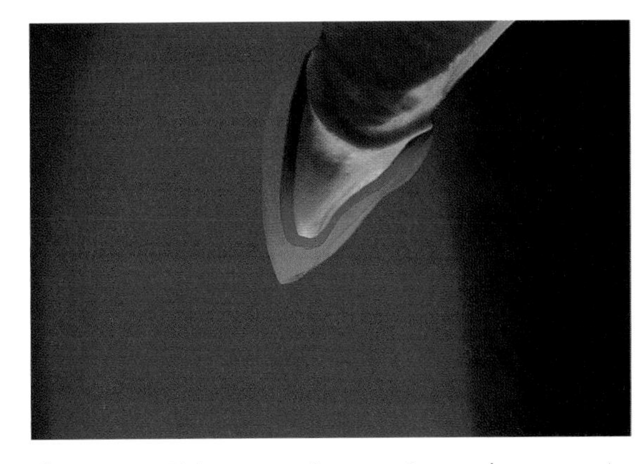

Figure 3.11 Bi-layer ceramic restorations: a dense ceramic core (blue) is veneered with an overlying porcelain (red).

with hydrofluoric acid, and adhesive cementation no longer a pre-requisite. However, bonding ceramics to tooth is still desirable, and the recently introduced adhesive resin cements are promising for achieving a chemical bond, similar to that with silane coupling agents to silica-based ceramics (see Chapter 10).

Aetiology of fractures

The major cause of failure of all-ceramic units is fracturing. Preventing fractures is not limited to material properties, but heavily reliant on correct clinical and laboratory protocols. These factors are often ignored, and fractures are blamed on the ceramic material. The reason for this is twofold:

- Clinical and laboratory techniques for metal–ceramics are relatively forgiving, allowing a degree of latitude
- There is always inertia to change from established materials and protocols such as metal–ceramic prostheses, which have become routine in the last four decades

When considering all-ceramic units, a paradigm shift regarding techniques is essential. Ceramic systems are unforgiving, demanding a different, more stringent protocol for long-term success. If this aspect is ignored, failure is inevitable. Furthermore, a balance is necessary: all-ceramic restorations are not indicated for every clinical situation, and for certain scenarios, metal–ceramics are more predictable. However, if judicially chosen and skilfully executed, all-ceramic restorations provide years of reliable service for aesthetically sensitive regions of the mouth.

Since fracture is the most prevalent cause of failure of all-ceramic units, a clear understanding of crack formation and propagation is mandatory. An inherently brittle substance, such as a ceramic, has innate microscopic flaws (cracks and pores) statistically distributed within the material. These are termed Griffith's flaws,[4] formed during fabrication and adjustments, and their propagation reduces fracture toughness of the material. Additionally, fracture toughness is time-dependent, reducing the strength of the ceramic over time.[5] If a ceramic is left undisturbed in an inert environment, the flaws are inconsequential. However, when exposed to a dynamic environment, for example the oral cavity, these flaws undergo so-called subcritical crack growth, eventually resulting in fractures. The humid environment, with or without normal functional and dysfunctional occlusal stresses, causes static fatigue and stress-corrosion, resulting in crack growth and eventual catastrophic fractures (Figs. 3.12 & 3.13).

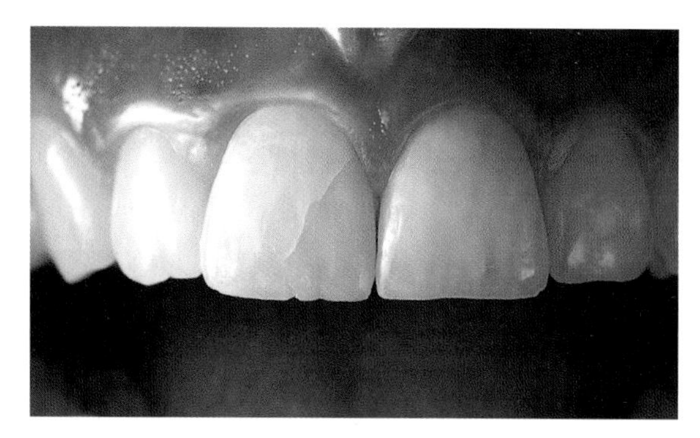

Figure 3.12 Catastrophic fracture of an all-ceramic crown on the maxillary right central incisor.

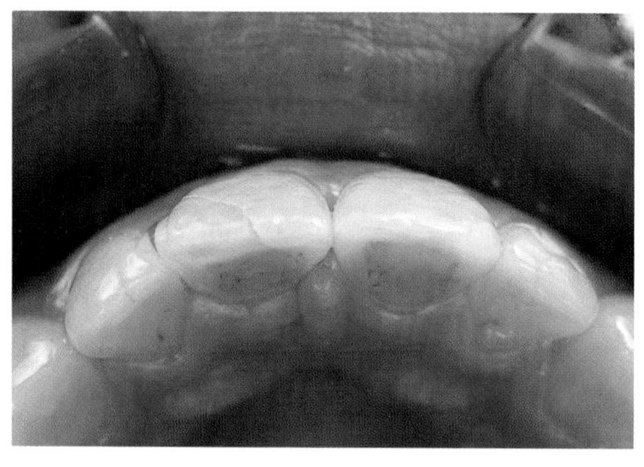

Figure 3.13 Catastrophic fracture of an all-ceramic crown on the maxillary right central incisor.

Definitions

- Fracture toughness – the resistance to fracture or crack propagation is measured as a material's fracture toughness, expressed as K_{IC}. The latter is the measure of the amount of energy required to initiate a fracture. The larger the K_{IC} value, the greater the force required for initiating a fracture, or put another way, the more resistant the material to fracture formation. Numerous methods are used to retard fracture within a ceramic material, including crack deflection, zone shielding, contact shielding, crack bridging and phase transformation (for zirconia ceramics). Many of these strengthening and toughening mechanisms are utilised in a variety of contemporary dental ceramics, with varying success, with the ultimate aim of increasing their fracture toughness[9]
- Modulus of elasticity (MOE) – measure of the elasticity or stiffness of a material. A low MOE (e.g. elastic band) implies greater flexibility and shock-absorbing capability, while a high MOE (e.g. porcelain) signifies brittleness and lower stress-handling ability

The average bite force is greatest in the first molar region and least in the incisor region. For the molar area, the force level ranges from 216–847 N, and for incisors from 108–299 N.[6] Clearly, in order for a ceramic to survive, it must be capable of resisting these stresses. As a general guide, in order for posterior restorations to survive, they should be capable of withstanding a mean load of approximately 1000 N.[7] Also, as mentioned above, if a flawed ceramic is placed in an aqueous milieu, it swells by imbibing water, which further degrades its fracture resistance.[8]

Dental ceramics

Dental ceramics are broadly divided into three categories, silica-based, alumina-based and zirconia-based. All varieties, with different fabrication processes, are used for intra- and extracoronal dental restorations. Table 3.1 compares mechanical properties, and Table 3.2 the fabrication processes of some popular all-ceramic systems.

Table 3.1 Average mechanical properties of contemporary dental ceramics.[10,11]

Ceramic	Flexural strength (MPa)	Fracture toughness – K_{IC} (MPa m$^{1/2}$)	MOE (GPa)	Hardness (GPa)
Feldspathic porcelain	95	0.9	60	Greater than 6.5
Empress 1	106–120	1.2–1.5	65	6.5
Empress 2	306–400	2.8–3.5	105	5.3
In-Ceram Spinell	238–377			
In-Ceram Alumina (slip)	594	4.4	265	11
In-Ceram Alumina (dry-pressed)	440	3.1–4.6	265	11
In-Ceram Zirconia (slip)	630	4.8–8	240	10.5
In-Ceram Zirconia (dry-pressed)	476	4.9	240	11
Procera alumina	450 (0.4 mm coping) to 687 (0.6 mm coping)	4.5–6		
DC-Zirkon (partially stabilised zirconia)	680	5.5	240	13
Procera AllZircon[12]	900–1200	9–10		Greater than 13

Table 3.2 Fabrication processes of some all-ceramic systems.

All-ceramic system	Platinum foil	Refractory dies	Lost wax	Wax template with milling	Strengthening mechanism	CAD/CAM
Feldspathic porcelain	Yes	Yes	–	Yes	–	–
Empress 1			Yes	–	Dispersion	CAD/CAM
Empress 2			Yes	–	Dispersion	CAD/CAM
In-Ceram Alumina			–	Yes	Infiltration	–
In-Ceram Zirconia			–	–	Infiltration	CAD/CAM
Procera			–	–	Densely sintered	CAD/CAM
Cercon			–	Yes	Phase transformation	CAM
Lava			–	Yes	Phase transformation	CAM
DC-Zirkon			–	Yes	Phase transformation	CAM

Silica-based ceramics

Feldspathic porcelains

Conventional, silica-based ceramics were the first types of porcelains used for fabricating dental restorations. These materials are highly aesthetic by mimicking natural dentition. The earliest method for fabricating all-ceramic inlays, veneers and crowns using feldspathic porcelains was using either a platinum foil or refractory dies. Whilst more expedient techniques have superseded these methods, they still have a place in contemporary dentistry. For example, minimal tooth preparation requiring thin cross-section veneers (less than 0.5 mm) are ideally fabricated on platinum foil or refractory dies. Refractory dies are also utilised for porcelain inlays.

The major drawback with feldspathic porcelains is low flexural strength according to ISO 6872, predisposing to fracture, with poor longevity.[13] However, they still have a place in contemporary aesthetic dental procedures, including PLVs and inlays/onlays (Figs. 3.14 & 3.15). However, due to inherent weakness, an adhesive technique using silane-coupling agents and resin luting agents for cementation is mandatory for gaining support from the underlying tooth structure. In addition, meticulous attention is necessary for tooth preparation, which should accommodate a uniform thickness of porcelain for PLVs (Figs. 3.16–3.19), and a minimum of 2 mm for sufficient bulk for inlays/onlays. Finally, many of the high-strength ceramic copings discussed below use silica-based porcelain for the veneer overlay.

IPS-Empress 1 (leucite-reinforced glass ceramic)

The IPS-Empress system was conceived at the University of Zurich, Switzerland in 1983, and commercially marketed by Ivoclar Vivadent in 1990.[14] The material is essentially a feldspathic silica-based ceramic, composed of 63% silicone dioxide and 19% aluminum oxide with the addi-

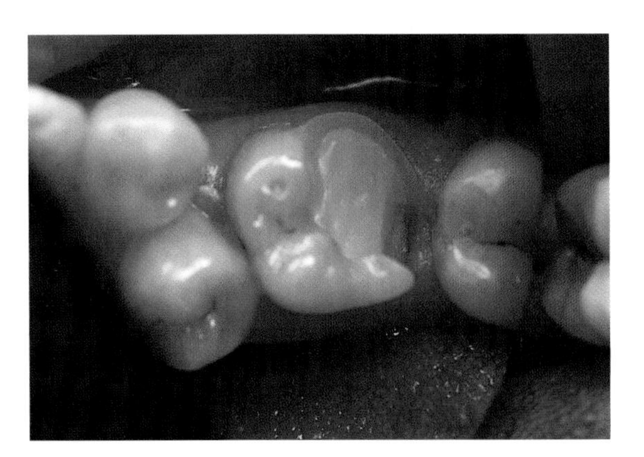

Figure 3.14 Cavity preparation for a feldspathic porcelain inlay in mandibular first molar.

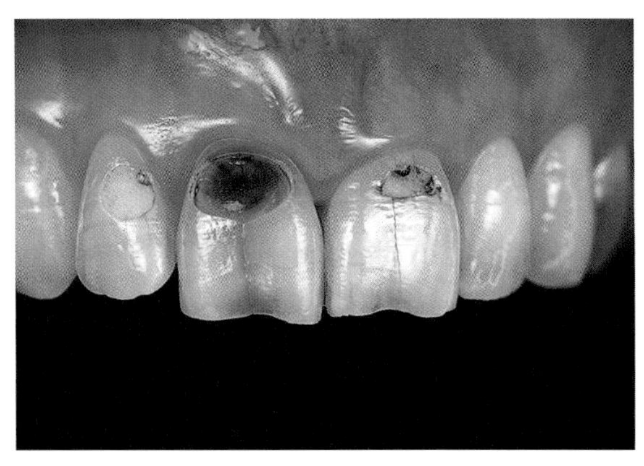

Figure 3.16 Feldspathic PLV case study: pre-operative status of maxillary centrals showing decay and worn, uneven edges.

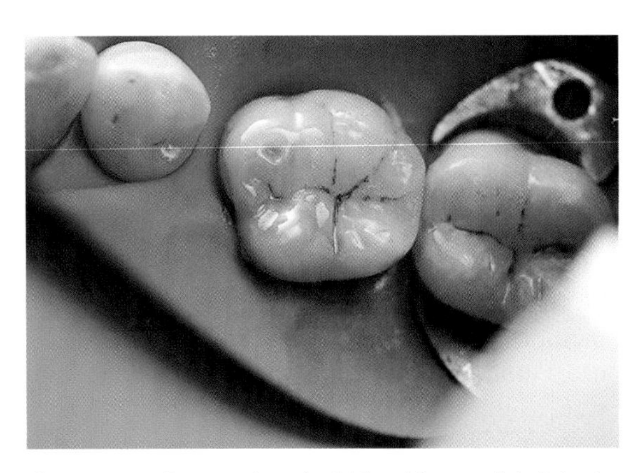

Figure 3.15 Cementation of a feldspathic porcelain inlay in mandibular first molar.

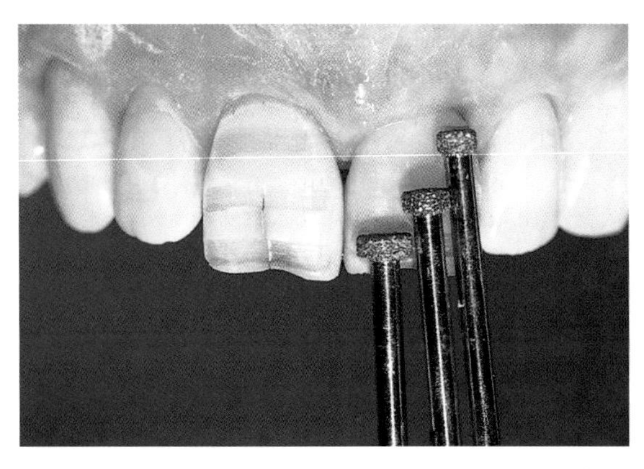

Figure 3.17 Feldspathic PLV case study: following decay and composite fillings removal, depth-cutting burs are used for precise tooth preparation.

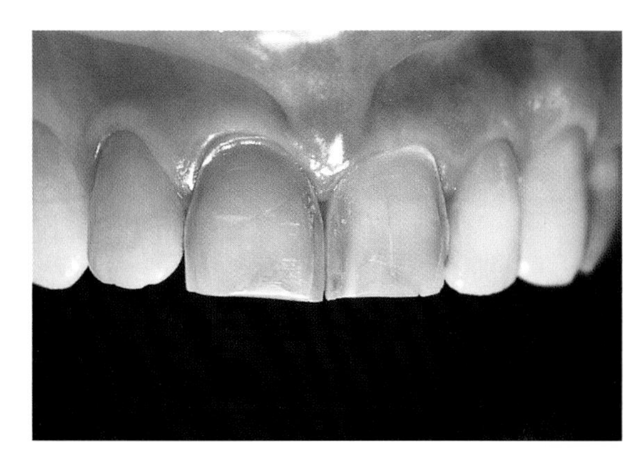

Figure 3.18 Feldspathic PLV case study: completed porcelain laminate tooth preparation, with underlying tooth substrate of an acceptable colour.

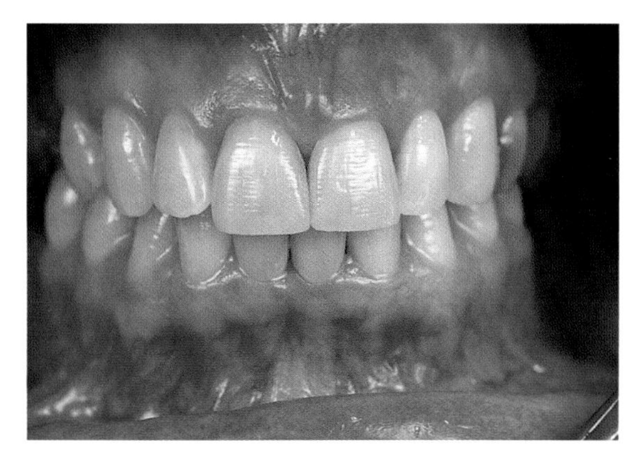

Figure 3.19 Feldspathic PLV case study: post-operative status showing restitution of aesthetics.

tion of leucite crystals to form a leucite-reinforced castable glass ceramic. The rationale for its development was to eliminate or minimise microporosities created during the sintering of all-ceramic materials.[15] These voids predispose to fracture initiation; fractures grow and eventually result in failure of the material. The incorporation of leucite crystals creates barriers to crack growth, preventing microcracks and improving flexural strength and fracture resistance by dispersion strengthening. In addition, the injection-moulding process with heat and pressure reduces shrinkage and further enhances the flexural strength. The flexural strength ranges from 95–180 MPa, and fracture toughness (K_{IC}) is approximately 1.3 MPa m$^{1/2}$.

Two methods are available for fabricating Empress 1 restorations. The first is using the lost-wax process, similar to that used for conventional porcelain fused to metal crowns. The shape of the restoration is carved in wax and the pattern invested and heated in a furnace. The mould of the restoration is then injected with the desired shade of an Empress ingot heated to 1200°C. The heat and pressure ensure accurate adaptation and marginal integrity. Following divesting, the restoration is finished using either the staining or the layering technique. The former is used for inlay/onlays by painting high chroma pigments for characterisation, followed by glazing to 'seal' the surface. The latter, layering technique, is used for crowns and laminates by veneering the pressed core with dentine and/or enamel porcelain.

The second method uses a computer-aided design/computer-aided manufacturing (CAD/CAM) process. Following tooth preparation, an impression is made or an intra-oral camera directly scans the cavity or crown preparation. Using appropriate software, the restoration is graphically designed and relayed to a milling machine, which cuts an Empress ingot to the desired shape. Once again, either the staining or the layering technique is used to complete the restoration.

Indications for Empress 1 are inlays/onlays and anterior single unit crowns (Figs. 3.20–3.23). Empress 1 is unsuitable for stress-bearing teeth and multiple splinted units or fixed partial dentures (FPD). The endearing qualities of Empress 1 are superb aesthetics, excellent marginal integrity and ease of fabrication. Furthermore, being a silica-based ceramic, the intaglio surface can be etched with hydrofluoric acid and bonded using silane and an adhesive cementation protocol. The ease of fabrication and the ability to bond restorations have contributed to the clinical success of Empress 1, even though the material is mechanically inferior to other dental ceramics.

IPS-Empress 2 (lithium disilicate glass ceramic)

Empress 2 (Ivoclar-Vivadent) was released in 1998, with superior mechanical properties com-

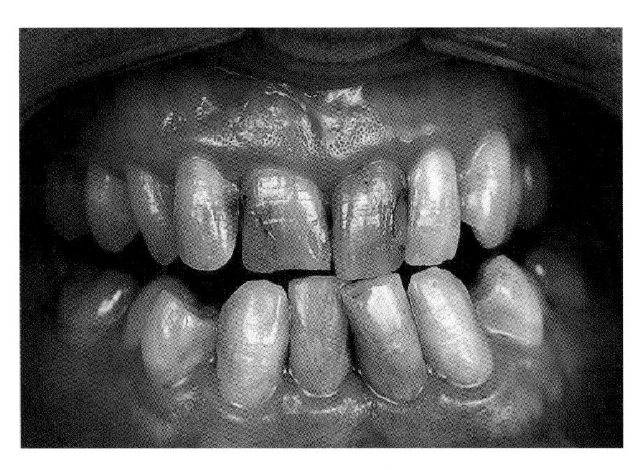

Figure 3.20 Empress 1 case study: pre-operative view showing discoloured, stained, heavily restored and chipped maxillary central incisors.

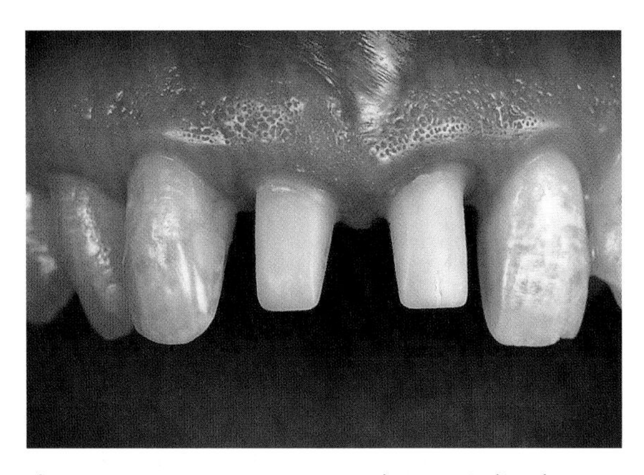

Figure 3.21 Empress 1 case study: two indirectly cast ceramic post-cores cemented into roots of maxillary centrals to improve colour and light transmission of tooth.

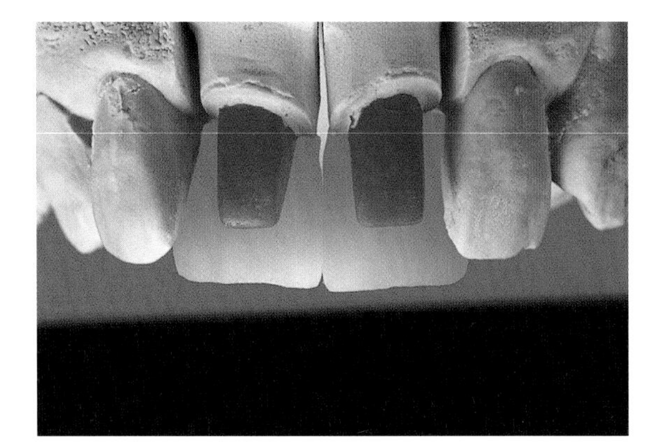

Figure 3.22 Empress 1 case study: tooth preparation-to-definitive crown relationship.

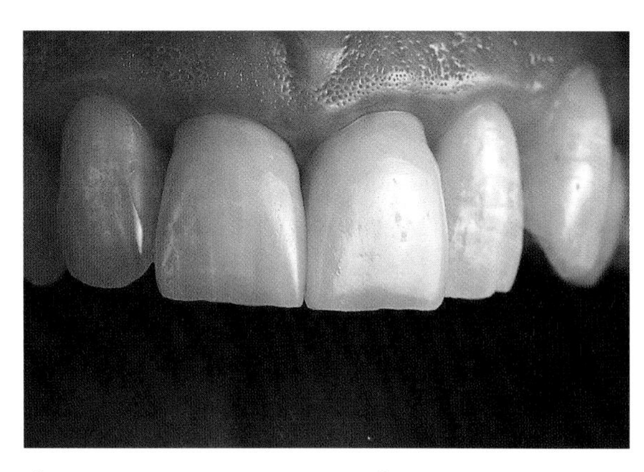

Figure 3.23 Empress 1 case study: post-operative status showing two cemented Empress 1 crowns with improved anterior aesthetics (laboratory work by David Korson, London).

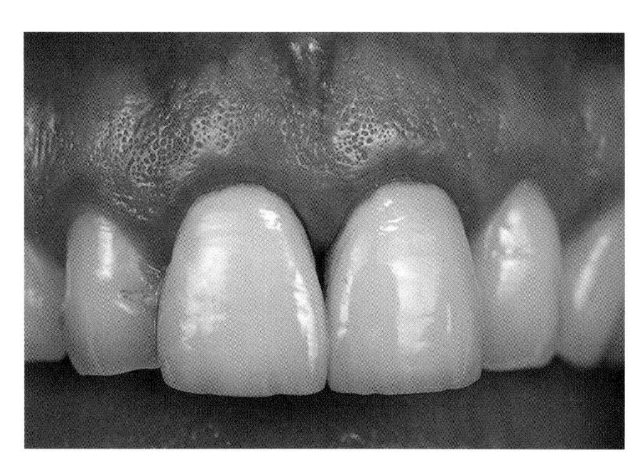

Figure 3.24 Empress 2 case study: defective metal–ceramic crowns on central incisors.

pared with Empress 1, but without compromising aesthetic qualities (Figs. 3.24–3.27). The flexural strength and K_{IC} range from 340–400 MPa and 2–3.3 MPa $m^{1/2}$, respectively. The fabrication process is identical to Empress 1, although different veneering porcelain (fluorapatite glass ceramic) is necessary for the Empress 2. Due to the mechanically stronger substructure, the manufacturer claims that gaining support from the underlying tooth, via adhesive cementation is not mandatory. The major drawback with Empress 2 is the extremely technique-sensitive laboratory protocol, which has resulted in numerous inci-

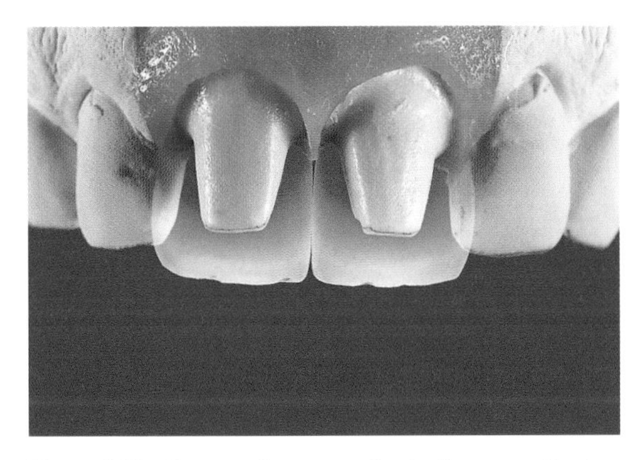

Figure 3.25 Empress 2 case study: tooth preparation-to-definitive crown relationship on soft tissue model.

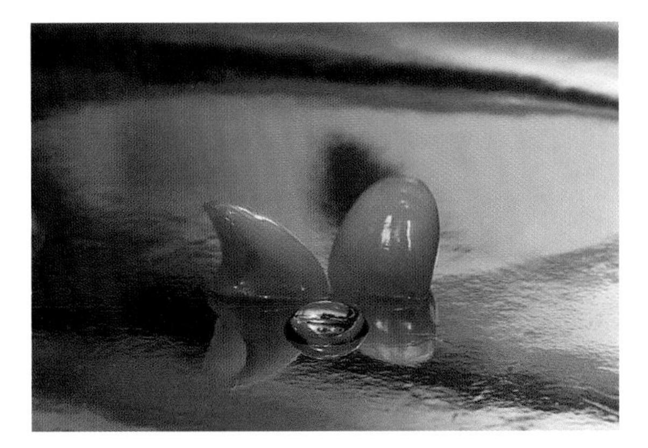

Figure 3.26 Empress 2 case study: completed Empress 2 crowns with correct lustre and texture.

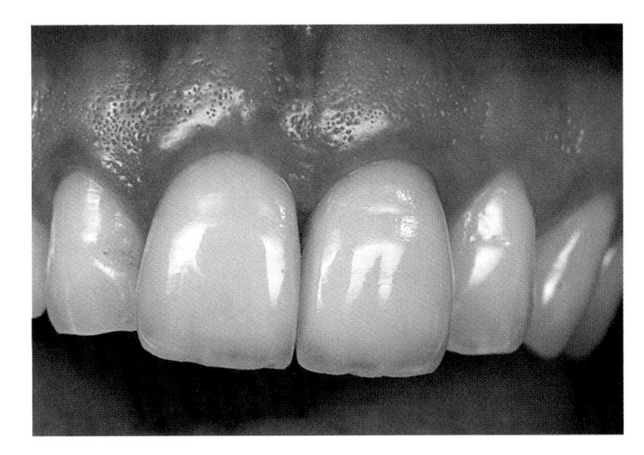

Figure 3.27 Empress 2 case study: post-operative view showing aesthetic enhancement and gingival health around the Empress 2 crowns on central incisors (laboratory work by Gerald Ubassy, France).

dences of de-lamination of the veneering porcelain from the underlying core. Another concern is its recommended use for FPDs, requiring connector dimensions between abutment and pontic of 4 mm × 4 mm. This means that the gingival embrasures should be of sufficient length with long contact points, which may not be anatomically possible, resulting in compromised periodontal health and poor aesthetics.

Alumina-based ceramics

In-Ceram Spinell (glass-infiltrated magnesium alumina)

In-Ceram Spinell (Vita) is twice as translucent as In-Ceram Alumina, specifically intended to allow the underlying natural tooth structure to 'shine though' the material. Its use is primarily for indirectly fabricated inlays and onlays, assuming an acceptable colour of the underlying tooth, allowing the restoration to disappear within the natural tooth. However, due to its reduced mechanical strength, In-Ceram Spinell is unsuitable for posterior crowns, but is highly aesthetic for single anterior crowns.[16]

In-Ceram Alumina (glass-infiltrated alumina)

In-Ceram Alumina (Vita) is a partially sintered porous alumina, which is subsequently infiltrated with molten glass. The flexural strength and K_{IC}, are 352–600 MPa and 2.7–4.49 MPa $m^{1/2}$,[17] respectively, superior to both classes of Empress. Optically, alumina is denser than leucite glass, but still exhibits excellent aesthetics (Figs. 3.28–3.31). Two methods for fabrication are possible. The dry-pressed method uses preprocessed ingots, allowing milling with or without CAM/CAM software. The slip method uses dispersed alumina in an aqueous solution, which is painted on to a specific plaster die. The laboratory process is protracted, involving numerous stages. To avoid de-lamination at the core–veneer interface, caution is required to avoid air particle abrasion of the core prior to veneering.[18]

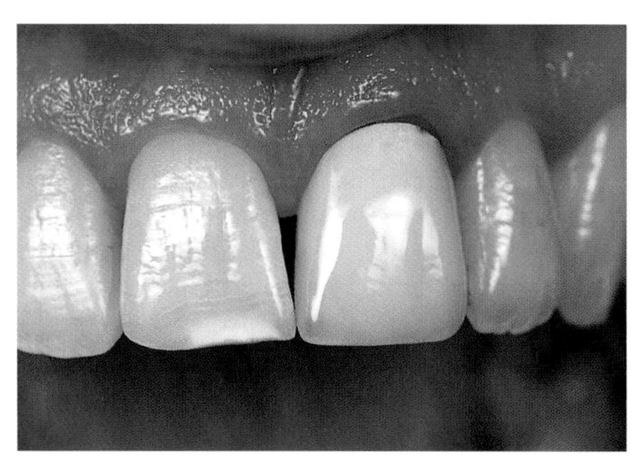

Figure 3.28 In-Ceram Alumina case study: defective metal–ceramic crown on left maxillary central incisor.

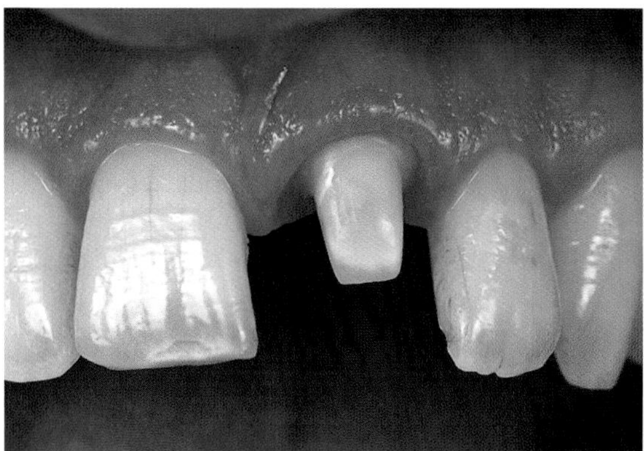

Figure 3.29 In-Ceram Alumina case study: tooth preparation.

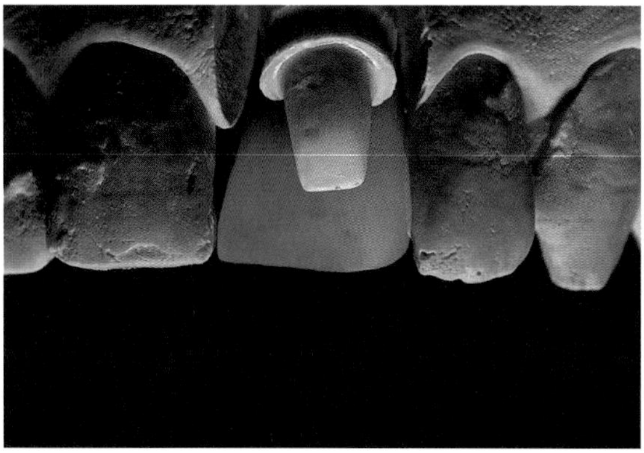

Figure 3.30 In-Ceram Alumina case study: tooth preparation-to-definitive crown relationship under ultra-violet illumination.

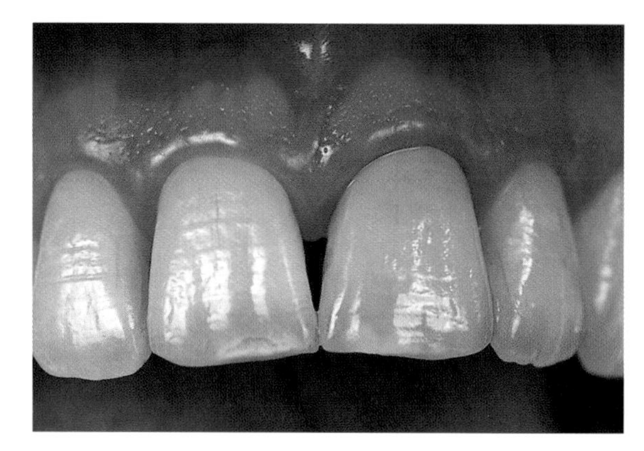

Figure 3.31 In-Ceram Alumina case study: cemented In-Ceram Alumina on left central incisor (laboratory work by Paul Sturridge, London).

Procera (pure densely sintered alumina)

To capitalise on the strength of alumina, the early 1990s saw the introduction of a pure, densely sintered alumina (99.9% aluminum oxide) core, called Procera.[19] The highly dense alumina possesses minimal microporosities, reducing fracture propagation, and improving mechanical properties. The occlusal stress needed to break a Procera coping is around 1500 N;[20] even after veneering with a low-fusing porcelain, such as AllCeram, the restorations still require a stress of 1300 N before fracture is imminent. As stated above, the recommended force resistance for posterior restoration is 1000 N. Therefore, a Procera coping is a suitable substructure for both anterior and posterior prostheses. Although strong, the aluminum oxide/low-fusing porcelain complex significantly reduces opposing natural tooth wear to 60 μm per annum, compared with feldspathic porcelain, which has annual wear rates in the region of 230 μm per annum.[21]

The fabrication process involves scanning a correctly trimmed plaster die of the tooth preparation (Figs. 3.32 & 3.33). Next, CAD/CAM software is used to design the substructure, and the digitised coping design is relayed via the Internet to Goteborg, Sweden or New Jersey, USA, where copings are manufactured in an industrial quality-controlled process, and subsequently returned to the ceramist. To compensate for shrinkage during sintering, the exact shrink-

Figure 3.32 Correctly trimmed plaster die with a hollow apical to finish line, allowing clear margin delineation for scanning and manufacture of alumina coping via a CAD/CAM process (Procera, Nobel Biocare).

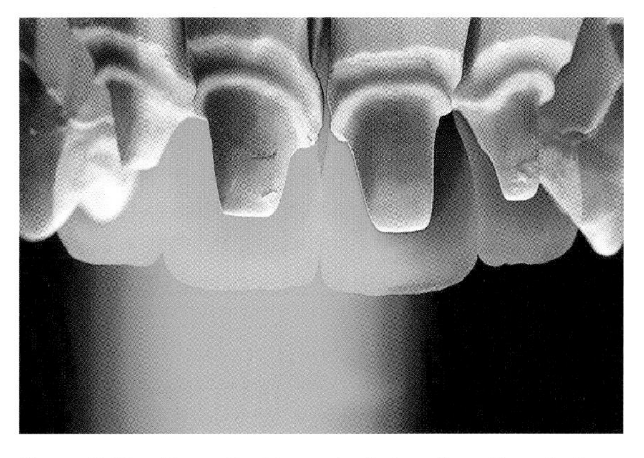

Figure 3.33 Correctly trimmed plaster die with a hollow apical to finish line, allowing clear margin delineation for scanning and manufacture of alumina coping via a CAD/CAM process (Procera, Nobel Biocare).

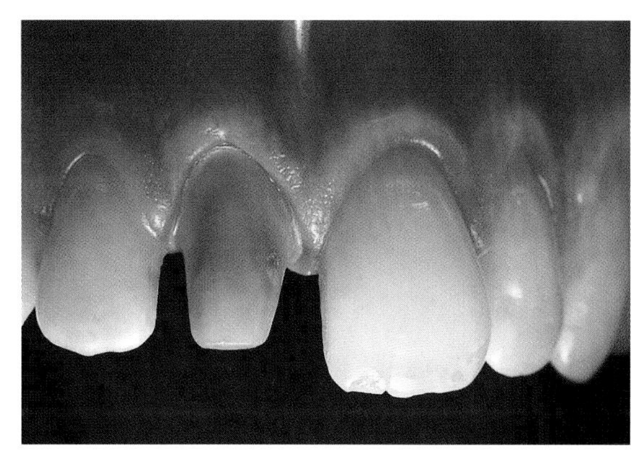

Figure 3.34 Discoloured right central incisor.

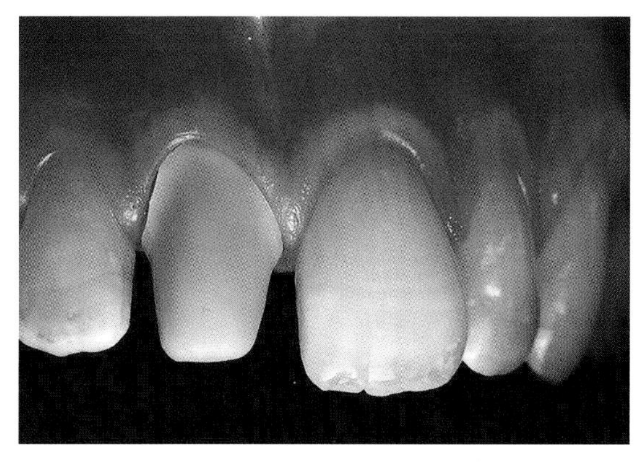

Figure 3.35 Masking ability of a ceramic core: the discolouration on the right central incisor is easily obscured by a Procera alumina coping.

age volume for each die is calculated, and an enlarged die is made to these dimensions to compensate for the anticipated contraction. The system offers a choice of coping thickness (0.25 mm, 0.4 mm or 0.6 mm), opacity (white or standard) and material (alumina or zirconia). A marginal integrity of 70 μm is achievable, within clinical accepted norms of 50–100 μm.[22]

The restoration is completed by veneering the coping with either silica- or alumina-based porcelain (Nobel Rhondo). A major advantage of a Procera coping is its ability to mask underlying tooth discolouration (Figs. 3.34 & 3.35).

Although translucent, allowing light transmission to the underlying tooth, the coping density is sufficient to conceal tooth discolouration or metallic cores.[23] Procera is classified as a high-strength ceramic with a flexural strength approaching 700 MPa, sufficient to support the weaker veneering porcelain, and obviating the need for an adhesive cementation protocol. This may be potentially advantageous because a variety of luting agents can be utilised, including zinc phosphate, glass ionomers and resin-modified glass ionomers (see Chapter 10). Finally, the longevity of Procera restorations is 7–10 years[24], comparable to conventional metal–ceramic crowns (Figs. 3.36–3.39).

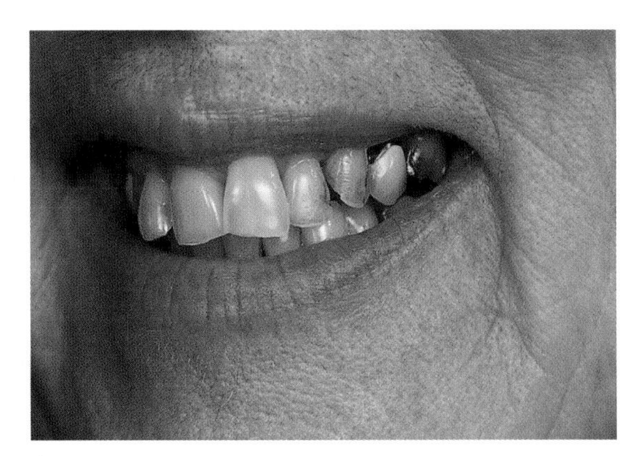

Figure 3.36 Procera alumina case study: palatal erosion of maxillary left lateral and canine has resulted in thin, fragile and unaesthetic enamel.

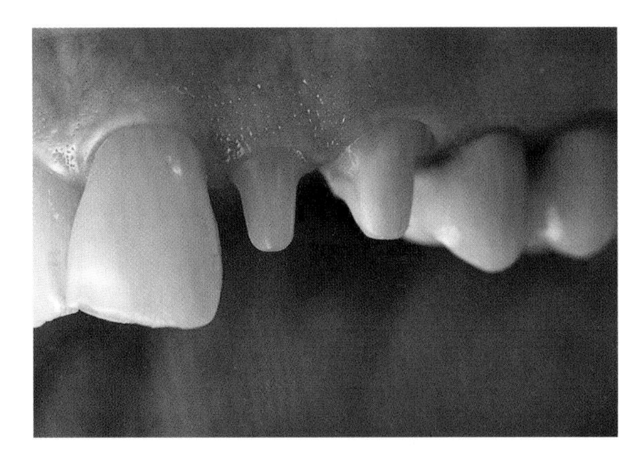

Figure 3.37 Procera alumina case study: tooth preparation with a chamfer finish line.

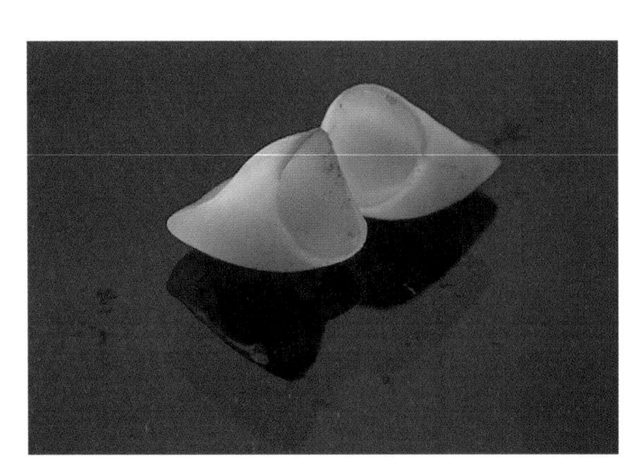

Figure 3.38 Procera alumina case study: two completed Procera crowns.

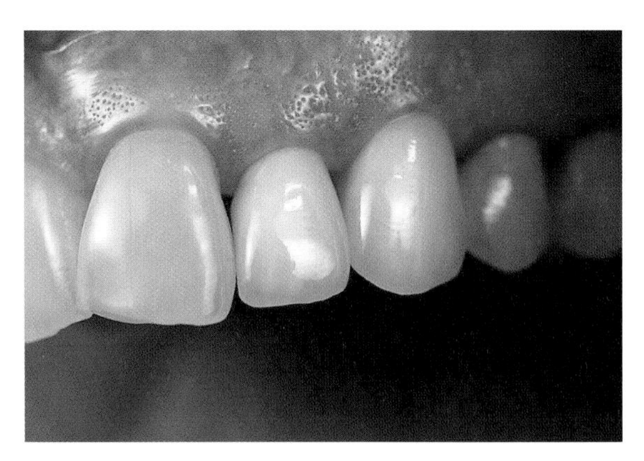

Figure 3.39 Procera alumina case study: cemented Procera crowns with enhanced aesthetics, preventing further enamel erosion (laboratory work by Jean-Marc Etienne, France).

Zirconia-based ceramics

The higher strength of zirconia, compared to alumina, is not solely related to phase transformation toughening, but varies according to complete sintering, porosity and addition of stabilising yttria. Zirconia is the strongest ceramic used in dentistry, and depending on a specific product, the flexural strength can exceed 1000 MPa. Although anterior crowns are possible, zirconia is primarily indicated for stress-bearing posterior crowns and FPDs (discussed below). Limitations of zirconia compared with alumina are poor light transmission (due to reduced glass content) and high value, resulting in an almost metallic optical opacity and radiopacity. Therefore, in situations where translucency is of paramount concern, for example anterior aesthetics, alumina is more suitable than a zirconia coping of comparable thickness.[25]

In-Ceram Zirconia

In-Ceram Zirconia (Vita) is a zirconia-reinforced glass-infiltrated alumina, which is basically In-Ceram Alumina toughened by the addition of 33 wt% of partially stabilised zirconia. As with In-Ceram Alumina, two methods of fabrication are available, slip or dry-pressed, and again, the latter is thought to be mechanically superior due to pre-processing by a controlled industrial process.

Yttrium-stabilised zirconia

Examples of commercially available materials include DC-Zirkon (Austenal), Procera AllZirkon (Nobel Biocare), Cercon (Dentsply/Ceramco), Lava (3-M ESPE) and Cerec (Sirona). For densely sintered materials, shrinkage is the major obstacle. This is circumvented by either milling a block of densely sintered material so that shrinkage is no longer a concern, or compensating for the anticipated dimensional changes. An example of a milling process is the DCS Precedent system (DCS Dental) that mills a pre-sintered ceramic block, while some processes combine milling and sintering. The Cercon and Lava methods use an enlarged framework of pre-sintered zirconia, which is milled and then fully sintered to the desired dimensions.

Longevity

Longevity of a restoration is the final aspect to consider before choosing an all-ceramic system. When assessing longevity, the two most frequently used words are survival and success rates. These are not synonymous, but two distinct evaluations. Survival rate implies that a particular restoration is functioning, albeit without all the initial desired parameters. Success, on the other hand, implies that the restoration is not only surviving but also successful, incorporating all initial treatment objectives.[26] For example, an all-ceramic bridge may fracture or delaminate, but is nevertheless surviving. Whilst it is healthy and functioning, it lacks aesthetics (the HFA triad – see Chapter 2). A truly successful outcome is presence of all three entities: health, function and aesthetics.

The mode of fracture of all-ceramic single units differs from that of bridges (FPDs). For crowns, the weakest part is the intaglio or fitting surface, which is subjected to the greatest tensile forces,[27] creating flaws in the core substructure eventually radiating to the veneering porcelain and causing de-lamination. Incorporating a dense, high-strength ceramic core below the veneering porcelain therefore reduces flaws at the intaglio surface. For a FPD, stress distribution is concentrated at the connector sites, making these the weakest parts, which are vulnerable to fracture.[28]

Numerous laboratory and clinical data and anecdotes are available supporting use of all-ceramic restorations, but the real tests are controlled clinical trials, which are lacking for many of the newer ceramic systems. It has been proposed that the minimal length of clinical trials should be 3–5 years, with a failure rate of less than 5%.[29] Currently, systems that conform to these broad guidelines are Empress 1, In-Ceram Alumina and Procera, demonstrating good short-term clinical performance for single unit prostheses.[30]

Metal–ceramic

Since their introduction in the 1960s, metal–ceramic crowns and bridges have shown remarkable clinical success. These restorations have the longest clinical use, and their survival rate is regarded as the gold standard, used as a guide for assessing success of all-ceramic systems. Table 3.3 lists clinical studies on the longevity of metal–ceramic restorations. Although limited in their conclusions, these trials act as a benchmark for evaluating all-ceramic longevity rates, certainly over a short-term period.

Table 3.3 Metal–ceramic restoration longevity rates.

Study	5 years	10 years	15 years
Leempoel *et al.*[31]		95%	
Kerschbaum *et al.*[32]	92%	79%	
Walton[33]		97%	
Walton[34]			85%

Variations of metal–ceramic crowns, such as galvano-ceramic systems, are also available as alternatives to conventional PFMs (porcelain fused to metal). However, long-term survival data is limited; a recent study claims success rates ranging from 92–96.5% after 7 years.[35]

Dicor and Cerestore

Dicor was the first castable all-ceramic system. Its indications, together with Cerestore crowns, were single anterior units. These systems gained popularity due to their simplified fabrication process using the lost wax technique, similar to metal–ceramic units. However, their reputation was tarnished due to high clinical failures, occurring at either the cement–core or core–veneering porcelain interfaces, and they are therefore currently obsolete.[36]

IPS-Empress 1

Since its inception in 1990, Empress has become a generic term for pressable ceramic restorations. Its success is due to ease of fabrication, by either the lost wax process or CAD/CAM machines, producing precise and accurate restorations. Numerous short-term clinical trails have reported positive performance, but only with meticulous clinical protocols and careful patient selection.[37,38,39] The success rate of Empress 1 crowns ranges from 92–99% for 3–3.5 years, with fracture as the primary cause of failure, followed by endodontic involvement and hypersensitivity.[40] These figures are predominantly limited to anterior crowns. A recent study over an 11-year period reports success rates of 98.92% for anterior crowns, but only 84.37% for posterior units, emphasising that Empress 1 crowns on posterior teeth are contraindicated.[41]

In-Ceram Alumina

This type of alumina ceramic, together with Empress 1, is one of the longest surviving all-ceramic systems, and therefore its longevity is a useful guide for assessing other systems. Over a 6-year period, the success-to-failure ratio for anterior and posterior units is 98.9% to 1.1%, and 99.2% to 0.8%, respectively.[42] The high success rate for both regions is promising, indicating that In-Ceram Alumina is suitable for single-unit anterior and posterior crowns.

Procera

Procera is a bi-layer ceramic system, and fractures can either be superficial (limited to the veneering porcelain) or global (involving the coping). The extent of the fracture determines whether the 'lesion' is salvageable, or a replacement is necessary. Minor fractures, not affecting health or function, can be readily repaired with composite resin. However, larger de-laminations, accompanied by sharp edges encouraging food impaction, require a remake.

Numerous studies have reported varying success rates for the Procera system. In a multicentre study over a 5-year period, the success rate ranged from 94–97%,[43] while in another study the success was 97.7% for 5 years and 92.2% for 10 years.[44] A recent study claims a 100% success rate after 5 years for anterior single units, and 95.15% for posterior crowns, averaging 96.7% for all regions of the mouth.[45] In another trial, Procera crowns over a 5-year period showed a success rate of 94%, and 87% of the patients rated their restorations more than 7/10 on an ordered analogue scale for aesthetics as well as for function.[46]

Although it is difficult to make comparisions of longevity reports from different studies, and bearing in mind a minimum success rate of 95% over 3–5 years, Table 3.4 shows success rates of single units of some all-ceramic systems.

Ceramic bridges (FPDs)

Due to superior aesthetics, ceramic systems have been proposed for bridges, especially for anterior regions of the mouth (Figs. 3.40–3.43). However, because of their relative infancy, the data about all-ceramic FPDs is confusing, depending on the

Table 3.4 Survival rates of single units of some all-ceramic systems.

System	3+ years	5+ years	10+ years
Empress 1 (anterior)	92–99%		98%
Empress 1 (posterior)			84%
In-Ceram Alumina (anterior)		99%	
In-Ceram Alumina (posterior)		99%	
Procera Alumina (anterior)		94–100%	92%
Procera Alumina (posterior)		95%	

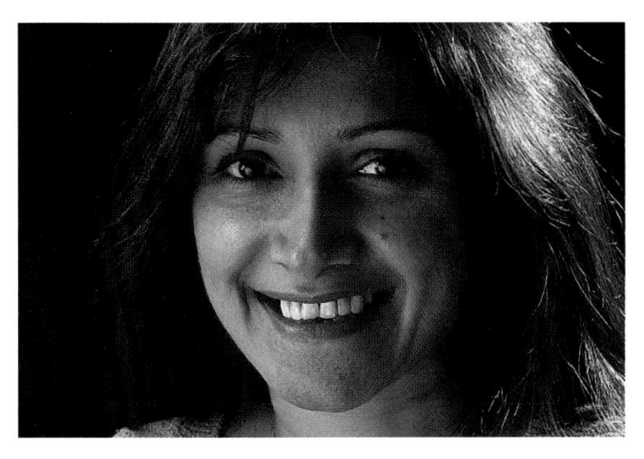

Figure 3.40 Procera alumina FPD case study: pre-operative facial view showing a worn, uneven incisal plane.

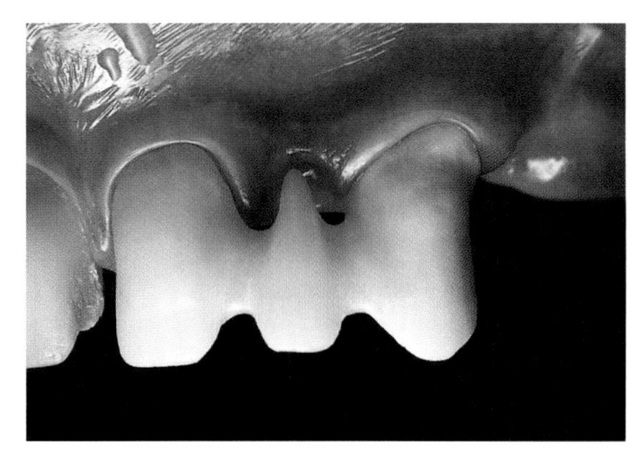

Figure 3.42 Procera alumina FPD case study: try-in of Procera alumina, three-unit FPD substructure spanning from left central to canine, with lateral as pontic.

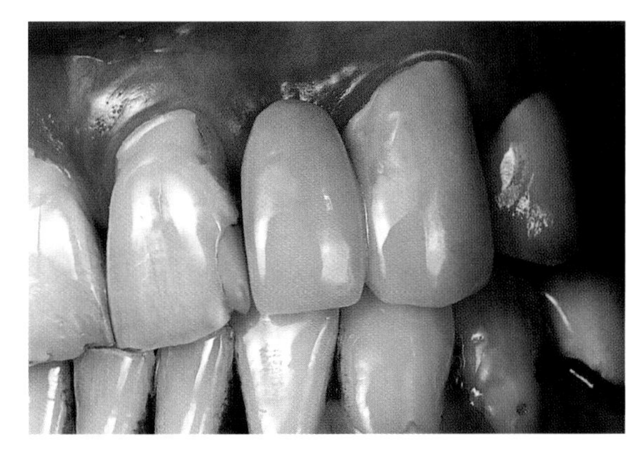

Figure 3.41 Procera alumina FPD case study: defective cantilever bridge from left maxillary canine replacing missing lateral.

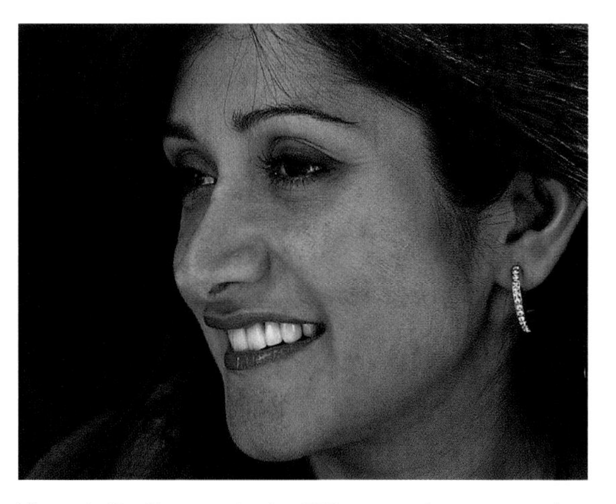

Figure 3.43 Procera alumina FPD case study: post-operative facial view showing incisal plane parallel to curvature of mandibular lip during a relaxed smile (laboratory work by Jean-Marc Etienne, France).

experimental methodology and sparse clinical trials.

To select a particular ceramic for a specific clinical scenario, it is useful to compare long-term failure possibilities. Using an in vitro method, such as finite element analysis, assesses stress distribution at a given load. This allows comparison of different ceramics, with predictions for long-term resilience, which are valuable for in vivo trials. Computational extrapolation of this data allows the calculation of a CARES/LIFE (Ceramic Analysis and Reliability Evaluation of Structure Life Prediction) index for time dependent reliability. With these methods, the long-term fracture resistance of Empress 1, 2 (Ivoclar-Vivadent, Schaan, Liechtenstein), In-Ceram Alumina (Vita, Bad Sackingen, Germany) and zirconia (3Y-PSZ zirconia, Metoxit, Thyangen, Switzerland) were evaluated. Both Empress 1 and In-Ceram Alumina exhibited high fracture probabilities if used for posterior all-ceramic bridge substructures after a 10-year period. The inference is, contrary to the manufacturer's claims, In-Ceram Alumina is unsuitable for posterior FPDs. Empress 2 was more promising, while zirconia showed the best results, with little fracture probability after 10 years of simulated stresses.[47]

Besides material properties, another critical factor for preventing fractures of FPDs is the surface area and design of the connectors between abutments and pontics. Ideally, the larger the surface area, the better the fracture resistance. However, if embrasure space is limited, large cross-section connectors are impractical, conflicting with oral hygiene access and/or aesthetics. This is particularly relevant for Empress 2 FPDs, which require an occlucogingival connector height of 5.0 mm (Figs. 3.44 & 3.45).[48] Since the core is stronger than the veneering porcelain, it may be prudent to leave a naked core at the tissue side of a connector for increased strength.[49] The opposing view is that FPD fracture resistance increases after veneering with the overlying weaker porcelain due to a stable bond between the two layers. Although many all-ceramic cores exceed the average threshold masticatory forces, even on posterior teeth,[50] life expectancies are not identical to clinical lifetimes as many factors are unaccounted for, such as the pulp, periodontal ligament or adhesive cement thickness.[51]

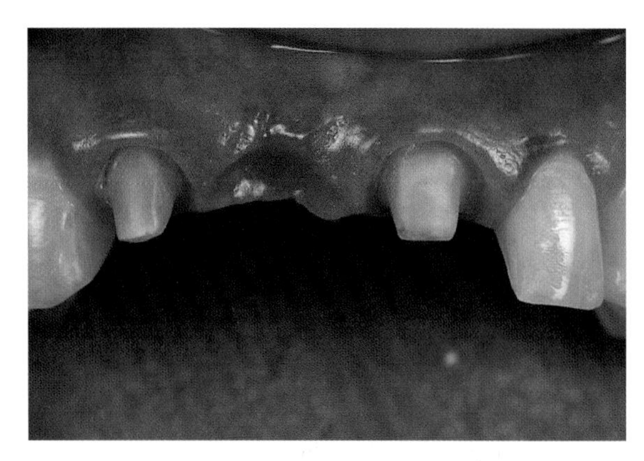

Figure 3.44 Tooth preparation for all-ceramic Empress 2, three-unit FPD, spanning from maxillary right lateral to left central with right central as pontic.

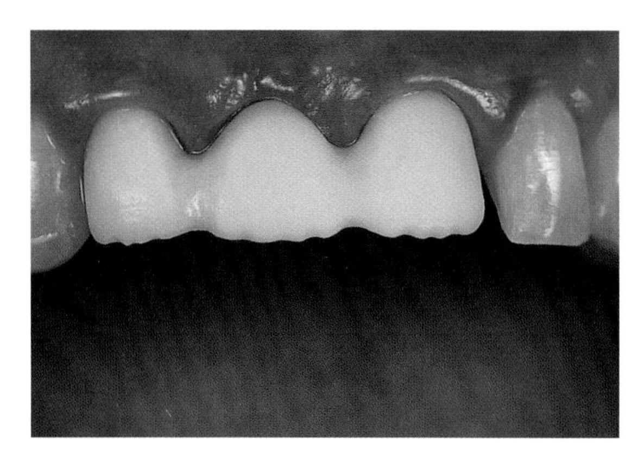

Figure 3.45 Try-in of Empress 2 substructure; notice the extremely long inciso-gingival connectors necessary for strength and resilience.

Probably the most promising ceramic for FPDs is zirconia, either infiltrated into an alumina matrix (In-Ceram Zirconia), or partially stabilised with yttria (DC-Zirkon, DSC Dental/Vita). Stabilised zirconia has the capacity to withstand occlusal stresses of around 2500 N, comparable to a conventional metal–ceramic FPD of similar dimensions. The main difference with metal–ceramics is that fractures are superficial, limited to the veneering porcelain, while for zirconia the fractures are global, encompass-

Table 3.5 Indications for choosing an all-ceramic system.

All-ceramic system	Inlays/ onlays	Veneers	Ant. single unit crowns	Post. single unit crowns	Ant. FPD	Post. FPD	Masks discoloured tooth
Feldspathic porcelain	Yes	Yes	Yes	No	No	No	No
Empress 1	Yes	Yes	Yes	No	No	No	No
Empress 2	Yes	Yes	Yes	Yes[1]	Possible[3]	No	Yes
In-Ceram Spinell	Yes	No	Yes	No	No	No	No
In-Ceram Alumina	No	No	Yes	Yes[1]	Yes	No	Yes
Procera	No	Yes[2]	Yes	Yes	Yes	No	Yes
In-Ceram Zirconia	No	No	Yes[4]	Yes	Yes[4]	Possible[5]	Yes
Procera Zirconia	No	No	Yes[4]	Yes	Yes[4]	Possible[5]	Yes
DC Zirkon	No	No	Yes[4]	Yes	Yes[4]	Possible[5]	Yes
Cercon	No	No	Yes[4]	Yes	Yes[4]	Possible[5]	Yes
Lava	No	No	Yes[4]	Yes	Yes[4]	Possible[5]	Yes

[1] Absence of occlusal dysfunction.
[2] Mask pronounced discoloration, e.g. tetracycline staining or metal post/core.
[3] Depending on occlusion and available embrasure space for connectors.
[4] Depending on colour of adjacent dentition: zirconia is brighter (high value) and has less light transmission than alumina.
[5] Promising, but sparse short- or long-term clinical longevity data.

ing the entire substructure, necessitating replacement of the entire prosthesis.[52]

Table 3.5 lists indications for choosing an all-ceramic system for a variety of clinical scenarios. Caution is necessary regarding all-ceramic FPDs until further clinical trials substantiate short- and long-term longevity.

CLINICAL PRACTICE

The above discussion has illustrated that the salient points regarding the choice of an all-ceramic system are its ability to withstand occlusal stresses and longevity. Fractures are the main cause of failure, occurring at any interface of the tooth/restoration complex including the following:

- Dentine: cohesive failure due to poor tooth preparation design
- Dentine–cement: adhesive failure of the DBA
- Cement: cohesive failure due to poor compressive strength of luting agent, e.g. glass ionomer (GI), resin-modified glass ionomer (RGI)
- Cement–ceramic core: adhesive failure, e.g. for Procera AllCeram, In-Ceram Zirconia, Dicor[53]
- Ceramic core: global failure for single crowns, initiating from the intaglio or fitting surface, and connector sites for FPDs
- Core–veneer: de-lamination, especially for Empress 2, Cerestore and In-Ceram Alumina
- Veneering porcelain: superficial fracturing or chipping due to inadequate support from the dense core. This is particularly significant when a uniform thickness ceramic core is fabricated of a tooth preparation with large inter-arch or inter-abutment spaces, resulting in an unsupported veneering overlay. Therefore it is essential that the core has sufficient height to support a uniform layer of the overlying weaker porcelain. This is achieved by waxing a short tooth preparation to the correct height, before core fabrication. With the Procera system, this can be achieved by

double scanning (inside–outside scanning) to ensure that the core is of sufficient height to support the overlying porcelain.

References

1. Oden, A., Wiatr-Adamczak, E. and Olsson, K. (1991) Aluminium release from alumina and aluminium plate. *Tandlakartindningen*, **83**, 634–636 (in Swedish)
2. Attanasi, R.C., Yaman, P., Lang, B., Razzoog, M. and Joarla, M.J. (1996) Evaluation of color stability of Procera All-Ceramic porcelain. *University of Michigan Abstract* 2134 IADR
3. Hacker, C.H., Wagner, W.C. and Razzoog, M.E. (1996) An in vitro investigation of the wear of enamel on porcelain and gold in saliva. *J Prosthet Dent*, **75**, 14–17
4. Griffith, A.A. (1924) The phenomenon of rupture and flaw in solids. *Philos Trans R Soc*, **221**, 163–189
5. Munz, D. and Fett, T. (1999) *Ceramics: mechanical properties, failure behaviour, material selection*. 1st edn. Springer, Berlin
6. Waltimo, A., Kemppainen, P. and Kononen, M. (1993) Maximal contraction force and endurance of human jaw-closing muscles in isometric clenching. *Scan J Den Res*, **101**, 416–421
7. Tinschert, J., Natt, G., Mautsch, W., Augthun, M. and Spiekermann, H. (2001) Fracture resistance of lithium disilicate-, alumina-, and zirconia- based three-unit fixed partial dentures: A laboratory study. *Int J Prosthodont*, **14**, 231–238
8. Castellani, D., Baccetti, T., Giovannoni, A. and Bernardini, U.D. (1994) Resistance to fracture of metal-ceramic and all-ceramic crowns. *Int J Prosthodont*, **7**, 149–154
9. Swain, M.V. (1989) Toughening mechanisms for ceramics. *Master Forum*, **13**, 237–253
10. Guazzato, M., Albakry, M., Ringer, S.P. and Swain, M.V. (2004) Strength, fracture toughness and microstructure of a selection of all-ceramic materials. Part II. Zirconia based dental ceramics. *Dent Mat*, **20**, 449–456
11. Raigrodski, A.J. (2005) All-ceramic full coverage restorations: concepts and guidelines for material selection. *Pract Proced Aesthet Dent*, **17(4)**, 249–256
12. Wagner, W.C. and Chu, T.M. (1996) Biaxial flexural strength and indentation fracture toughness of three new dental core ceramics. *J Prosthet Dent*, **76**, 140–144
13. Oilo, G. (1988) Flexural strength and internal defects of some dental porcelains. *Acta Odont Scan*, **46**, 313–322
14. Dong, J.K., Luthy, H., Wohlwend, A. and Scharer, P. (1992) Heat pressed ceramics: technology and strength. *Int J Prosthodont*, **5(1)**, 9–16
15. Probster, L., Geis-Gerstorfer, J., Kirchner, E. and Kanjanttra, P. (1997) In vitro evaluation of a glass-ceramic restorative material. *J Oral Rehabil*, **24(9)**, 636–645
16. Fradeani, M., Aquilino, A. and Corrado, M. (2002) Clinical experience with In-Ceram Alumina and Spinell crowns: 5-year follow-up. *Int J Periodont Rest Dent*, **22(6)**, 525–533
17. Jung, Y.-G., Peterson, I.M., Pajares, A. and Lawn, B.R. (1999) Contact damage resistance and strength degradation of glass-infiltrated alumina and spinel ceramics. *J Dent Res*, **77**, 804–814
18. Carrier, D.D. and Kelly, J.R. (1995) In-Ceram failure behaviour and core-veneer interface quality as influenced by residual infiltration glass. *J Prosthodont*, **4**, 237–242
19. Andersson, M. and Oden, A. (1993) A new all-ceramic crown. A dense-sintered, high purity alumina coping with porcelain. *Acta Odontol Scan*, **51**, 59–64
20. Craig, R.G., O'Brian, W.J. and Powers, J.M. *Dental Material Properties and Manipulations*. 6th edn. Mosby, St Louis
21. Hacker, C.H., Wagner, W.C. and Razzoog, M.E. (1996) An in vitro investigation of the wear of enamel on porcelain and gold in saliva. *J Prosthet Dent*, **75**, 14–17
22. May, K., Russel, M., Razzoog, M. and Lang, B. (1998) Precision of fit of the Procera AllCeram crown. *J Prosthet Dent*, **80(4)**, 394–404
23. Oden, A. and Razzoog, M.E. (1997) Masking ability of Procera AllCeram copings of various thickness. *J Dent Res*, **76**, 310

[24] Oden, A., Andersson, M., Krystek, I. and Magnusson, D. (1996) A 5-year clinical follow-up study of Procera AllCeram crowns. Thesis, University of Umea
[25] Sadan, A., Blatz, M.B. and Lang, B. (2005) Clinical considerations for densely sintered alumina and zirconia restorations: Part 1. *Int J Periodontics Restorative Dent*, **25**, 213–219
[26] Malament, K. and Socransky, S. (1999) Survival of Dicor glass-ceramic dental restorations over 14 years. Part II: Effect of thickness of Dicor material and design of tooth preparation. *J Prosthet Dent*, **81**, 662–667
[27] Proos, K.A., Swain, M.V., Ironside, J.V. and Steven G. (2002) Finite element analysis studies of an all-ceramic crown on a first premolar tooth. *Int J Prosthodont*, **15**, 404–412
[28] Guazzato, M., Proos, K., Sara, G. and Swain, M.T. (2004) Strength, reliability, and mode of fracture of bilayered porcelain/core ceramics. *Int J Prosthodont*, **17**, 142–149
[29] Scherrer, S.S., De Rijik, W.G., *et al.* (2001) Incidence of fractures and lifetime predications of all-ceramic crown systems using censored data. *Am J Dent*, **14**, 72–80
[30] Donovan, T.E. and Cho, G.C. (2003) The role of all-ceramic crowns in contemporary restorative dentistry. *J Calif Dent Assoc*, **31**(7), 565–569
[31] Leempoel, P.J., Eschen, S., De Haan, A.F. and Van't Hof, M.A. (1985) An evaluation of crowns and bridges in a general dental practice. *J Oral Rehabil*, **12**, 515–528
[32] Kerschbaum, T., Paszyna, C., Klapp, S. and Meyer, G. (1991) Failure time and risk analysis of fixed partial dentures. *Dtsch Zahnarztl Z*, **46**, 20–25
[33] Walton, T.R. (1999) A 10 year longitudinal study of fixed prosthodontics: clinical characteristics and outcome of single-unit metal-ceramic crowns. *Int J Prosthodont*, **12**, 519–526
[34] Walton, T.R. (2002) An up to 15-year longitudinal study of 515 metal-ceramic FPDs: part 1. Outcome. *Int J Prosthodont*, **15**(5), 439–445.
[35] Erpenstein, H., Borchard, R. and Kerschbaum, T. (2000) Long-term clinical results of galvano-ceramic and glass-ceramic individual crowns. *J Prosthet Dent*, **83**(**5**), 530–534
[36] Thompson, J.Y., Anusavice, K.J., Naman, A. and Morris, H.F. (1994) Fracture surface characterisation of clinically failed all-ceramic crowns. *J Dent Res*, **73**, 1824–1832
[37] Sjogren, G., Lantto, R., Granberg, A., Sundstorm, B.O. and Tillberg, A. (1999) Clinical examination of leucite-reinforced glass-ceramic crowns (Empress) in general practice: a retrospective study. *Int J Prosthodont*, **12**(**2**), 122–128
[38] Fradeani, M. and Aquilano, A. (1997) Clinical experience with Empress crowns. *Int J Prosthodont*, **10**(**3**), 241–247
[39] Sorensen, J.A., Choi, C., Fanuscu, M.I. and Mito, W.T. (1998) IPS Empress crown system: Three-year clinical trial results. *J Calif Dent Assoc*, **26**(**2**), 130–136
[40] Brochu, J.-F. and El-Mowafy, O. (2002) Longevity and clinical performance of IPS-Empress ceramic restorations – a literature review. *J Can Dent Assoc*, **68**(**4**), 233–237
[41] Fradeani, M. and Redemagni, M. (2002) An 11-year clinical evaluation of leucite-reinforced glass-ceramic crowns: a retrospective study. *Quintessence Int*, 33, 503–510
[42] Segal, B.S. (2001) Retrospective assessment of 546 all-ceramic anterior and posterior crowns in a general practice. *J Prosthet Dent*, **85**(**6**), 544–550
[43] Oden, A., Andersson, M., Krystek-Ondracek, I. and Magnusson, D. (1998) Five-year clinical evaluation of Procera AllCeram crowns. *J Prosthet Dent*, **80**, 450–456
[44] Odman, P. and Andersson, B. (2001) Procera AllCeram crowns followed for 5 to 10.5 years: a prospective clinical study. *Int J Prosthodont*, 14, 504–509
[45] Fradeani, M., D'Amelio, M., Redemagni, M. and Corrado, M. (2005) Five-year follow-up with Procera all-ceramic crowns. *Quintessence Int*, **36**, 105–113
[46] Naert, I., Van der Donck, A. and Beckers, L. (2005) Precision of fit and clinical evaluation of all-ceramic full restorations followed between 0.5 and 5 years. *J Oral Rehabil*, **32**(**1**), 51–57

[47] Hannink, R.H.J., Kelly, P.M. and Muddle, B.C. (2000) Transforming toughness in zirconia-containing ceramics. *J Am Ceram Soc*, **83**, 461–487

[48] Sorrensen, J.A., Cruz, M., Mito, W.T., Raffeiner, O., Meredith, H.R. and Foser, H.P. (1998) A clinical investigation on three-unit fixed partial dentures fabricated with lithium disilicate glass-ceramic. *Pract Periodontics Aesthet Dent*, **11**, 95–106

[49] McLaren, E.A. and White, S.N. (2000) Glass-infiltrated zirconia/alumina-bases ceramic for crowns and fixed partial dentures: Clinical and laboratory guidelines. *Quintessence Dental Technology 2000*. pp 63–76. Quintessence, Chicago

[50] Pallis, K., Griggs, J.A., Woody, R.D., Guillen, G.E. and Miller, A.W. (2004) Fracture resistance of three all-ceramic restorative systems for posterior applications. *J Prosthet Dent*, **91**, 561–569

[51] Fischer, H., Weber, M. and Marx, R. (2003) Lifetime prediction of all-ceramic bridges by computational methods. *J Dent Res*, **82(3)**, 238–242

[52] Pauli, C. (1996) Biegefestigkeit dreigliedriger metal- und vollkeramischer Oberkieferseiten-zahnbrucken. *Zahnarztl Welt/Ref*, **105**, 626–632

[53] Kelly, J.R., Giordano, R., Pober, R. and Cima, M.J. (1990) Fracture surface analysis of dental ceramics: clinically failed restorations. *Int J Prosthodont*, **3**, 430–440

4 Colour and shade analysis

A thing that is not understood often becomes the focus of mystery, fear, indifference or abject rejection. Colour, although a part of nearly every human activity, is one of those things that is poorly understood and shrouded by misconceptions. Much of the scientific literature on colour is riddled with mathematical formulae, which, useful in a technical or industrial laboratory, have little meaning to everyday situations. The dental literature usually reports results of the particular aspect of colour under scrutiny, without discussing fundamental principles. The aim of this chapter is to 'open the doors of perception' so that the entire dental team can comprehend and use colour in daily practice. The first section deals with fundamental concepts, including definitions, measurements (both quantitative and qualitative), sensation and perception of colour. The second section explains variables influencing shade selection and how to circumvent pitfalls during ocular assessment, and concludes with digital colour devices for dental shade analysis.

SCIENTIFIC RATIONALE

Sight is the spearhead of human senses. Vision takes precedence over all other senses: hearing, smell, touch and taste. If there is a sensory conflict between the senses, vision is the ultimate arbitrator, a phenomenon known as visual capture. Colour vision is a part of the visual experience and one of the most complex processes occurring in the brain. Colour realisation is the result of three processes: stimulation, sensation and perception. It is important to clarify that these three processes are not synonyms to describe the same event, but distinct sequential events occurring during colour detection. An explanation of colour involves many branches of science, including physics, chemistry, physiology and psychology. The process by which radiant energy (light) relates to a psychological experience (colour) is termed psychophysics.

Colour perception involves the presence of three entities: a light source (illuminant), an

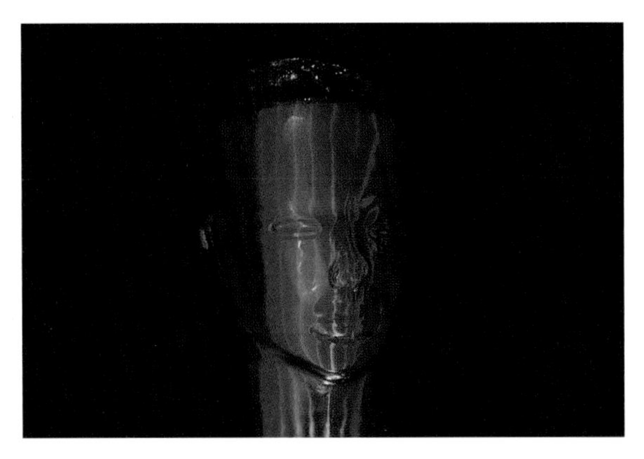

Figure 4.1 A glass sculpture illuminated by colours of the visible spectrum as an allegorical illustration that colour experience is in the mind of the beholder.

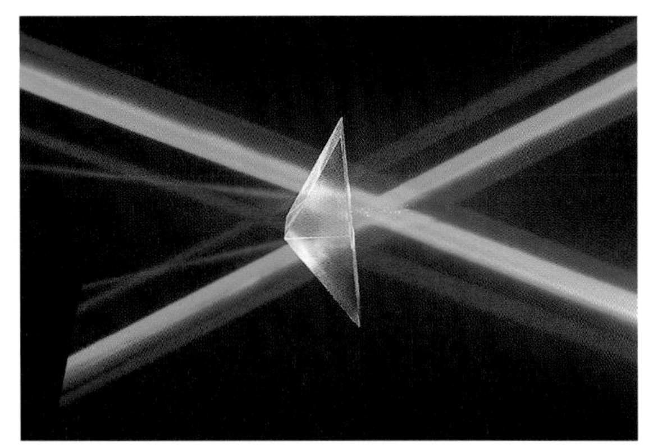

Figure 4.2 A variation of the seminal Isaac Newton experiment showing that a glass prism splits white light into colours of the visible spectrum.

object and a detector (ocular or instrumental). The preceding statement implies that all three items should be present before colour is perceived. This is not always necessary, and contrary to popular belief, it is possible to perceive colour without a stimulus or a sensation. Ultimately, colour experience is in the mind of the beholder, it is not an innate property of an object or the eyes (Fig. 4.1). Although an illuminant/object/detector does lead to colour perception, it is important to realise this is only one type of colour experience, known as conscious colour perception. Other types of colour experiences are subconscious colour perception, e.g. recalling a memory or dreaming,[1] and paraconscious perception, e.g. during a psychedelic experience under the influence of hallucinatory drugs (in both these states of mind, neither illuminant nor object is present to illicit a response). In the discussion that follows, colour experience is confined to conscious colour perception.

The stimulus for colour

The first part of the stimulus/sensation/perception triad is the physical stimulus of colour. Radiant energy (light) is a narrow band of the electromagnetic spectrum, on the one extreme comprising long waves of radio broadcasting to the other of shorter gamma radiation waves. The visual system of the eye is only capable of detecting wavelengths ranging from 380 nm (violet) to 780 nm (red).[2] According to Isaac Newton,[3] light has no colour, it is only when it interacts with an object that colour is produced. This was depicted in his famous experiment of splitting light by a prism into the colours of the visible spectrum, comprising red, orange, yellow, green, blue, indigo and violet (Fig. 4.2). As previously stated, the parts which comprise the stimulus for colour are the illuminant (light source), an object and a detector.

The illuminant

The quality of light is determined by its colour temperature, measured in Kelvin (K); this varies from a cool blue sky (9000 K) to candle light (2500 K). In 1931, CIE (Commission Internationale de l'Éclairge or International Commission on Illumination)[4] recommended use of standard light sources A, B, and C, which were supplemented in 1971[5] to include illuminant D_{65}. These light sources are distinguished by their spectral power distribution curves and are utilised for colour determination under specific conditions. For example, Standard Illuminant A represents incandescent light with a colour temperature of 2856 K, Standard Illuminant C is average daylight at 6774 K without ultraviolet radiation, and Standard Illuminant D_{65} is daylight at 6540 K including the wavelengths of ultraviolet radiation. A distinction is required between a source and an illuminant. To be precise, a source is a physically realisable light (e.g. a dental operating light), an illuminant may or may not be realisable, but if an illuminant is converted into a physical form, it is then termed a standard source. For the purpose of this discussion, the terms source and illuminant are interchangeable. The colour of an object appears different depending on the illuminant. This property of light sources to influence the colour of objects is termed colour rendition (Figs. 4.3 & 4.4).

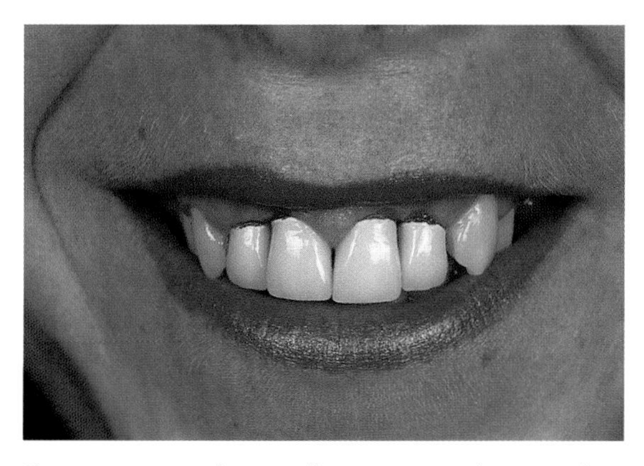

Figure 4.3 Incandescent illumination renders a yellow appearance to this dentofacial composition.

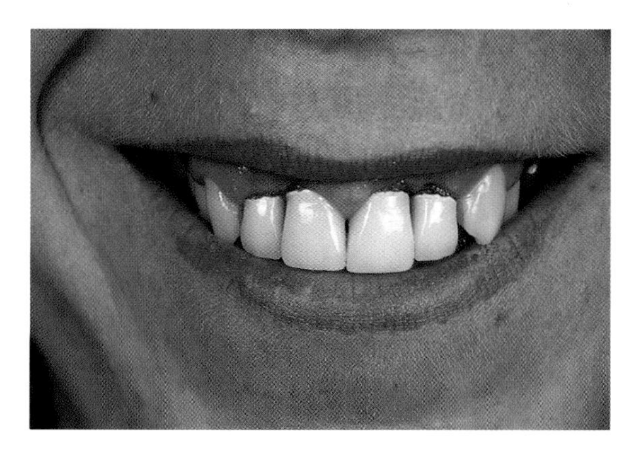

Figure 4.4 Same image as Figure 4.3, but viewed by light with a colour temperature of 5600 K (simulated daylight), producing a more realistic colour rendition.

The object

Similar to a cube having three dimensions, length, width and depth, colour also possesses three dimensions: value, hue and chroma. The value is the quantity of light reflected by an object compared to a pure white diffuser (reflecting 100%), and a black absorber (absorbing all incident light with no reflection). If a material reflects most of the light falling on its surface, it appears bright, i.e. it has a high value. Conversely, a dark object absorbs most of the incident light and appears dull, i.e. has a low value. Between these two extremes is a gradation of value termed the grey-scale. The tomato in Figure 4.5 shows a reflectance of 14%, compared to the 100% white diffuser on the left, and a black absorber with 0% reflectance on the right.

The second dimension of colour is hue or wavelength of light; this is dependent on the spectral reflectance (of the visible spectrum) from an object. For example, Figure 4.6 shows that when white light strikes the surface of a tomato (in this case separated into the colours of the spectrum for clarity), all colours are absorbed expect red. The tomato therefore appears red because the spectral reflectance is limited only to the red wavelength (i.e. the tomato reflects only the red part of the white light). An opaque object (such as the tomato) reflects a specific

Figure 4.5 The value of the white diffuser on the left is 100%, and that of the black absorber on the right is 0%. The tomato has a reflectance of 14%, reflecting only 14% of the incident light falling onto its surface.

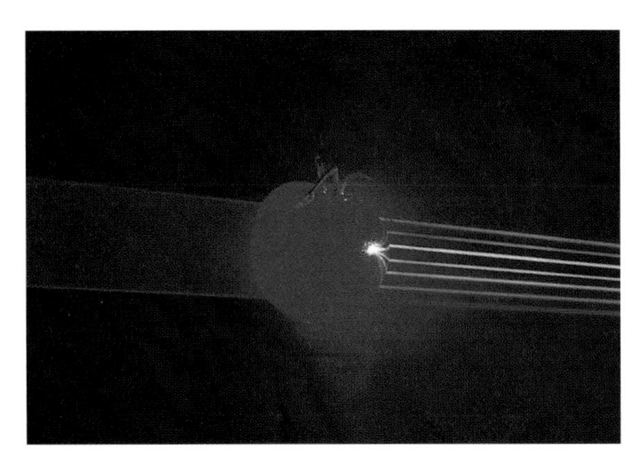

Figure 4.6 A tomato appears red because it absorbs all the colours of the visible spectrum (right side) except those in the red wavelength region (left side).

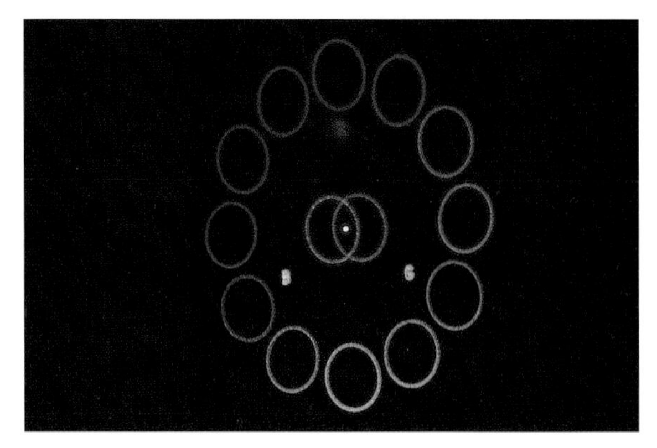

Figure 4.8 Graphical representation of the three primary colours: red, green and blue.

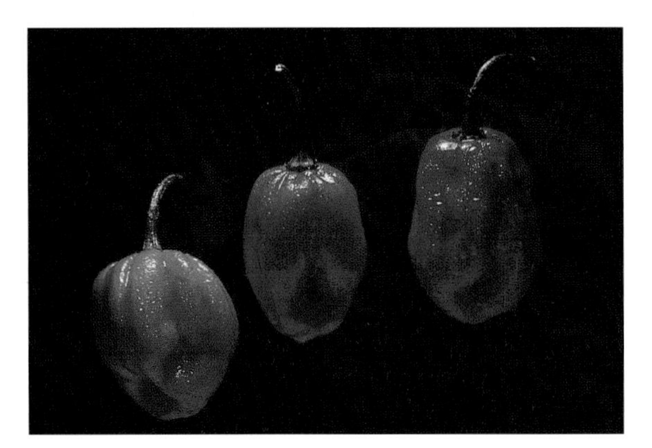

Figure 4.7 Three red peppers of the same hue [red] but varying chroma (depth of colour) increasing from left to right.

wavelength of the visible spectrum and produces a spectral *reflectance* curve, while a transparent coloured object (e.g. coloured glass) creates a spectral *transmittance* curve. A translucent object, such as a tooth, produces both spectral reflectance and transmittance curves. These spectral curves are analogous to the power distribution curves of illuminants.

Chroma is the last component of colour. The three peppers in Figure 4.7 have the same hue, but with an increasing colour intensity from left to right. The pepper on the left is least saturated and appears pale, i.e. it has a low chroma. The middle is more saturated, while the third on the right is the most saturated, having a vivid appearance, with the highest chroma.

Colour is numerically quantified by its three dimensions: hue, value and chroma. Quantifying colour is similar to determining the dimensions of an object, where a ruler is equivalent to a colour-measuring instrument (colorimeter or spectrophotometer), length to a colour space, and the scale, such as imperial (inches) or metric (metres) to colour co-ordinates of a specific colour space. The two popular devices for objective measurement of colour are the colorimeter and spectrophotometer. The colorimeter uses the tri-stimulus method, comprising three coloured filters corresponding to selective spectral sensitivities to the three primary colours, red, green and blue (Fig. 4.8). The readings X, Y and Z are the amount of the three primary colours for a given object, which are converted to a specified colour space. The spectrophotometer, on the other hand, measures the spectral distribution (reflectance or transmittance) of an object rather than just three colours. This method is more descriptive and is capable of ascertaining colour using different illuminants. The readings of a spectrophotometer curves (spectral reflectance or transmittance) can either be plotted, or converted to colour co-ordinates for particular colour spaces.[6]

Many colour spaces and co-ordinates are available to quantify colour, but for brevity, the Munsell[7] and the CIEL*a*b* (1976), are described. The benchmark is the Munsell System, conceived in 1905 by the American artist A.H.

Munsell. This is fabricated from paper colour strips corresponding to three colour co-ordinates: the Munsell Hue, Munsell Value and Munsell Chroma, and later modified to the Munsell Re-notation System.[8,9] These systems express a colour by a letter and number combination according to the Munsell Colour Charts. This notation is also used for the Vitapan 3D-Master shade guide (Vita) (Fig. 4.9).

The initial CIE colour space introduced in 1931 with the Yxy coordinates proved inadequate because colours were represented only in two dimensions (hue and chroma), and the perceived colours had no correlations to visual perception. In 1976, CIE modified their colour space to the L*a*b*, where L* indicates lightness (value), and a* and b* are the chromaticity co-ordinates. The CIE L*a*b* colour space is best visualised using a sphere (Fig. 4.10). The vertical axis representing L*, the top is white (value of 100%) and the bottom black (value of 0%). In the a* direction, +a* corresponds to red, while -a* is the complementary colour green and for the b* co-ordinate, +b* is yellow, and -b* denoting the complementary colour blue. Chroma is the radial axis traversing from the centre to the periphery of the sphere. The centre of the sphere has low chroma, and the periphery high chroma colours. The colour space representing natural teeth is located between the +a* and +b* co-ordinates, in the red, red – yellow (orange) and yellow wavelengths of the spectrum (Fig. 4.11).

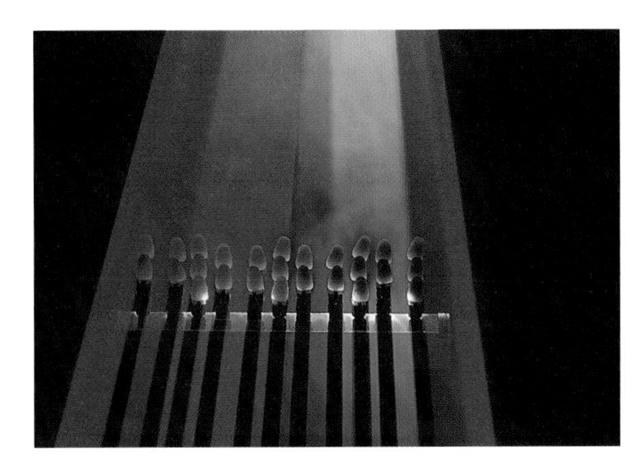

Figure 4.9 The Vitapan 3D-Master shade guide.

Sensation (the detector)

The third part of the stimulus for colour is the spectral response of the detector, in this case the eye. Visual sensation is a chemical, electrical and physiological process. An elementary description is conversion of physical energy (light) into neural messages, a process termed transduction.

Radiant energy enters the eye via the cornea and is focused on to the retina by the lens. The lens changes its curvature (accommodation) to focus light rays through an aperture of the iris

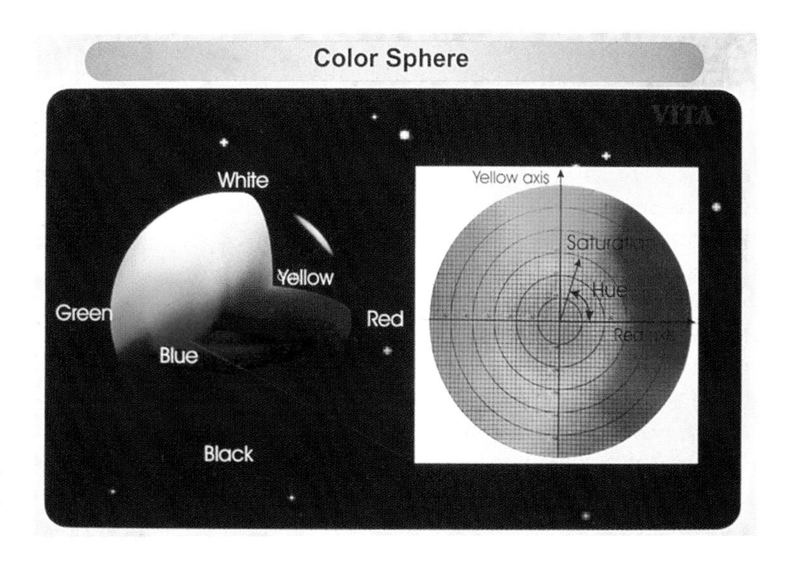

Figure 4.10 The CIE L*a*b* colour space depicted by a sphere (image courtesy of Vita).

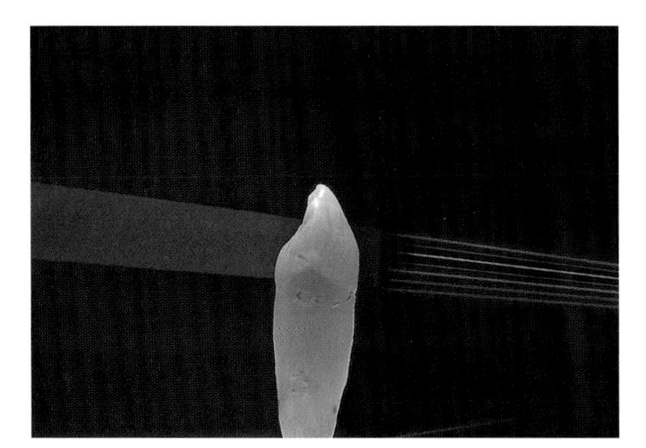

Figure 4.11 A natural tooth absorbs all the colours of the spectrum (right side) except those in the yellow, orange and red wavelengths (left side).

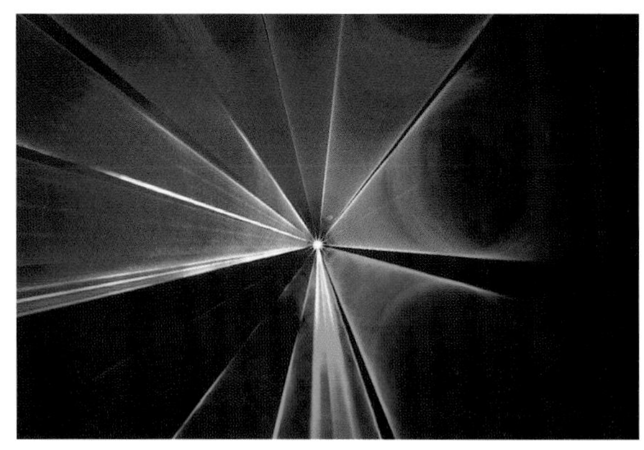

Figure 4.13 Colours of the visible spectrum converging onto the fovea in the eye, where chromatic vision is feasible.

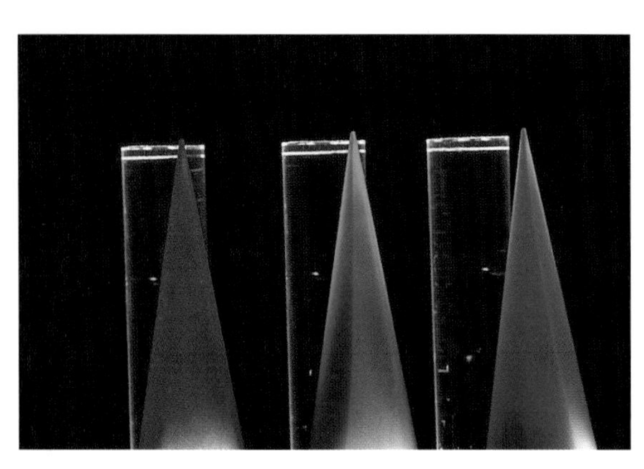

Figure 4.12 Pictorial representation of rods and cones in the retina of the eye. The cones are responsible for chromatic vision, responding to one of the three primary colours, red, green or blue. The rods (in the background), are responsible for achromatic vision, lightness and darkness.

known as the pupil. The black appearance of the pupil is attributed to the fact that most of the light entering the eye is absorbed by light sensitive pigments in the retina[10] (similar to light falling on a black surface). Visual acuity (sharpness) occurs at the centre of the lens where spherical and chromatic aberrations are negligible.

The retina is a mosaic of two types of photosensitive cells, called rods and cones (Fig. 4.12). The cones are responsible for chromatic vision, and contain photosensitive pigments with spectral sensitivities to the three primary colours, corresponding to wavelengths 448 nm (blue), 528 nm (green) and 567 nm (red).[11] When stimulated by light, the pigments undergo photodecomposition to create an electrical impulse for nerve excitation. Most of the 6 million cones are clustered in the fovea, a depression in the retina with a surface area of 1 mm^2 at the retina's central focal point (Fig. 4.13). The field of view of the fovea is 2°, and moving peripherally, the cones mingle with rods. The cones have a direct one-to-one neurone link, which accounts for their ability to convey precise information to the optic nerve, resulting in sharp images.

The rods have a maximum distribution about 20° from the fovea. Their photosensitive pigment (rhodopsin) has a maximum relative spectral sensitivity to only one wavelength of 510 nm (green), resulting in achromatic vision. The rods have no 'hotline' to the optic nerve and impulses from a group of rods converge on to a single neurone. An advantage of this neural arrangement is that rod vision is possible under dim lighting conditions, but the disadvantage is that the resulting image is blurred compared to that of cone vision.

In dentistry, the rod and cone distribution of the retina is significant during shade determination. The clinician should concentrate, or stare at the tooth and shade tab to assess hue and chroma which activates cone (chromatic) vision within the 2° foveal locus. To ascertain brightness (value), the observer needs to look aside in order to engage rod vision located at a 20° radius from the foveal locus.

The difference threshold for colours in the human eye is low enough to discriminate 7 million colour variations.[12] There are two main theories to explain colour vision. The first is the Young–Helmholtz trichromatic theory, which stipulates that the retina has three types of receptors, each sensitive to one of the three primary colours, red, green, and blue (Fig. 4.14).[13,14] This relies on the additive mixtures on colours, for example when red and green lights are mixed, yellow is produced. Most dichromatic colour blindness is an inability to distinguish reds and greens, and affects 1 in 50 of the population, predominately men, since the defect is genetically sex-linked. In dichromats however, yellow (mixture of red and green) is still discernible, a finding that is in direct conflict with the Young–Helmholtz theory. The limitation of the Young–Helmholtz theory is that it only explains colour reception at one site (the retina), and is termed a single-stage theory.

Hering's opponent-process theory proposes that post-retinal analysis of visual information occurs en route to the brain. This further analysis comprises opponent colours, red–green, blue–yellow and white–black, e.g. some of the neurones are turned 'on' by yellow, but turned 'off' by blue.[15] This means that if a colour is detected at a particular site of the retina, the opposing colour cannot be detected at the same time, i.e. it is not possible to detect a yellowish-blue. Together, the Young–Helmholtz and Hering's theories offer a better explanation of colour sensation, termed a multi-stage theory.[16]

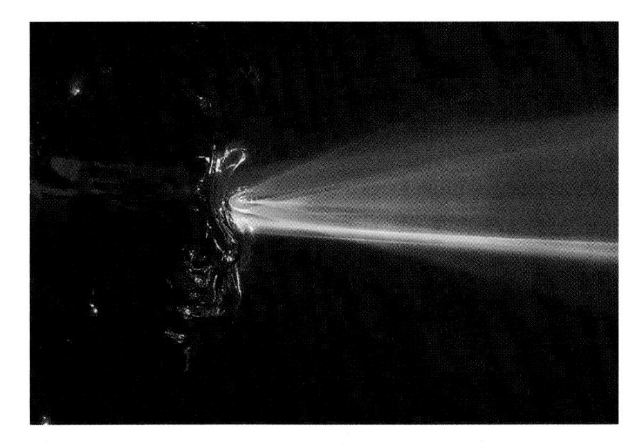

Figure 4.14 A glass sculpture demonstrating the Young–Helmholtz trichromatic theory, which stipulates that the eye has receptors for only the three primary colours, red, green and blue.

Exploitation of the opponent-process theory in dentistry can be used to resolve severely discoloured teeth using porcelain laminate veneers. Patients exhibiting tetracycline staining are often prescribed veneers with an opaque masking porcelain to conceal the discolouration, resulting in artificial, high-value prostheses. To create a more natural appearance, veneers can be fabricated using porcelains with modifiers of a complementary colour to tooth discolouration. In this way post-retinal processing of the neural information will counteract tooth discoloration by the porcelain veneers, e.g. an orange stained tooth would require a green porcelain modifier (although not a true complement, it serves the intended aesthetic function in ceramics).[17] Dental luting cements also employ the same theory for improving the colour of a translucent all-ceramic restoration.

Synopsis of the stimulus for colour

The three items constituting the stimulus for colour are the illuminant, the object and the detector (eyes). Each forms a spectral curve: the illuminant is represented by a spectral power distribution curve, the object by its spectral reflectance (or transmittance) curve and the eye by its spectral response curve. It is the product of these three curves that forms the stimulus for colour, which in finally interpreted by the brain. The next part describes how the cerebral apparatus interprets and decodes this chromatic graffiti.

Perception

The psychological process of vision resides in the brain, involving decoding neural data from the eyes. Retinal information reaches the visual

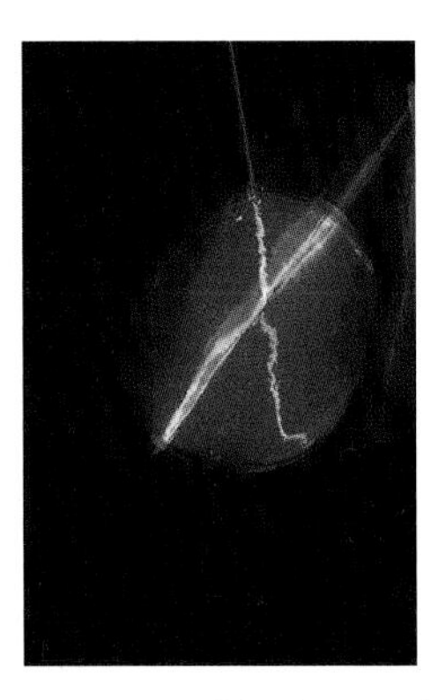

Figure 4.15 Superior view of the human skull, showing that a light flashed to the right eye (yellow beam) is relayed to the left visual cortex located in the occipital lobe and vice versa for the left eye (pink beam).

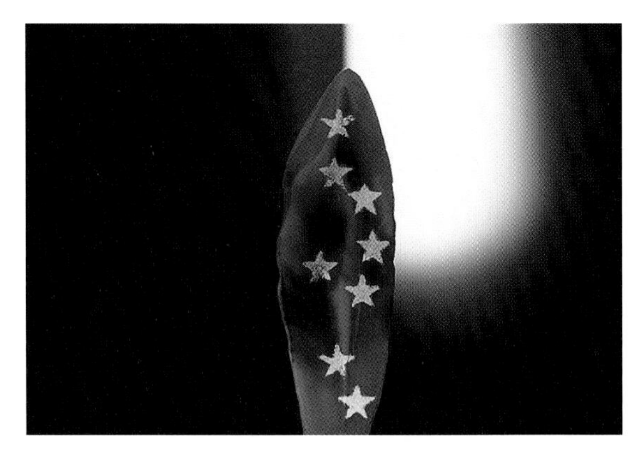

Figure 4.16 An individual with a severed corpus callosum can not interpret this image of a tooth as a surreal representation of the American flag.

cortex, situated in the occipital lobe, via the optic nerve by traversing the thalamus. During transit, the information is continuously processed until it reaches the higher centres of the brain, comprising the right and left cerebral hemispheres. The right eye relays information to the left hemisphere and vice versa (Fig. 4.15). The visual cortex is one of the major sites responsible for processing visual data, and is part of the cerebral cortex. Three-quarters of the cerebral cortex is comprised of the association areas that interpret, integrate and act on information from the sensory organs. Cerebral information processing is a two-way conduit, bottom-up processing from the senses to the brain, and top-down processing from the brain to other parts of the body for eliciting a response in reaction to an input.

The right and left cerebral hemispheres perform different analytical computations. In a right-handed individual, the left hemisphere is 'dominant' and responsible for cognitive tasks. Although the right is regarded as the 'minor' hemisphere, it boasts perceptual and visual spatial superiority. This means that if an image is flashed to the right hemisphere, it is recognised quicker than if flashed to the left hemisphere. A bundle of neural tissue called the corpus callosum, besides a physical link between the two hemispheres, is also an important communication channel. If the latter is incised (e.g. in neural surgery to treat epilepsy), the brain sees an object, but cannot recognise it. In an individual whose corpus callosum is severed, the image in Figure 4.16 is perceived as shapes and colours without any significance. However, in a person with an intact corpus callosum, the left hemisphere senses shapes and colours and relays this information to the right hemisphere, which conceptually perceives the image as a surreal representation of the American flag.

The image formed on the retina by the ocular apparatus is incomplete. In fact the retina does not see the object as it appears, but rather a symbolic representation of it, which is termed an implicit representation. This image is a $2\frac{1}{2}$-dimensional sketch, more than two dimensions because orientation is conveyed, but not three-dimensional because depth is not explicitly represented.[18] The brain carries out complex computations, using past experiences (either its own or atavistic references), biases, etc. to convert an image into a three-dimensional explicit representation.[19] The mind is unaware of this computational aspect of visual consciousness, but responsive to its result.[20]

From the above, it is apparent why individuals discern a particular colour differently. Additionally, the brain perceives the world not as it is, but as our mind wants it to be. A clinician, during tooth shade analysis, is tainted by past experiences, which may not be identical to those of the patient or the ceramist. These conflicts are inevitable, but awareness of biases and idiosyncrasies prevents disagreements and avoids clinician/patient/ceramist conflicts.

Tooth colour determination

The variables affecting tooth colour determination are broadly divided into:

- Physical
- Physiological
- Psychological
- Dental

Physical variables

The illuminant

It is well established that the quality of illumination affects colour perception, a phenomenon known as colour rendition. In order to achieve reliable and repeatable shade assessment, the illumination must be standardised with respect to quality and quantity. The light qualities most conducive to colour discrimination are Cloud Diffused North Noon Daylight, possessing a uniform spectral power distribution[21] with a colour temperature of 6500 K[22], CIE Standard Illuminant C or D_{65}. The quantity or intensity of light should be 1500 lux[23], which is equivalent to four 220 W fluorescent tubes at a distance of 2 metres.[24] Also, the light source should not be directional, but uniformly diffuse to avoid specular reflection.[25] Many proprietary devices satisfy these criteria, and their use is mandatory to circumvent shade discrepancies.

Metamerism

The stimulus for colour is a product of spectral curves belonging to the illuminant (spectral power distribution), the object (spectral reflectance or transmittance) and observer (spectral response). Metamerism is a phenomenon that describes why the colour of a pair of objects is differently perceived when one factor is changed, while the other two remain constant. There are two types of metamerism: object and observer metamerism.

Object metamerism is the comparison of a pair of objects that have the same colour under a given illuminant, but when the illuminant is

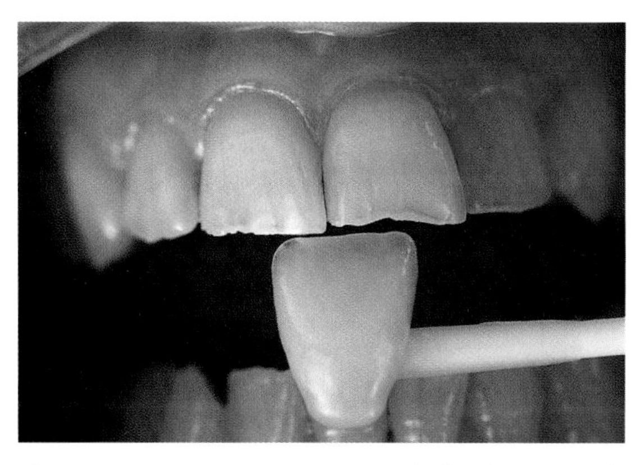

Figure 4.17 Metamerism: a custom shade tab is a match with this patient's dentition with flash illumination of colour temperature 5500 K.

changed, their colours no longer match. This is because the objects have different spectral reflectance curves, but if they match for a given source they must share the same colour co-ordinates (e.g. CIE tri-stimulus values).These two statements seem contradictory but are not; the reason is that a spectral reflectance curve contains more information than the colour co-ordinates derived from it. In order for two objects to match for any lighting condition, i.e. to be an invariant pair, their spectral reflectance curves must be identical. The significance of object metamerism is that if a restoration (crown or filling) matches the surrounding or adjacent teeth under the halogen dental operating light, it may not match when viewed by daylight (Figs. 4.17 & 4.18). It is therefore advisable to perform dental procedures using daylight-corrected illumination to avoid metamerism.[26]

Observer metamerism, either visual or instrumental, is if the illuminant remains constant but the observer changes. In humans, this is dependent on the different physiological spectral response sensitivities of cones in the eyes. In dentistry, this is manifested when a restoration is perceived to be a colour match by both patient and clinician, but not by the patient's family and friends. To avoid this scenario, it is desirable to request that relatives or close friends accompany the patient during the shade assessing appointment.

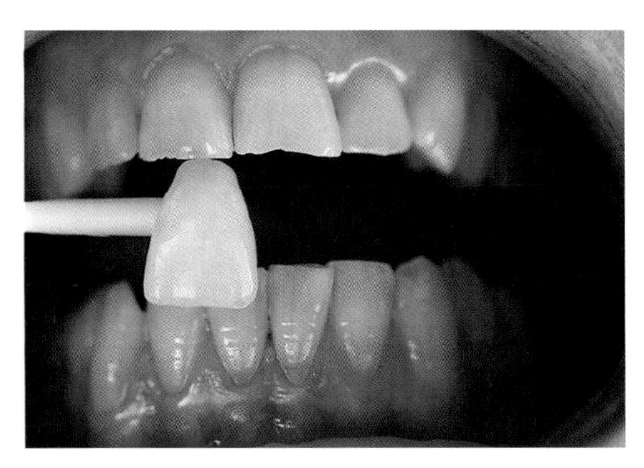

Figure 4.18 Metamerism: the custom shade tab from Figure 4.17 is too bright (high value) when viewed with daylight of colour temperature 6500 K.

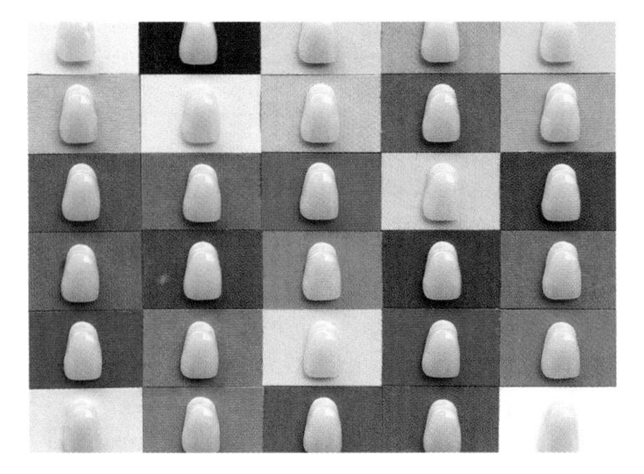

Figure 4.19 The context (background) influences the perceived colour of an object. All the shade tabs in this picture are identical (Vitapan 3L1.5), but are perceived differently depending on the background colour. The correct shade assessment is the tab with the neutral grey background.

The ambient environment

The context in which an object is viewed also influences its perceived colour, e.g. an object with bright surroundings will appear duller. Also, according to the opponent-process theory of post-retinal processing of visual information, looking at a red object will increase ocular sensitivity to green. Figure 4.19 demonstrates that a tooth tab of the same shade is perceived differently, depending on the coloured backdrop. The dental surgery is a haven for a multitude of coloured items, including the interior decor, equipment, patient's complexion, clothing and cosmetic adornment, etc., with conflicting visual stimuli.[27] It may therefore be necessary to create a chromatic microcosm with correct lighting with an ideal background using a Munsell neutral grey N 7/0 card,[28] and limit shade determination to this designated area.

Physiological variables

In advancing years the lens of the eye diminishes its capacity to change shape (accommodate) with diminishing focusing capabilities. Furthermore, cataract changes cause murkiness and yellowing of the lens. These degenerative processes cause spherical and chromatic aberrations, with 'yellowing' of the vision.[29] An affected operator tends to provide restorations that are yellower, which can be counteracted by allowing younger members of staff to participate in colour assessment.

If vision is not concentrated on the fovea of the eye, the location of the majority of cones, it is termed peripheral with a diminished ability to discern colours. If this so-called indirect vision is more than 40 μm from the fovea, total colour blindness occurs. An operator who has constant difficulty matching colours is advised to seek an optician consultation to ascertain whether he/she suffers with indirect vision.

Hue bias is differing tolerance for a specific colour, an occupational hazard affecting dentists and ceramists. The result is increased tolerance to yellow and reduced sensitivity to red (a colour rarely seen in natural teeth). Both dentist and ceramist therefore demonstrate a red hue bias.[30,31] If a restoration has a mismatch with a red hue, it is more likely to be rejected than a mismatch with a yellow hue. Clinical relevance of hue bias is that a prosthodontist or ceramist may consider a restoration as acceptable, but it may be rejected by the patient as being too yellow.

Psychological variables

Psychological variables are the most complex and least understood variables of colour realisation. Before describing cerebral processes specific to colour, it is necessary to outline basic functions of all sensory organs.

Stimulus detection

For a sense organ to detect a stimulus, the latter must be of a minimum magnitude, termed an absolute threshold, described by the signal detection theory, which states **when** a signal is detectable.[32] An individual's temperament greatly influences whether or not a signal is detected, influenced by expectations, experience, motivations, fatigue, the task at hand, time of day or even regular exercise. Many inter- and intra-operator disagreements of a particular shade are attributed to these variables.

Discriminating two stimuli simultaneously, for example matching a shade tab with a natural tooth, involves a process called difference threshold or just noticeable difference (JND).[33] Practically, a minimum difference is necessary to discern two different stimuli. This is the distinction between what is a clinically *acceptable* colour match, as opposed to what is a clinically *perceptible* colour match. The minimum colour difference perceptible by the human eye ranges from ΔE^* 0.3–0.5 (where ΔE^* is colour difference defined by CIE). However, acceptable thresholds are much higher at ΔE^* 1.1–2.1, allowing greater latitude if restorations are not an absolute match with the surrounding dentition, but are nevertheless acceptable.

Adaptation

Sensory adaptation is diminished sensitivity by a sense organ of a perpetual or unchanging stimulus. For example, one is not aware of the sensation of wearing shoes throughout the day, freeing the brain to concentrate on other stimuli. It can be argued, if one stares at an object with undivided attention, why it does not disappear? The reason for this is that eye quiver and regular blinking guarantee that the retinal image is continually changing.

Another form of adaptation is the phenomenon of chromatic adaptation or colour constancy. If a white card is viewed in sunlight and then by indoor incandescent light, it is perceived as white under both lighting conditions. This is one of the most enigmatic cerebral processes, and further endorses the fact that ultimately, it is the brain that 'manufactures' the perception of colour. The reason why the card maintains its chromatic status quo is that the brain 'stores' the colour of the card in short-term memory, and, upon seeing the card for a second time (with a different colour temperature light source), recalls its initial memory of the card, and automatically assumes it is white. The technique to overcome this obstacle with shade assessment is as follows.

In order to detect a stimulus the image must be visible for a minimum of 60–70 milliseconds.[34] Below this minimum threshold, it is impossible for the brain to interpret an image or its colour. Further exposure, up to a maximum of five seconds, is possible without the influence of chromatic adaptation.[35] This time interval during which colours can be accurately perceived is called the chromatic assessment period (CAP). Shade determination should therefore be carried out within the CAP. Concentrating on a tooth for protracted periods, in the hope of gaining further chromatic information is futile and compromises shade analysis.

Brightness or lightness constancy is similar to colour constancy (chromatic adaptation), i.e. the brain perceives the value of an object in relation to its context (background).[36] In Figure 4.20 a tooth of the same value appears lighter in front of a black compared with a white background. The clinical relevance of brightness constancy is that a tooth appears lighter with the darker oral cavity as the backdrop. To counteract this illusion, value determination should be performed with a neutral grey background.

Dental variables

Tooth colour is not uniform across the populous, and even varies from tooth to tooth in a given individual. After the age of 35, teeth become increasingly saturated with deeper chroma, especially in cervical regions. The value also decreases as the enamel overlay becomes more

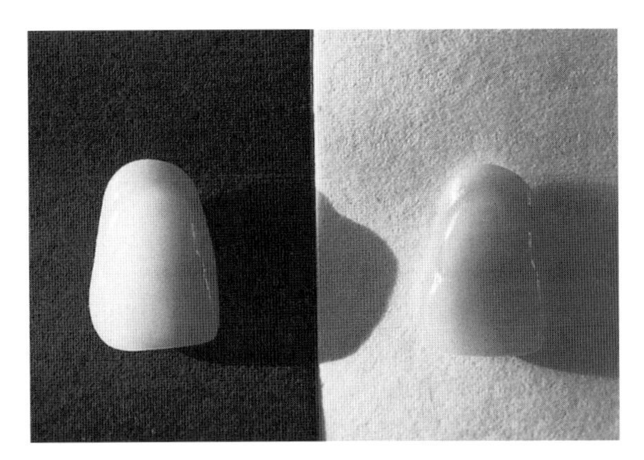

Figure 4.20 Brightness or lightness constancy is demonstrated by placing a tooth tab of the same value (Vita Value group 4), which appears brighter in front of a black (left), than the white (right) background.

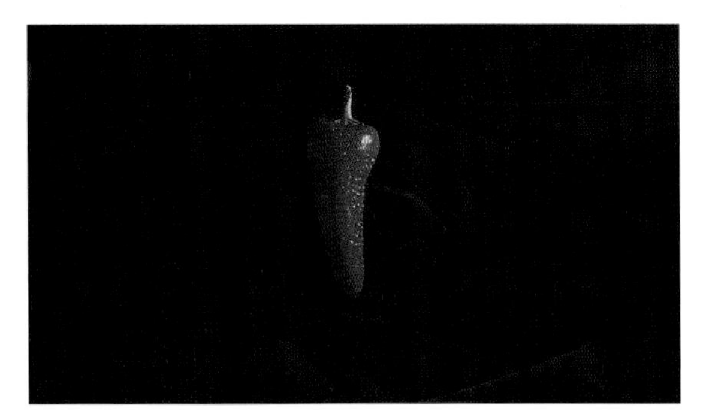

Figure 4.21 The hue, value and chroma of the red chilli are clearly discernible when viewed without an optical barrier.

translucent. Inter-arch differences include yellower maxillary anterior teeth compared to the mandibular antagonists. An interesting variation is that the maxillary canines are redder than those in the mandible. Intra-arch differences include lower value, yellower, and higher chroma canines compared to the adjacent incisors, which have the highest value of all teeth. These variations should be borne in mind during extensive prosthodontic treatment, especially when no surrounding teeth are present to act as reference or guides for the proposed prostheses.[37]

Shade matching of natural teeth to artificial prostheses

To obtain an absolute match (invariant match) for all illumination and viewing conditions, a natural tooth and artificial restoration must have identical physical properties and spectral reflectance curves. Matching materials of different compositions results in a close match, under limited lighting and viewing conditions, which is termed a conditional match. Most visual shade determination in dentistry is a conditional match that is clinically acceptable (see above discussion on perceptibility vs. acceptability).

Multi-layered structure of natural and artificial teeth

The difficulty of dental shade selection is that the operator has to negotiate a multi-layered structure of varying thickness, opacities and optical surface characteristics. This introduces complexities far greater than assessing colour of a uniformly turbid opaque object. Natural teeth, as well as restorative materials that aim to emulate their structure, are multi-layered, which has an impact on the way they are perceived.

The basic hue of a tooth is determined by the colour of underlying dentine, while value is a quality of the enamel overlay. Chroma is essentially the saturation of colour in dentine, but is influenced by the value and thickness of enamel. For accurate colour analysis, it is important to grasp the concept of visual interaction between dentine and enamel. The following model explains how chromaticity of a tooth is affected by its heterogeneous structure. The three dimensions of colour (hue, value, chroma) of a red pepper shown in Figure 4.21 can be gauged with relative ease. The situation becomes complicated when the red pepper is viewed through sheets of glass of varying translucency. As translucency of the glass decreases its value increases, chroma decreases, but the hue is unchanged (Figs. 4.22 & 4.23). The preceding analogy is identical to the dual layering found in natural teeth, the red pepper representing dentine, and glass sheets the

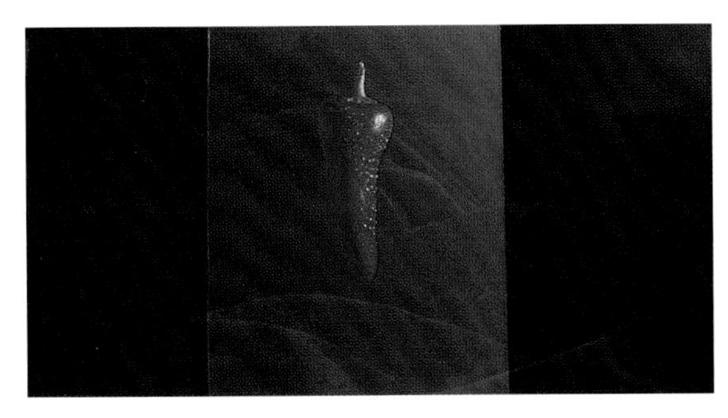

Figure 4.22 A glass sheet is placed in front of the pepper in Figure 4.21, the chroma appears to decrease but its hue remains constant.

Figure 4.23 When a glass sheet of increasing opacity (decreasing translucency) is placed in front of the pepper in Figure 4.21, the chroma appears to decrease further still, but its hue remains constant. The increasing value of the glass (i.e. its brightness) is directly proportional to its increasing opacity.

enamel overlay. Young dentition is characterised by highly opaque, bright (high value) enamel, which obscures the underlying dentine. In advancing years the enamel becomes progressively more translucent and dull (low value), revealing the underlying dentine strata. The multi-layered enamel/dentine is a major obstacle for instrumental reading of tooth colour, since the value of enamel and its surface lustre often complicate colour evaluation of the underlying dentine.

Other optical variables influencing colour

Having established fundamentals of colour theories, other optical variables influencing colour are fluorescence and opalescence, discussed below. Properties of dental porcelains including chromatic reactivity and adaptability, optical purity and chromatic stability can be found elsewhere in texts dealing with dental materials.[38]

Fluorescence

Incandescence is the inherent ability of an object, animate or inanimate to emit visible light. An example of an incandescent creature is the glowworm, while an artificial source is any household bulb. Luminescence is the light emission from an object other than that due to incandescence. This implies that the object does not inherently emit light, as with an incandescent entity, but an external light source is necessary to elicit an emission. Examples include luminescent road signs, which 'glow' when car headlights strike their surface. Fluorescence is a particular type of luminescence, described as visible light emission from an object or surface in the presence of ultraviolet illumination. The degree of brightness from a fluorescent object is often termed its luminescent intensity.

Natural teeth have the capability to emit visible light when exposed to ultraviolet light and therefore exhibit fluorescence (Fig. 4.24).[39] Irrespective of their shade under white daylight, natural teeth fluoresce at a peak wavelength of 450 nm gradually decreasing to around 680 nm.[40] The salient point to note is that fluorescence of teeth is independent of their perceived colour under white light. This is a crucial factor during manufacturing of dental porcelains, which endeavour to simulate optical characteristics of natural teeth. Ultraviolet light is not exclusively limited to nocturnal social venues such as clubs and discos, but is also prevalent in natural daylight. Since industrial pollutants are constantly depleting the protective ozone layer, the amount of ultra-violet entering the atmosphere is ever increasing. Fluorescence makes teeth appear brighter and whiter, and therefore alters their

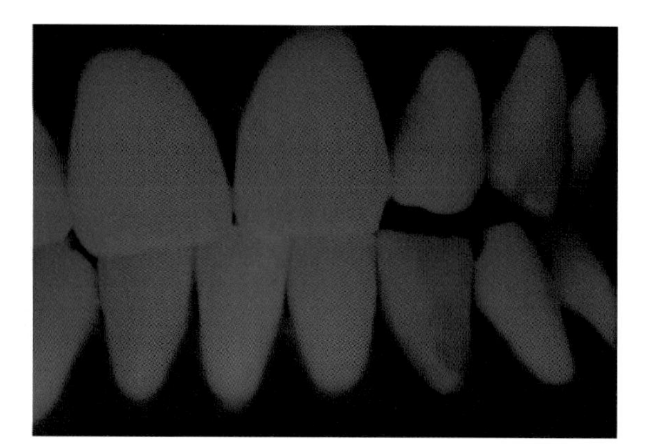

Figure 4.24 Natural teeth fluorescence when viewed by ultraviolet illumination.

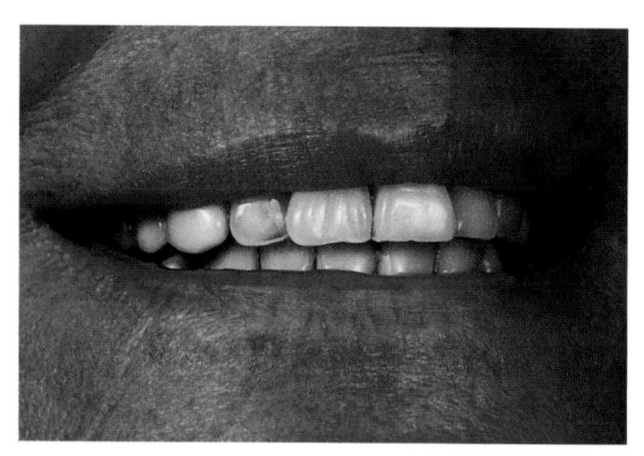

Figure 4.25 Opalescence: with reflected light, teeth have a bluish tint (see incisal edge of right maxillary lateral incisor).

visible colour under natural daylight. It is often stated that fluorescence is the property that confers vitality to natural teeth. The latter is one of the culprits for apparent mismatching of dental shade tabs with natural teeth. The reason is that, although the visible colour of the tooth coincides with its porcelain analogue, the definitive restorations fails to harmonise with adjacent natural counterparts due to different degrees of fluorescence. The fault lies in the fact that although a shade tab may match a given tooth, its fluorescence spectrum and luminescent intensity are dissimilar.

Opalescence

Radiant visible light contains photons ranging from 380–780 nm. Certain materials, e.g. the semi-precious opal gem, possess the ability to transmit and refract photons of larger wavelengths, while reflecting or scattering photons of a smaller wavelength. The result is that when opalescent objects are viewed by incident white light a bluish appearance is apparent. Conversely, when viewed by transmitted light they appear orange–amber. Dental enamel also possesses opalescence, and when viewed by incident light its appearance is bluish (Fig. 4.25), but by transmitted light it glows with an orange–amber aura (Fig. 4.26). Similar to fluorescence, optical purity is also advantageous for emulating opalescence with enamel porcelain.

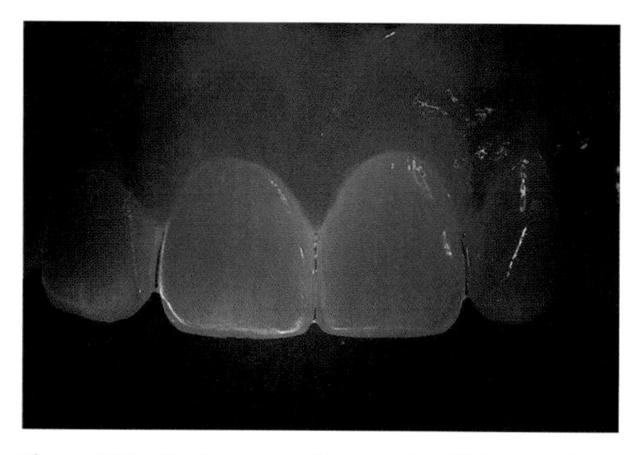

Figure 4.26 Opalescence: with transmitted light, teeth have a orange–amber aura (see incisal edges of maxillary central incisors).

Shade guides

Clinical conditions permitting, an ideal way to evaluate dentine hue and the enamel overlay independently is to half prepare a tooth (Fig. 4.27). This allows individual analysis of dentine and enamel as well as the thickness of each layer. This information is extremely valuable for the ceramist to emulate both shade and thickness of the dentine and enamel porcelain layers of a restoration.

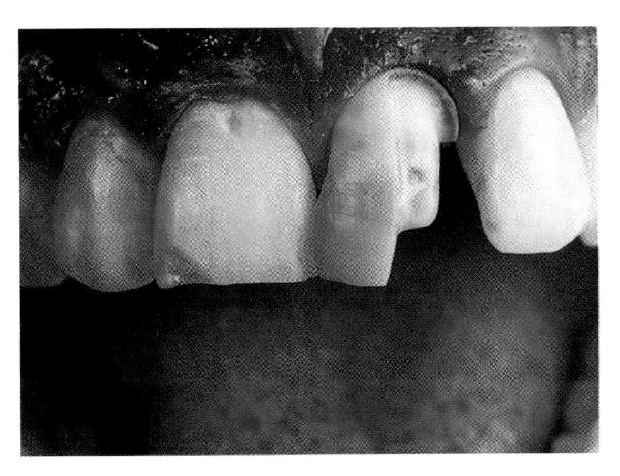

Figure 4.27 Half crown preparation on the left maxillary central incisor for independent assessment of dentine and enamel colour.

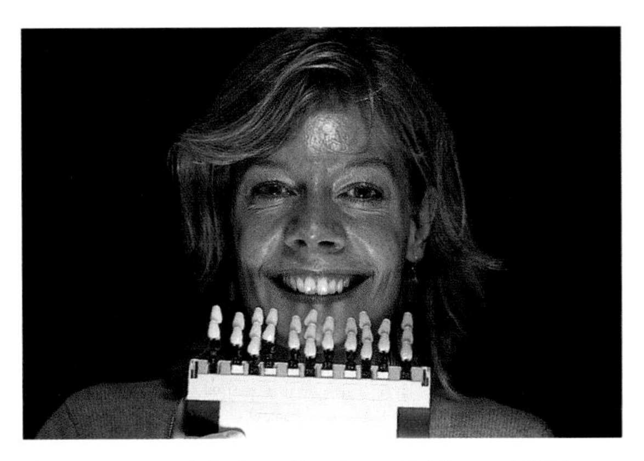

Figure 4.28 Facial view of patient with Vitapan 3D-Master photographed using light of 5500 K.

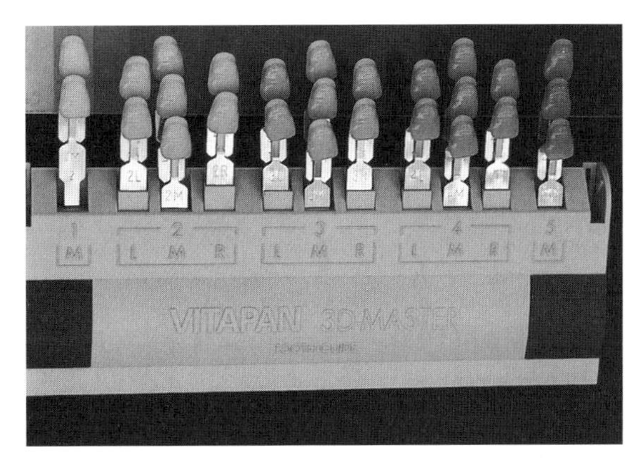

Figure 4.29 The value groups in the Vitapan 3D-Master are numbered 1 to 5 with all tabs within a group having the same value. The grey-scale in the background depicts decreasing value from left to right.

Types of shade guide

The most popular shade guides currently used for dental colour analysis are:

- Vita Classic (Vita, Bad Sackingen, Germany)
- Vitapan 3D-Master (Vita)
- Chomascop (Ivoclar-Vivadent, Schaan, Liechtenstein)
- Custom or specific chroma and value guides

Vita shade guides

The ubiquitously used, and universally quoted shade guide is the Vita Classic, categorising hues with the letters A (orange), B (yellow), C (yellow – grey) and D (orange – grey or brown). Within each hue, the numbers are used to denote chroma and value. For example 1 is high value with low chroma and 4 is low value with high chroma. This system of shade analysis, although inaccurate, is indelibly fixed in clinical and laboratory practice.

In the early 1990s, Vita introduced the 3D-Master shade guide (Fig. 4.28), with the aim of accurately assessing shade according to the three components of colour: hue, value and chroma. Unlike the majority of dental shade guides, the 3D-Master attempts a three-dimensional analysis of tooth colour. The colour space occupied by the guide is similar to natural dentition, between the a* (red) and b* (yellow) colour co-ordinates of the CIE L*a*b* system. The tabs are arranged systematically and logically, rather than randomly as in the Classic guide. Two 3D-Master guides are available, Red and Blue, both fabricated from dental porcelains. The Red guide is made purely of dentine porcelain, allowing accurate assessment of the basic dentine colour (Fig. 4.28), while the Blue incorporates cervical and incisal porcelains for a more realistic representation of the multi-layers of natural teeth (Fig. 4.29).

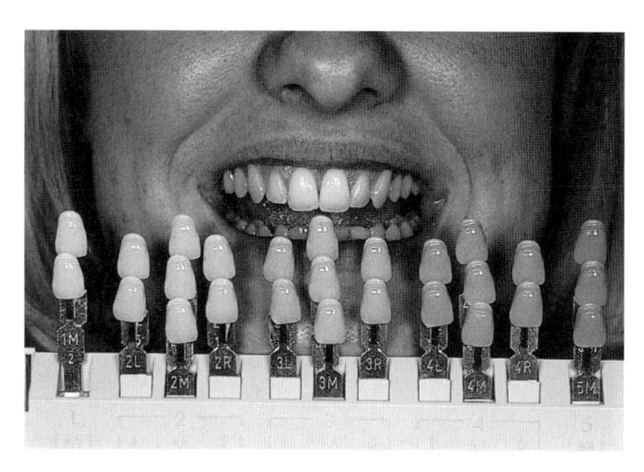

Figure 4.30 Shade matching using the Vitapan 3D-Master guide. Step 1: ascertain the value group that corresponds to the tooth. In the case illustrated, the value group of the maxillary central incisors = 2.

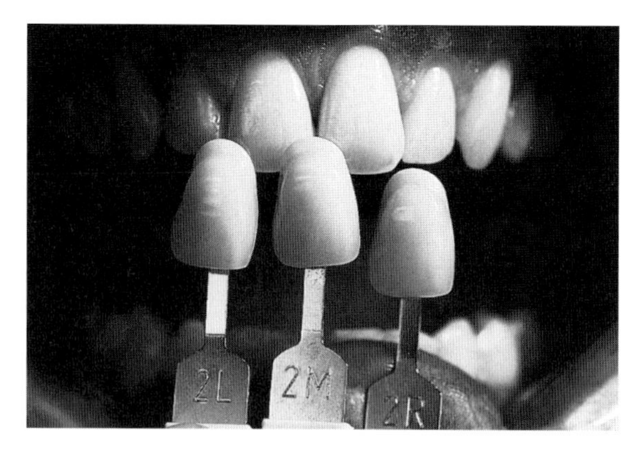

Figure 4.32 Shade matching using the Vitapan 3D-Master guide. Step 3: select hue from the L, M or R tabs, here M is chosen to be the nearest match. The final shade prescription is written as 2M2.

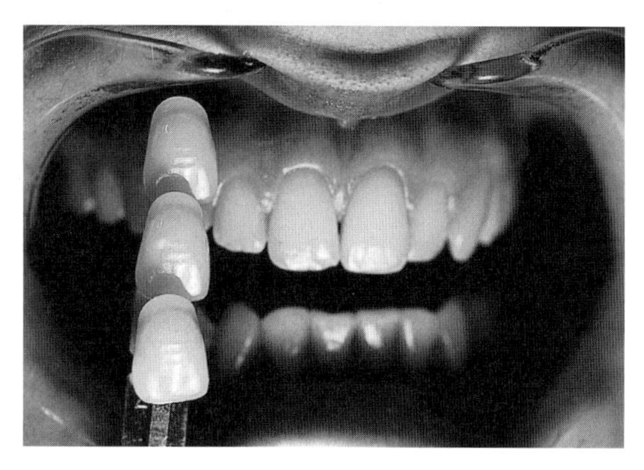

Figure 4.31 Shade matching using the Vitapan 3D-Master guide. Step 2: using the M tab, the chroma = 2.

Vita Value, Vita Chroma and Vita Hue, similarly to the Munsell hue, value and chroma colour co-ordinates, represent the three dimensions of colour. The tabs are grouped into five categories, sequentially numbered, with an increasing value (1, 2, 3, 4 and 5). All tabs within a value group have the same brightness (Fig. 4.30). In a given value group, the chroma increases from top to bottom (Fig. 4.31). All groups, with the exception of 1 and 5, are designated three letters, L, M and R, corresponding to varying hue. For example L (light) is indicative of a yellow, M (medium) of a yellow–red or orange, and R (red) of a red hue (Fig. 4.32). Documentation for the 3D guide is analogous to the Munsell Renotation System, comprising a number/letter/number configuration. The first number indicates the value group (1 to 5), the letter is the hue (L, M or R) and the second number the chroma (1, 2 or 3). For example 2M2 corresponds to the second value group, the M hue sub-group and a 2-chroma level. For an intermediate tooth shade, a combination of two tabs is used for the final colour prescription.

Chomascop guide

The Chomascop uses numbers to distinguish hue, e.g. 100 (white), 200 (yellow), 300 (orange), 400 (grey) and 500 (brown). Chroma is indicated by another set of numbers, 10 are high value with low chroma, while 40 is low value with high chroma (Fig. 4.33). This system is particularly useful when fabricating Empress restorations, since the Empress ingots correspond to the Chomascop shade guide. A conversion chart is available to convert Chromascop shade tabs to the Vita Classic shades.

Custom guides

Finally, if the tooth colour fails to concur with any of the shade guide tabs, porcelains can be used to fabricate a custom shade tab. If extremes of value and chroma are required, specific detailed chroma and value guides are available

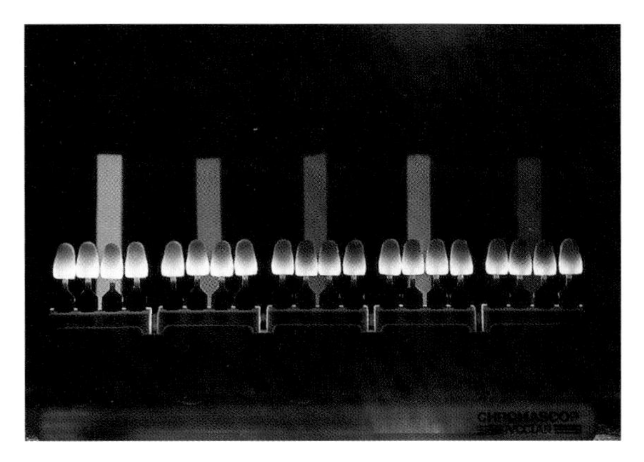

Figure 4.33 The Chomascop shade guide.

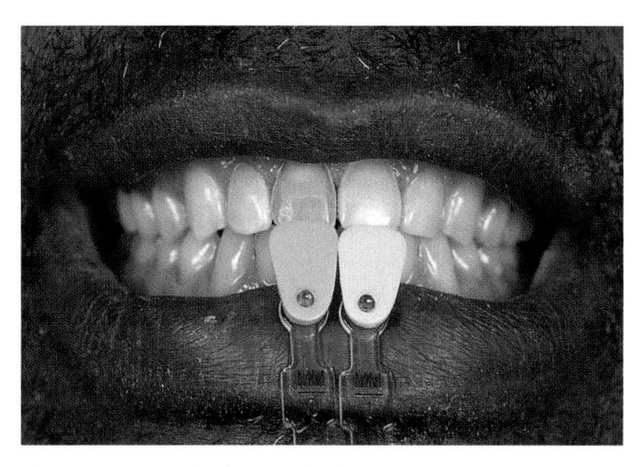

Figure 4.35 High chroma shade tabs.

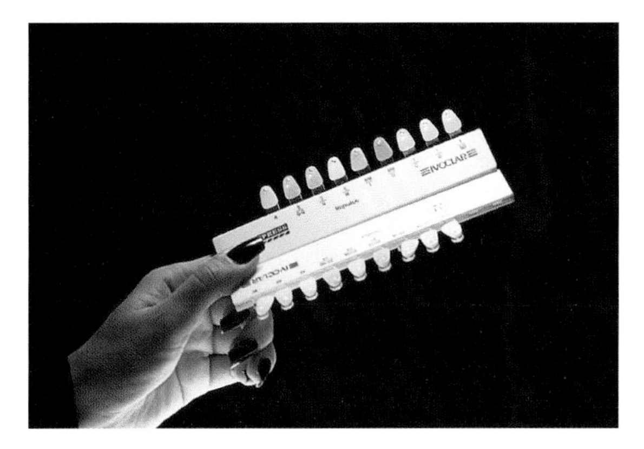

Figure 4.34 Accessory chroma and value shade tabs.

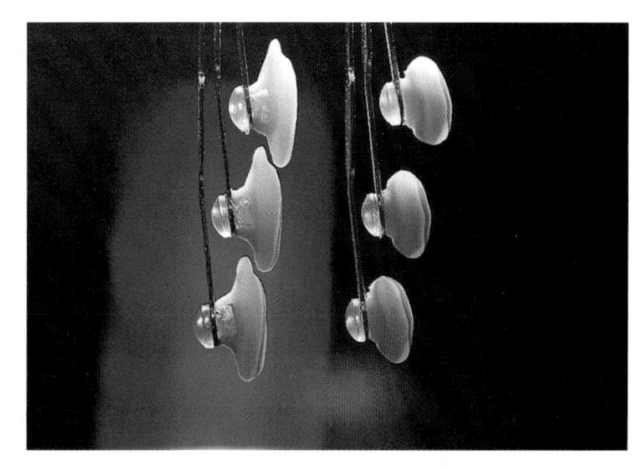

Figure 4.36 Unlike enamel of natural teeth, the enamel thickness is uniform for all shade tabs in the Vitapan 3D-Master guide. The left tabs are sectioned in a sagittal plane, and the right in a mesial-distal plane.

(Figs. 4.34 & 4.35). These may be necessary with aged teeth of deep chroma, or youthful teeth with high values.

Limitations of shade guides

Limitations of shade guides are failure to account for the variability found in natural teeth:

- Degree of fluorescence[41]
- Degree of opalescence
- Degree of enamel translucency[42]
- Enamel thickness (Fig. 4.36)
- Enamel texture and lustre
- Objectivity

Instrumental assessment

The main advantage of instrumental colour assessment is eliminating subjectivity. However, colour is not entirely an objective entity, and its perception is heavily tainted by cerebral interpretation. Limitations of digital analysis have already been mentioned in the colour theories section. Nevertheless, for comparative purposes, instrumental shade analysis is useful, and no doubt will play a significant role in the future.[43] Three basic types of device are used for instrumental or digital shade analysis.

Spectrophotometer

The most accurate device for colour analysis is a spectrophotometer, which produces spectral reflectance and/or transmission curves. The disadvantages are complex technology, requiring extensive extrapolation of data, and high cost. Additionally, an object must be placed inside a spectrophotometer, which obviously presents a difficulty with natural teeth.

Proprietary products include SpectroShade (MHT Optic Research, Niederhasil, Switzerland) and Easyshade (Vita, Bad Sackingen, Germany).

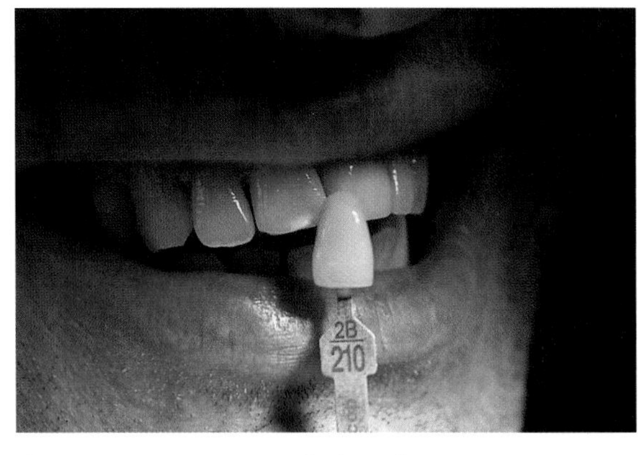

Figure 4.37 Pre-operative shade analysis.

Colorimeter

The colorimeter is based on the principles the Young–Helmholtz theory of human vision, having 'cells' that are sensitive to the three primary colours. Whilst this method is not as accurate as a spectrophotometer, the data is relatively easy to manipulate and user friendly.

Proprietary products include ShadeVision (X-Rite, Grandville, MI), ShadeEye NCC (Shofu, San Marcos, CA) and Digital Shade Guide (Rieth, Schorndorf, Germany).

Digital camera and red, green, blue (RGB) devices

The final, and probably the least accurate method is using a RGB or digital camera for colour analysis. These devices analyse a captured digital image for colour and chromatic mapping. Hence, software interpretation is heavily reliant on the quality of the captured image, which is essentially the weak link. However, in theory, using high-quality glass optics with elaborate sensors, the analysis may be acceptable.

Proprietary products include ShadeScan (Cynovad, Montreal, Canada) and ikam (DCM, Leeds, UK).

CLINICAL PRACTICE

The aim of shade analysis is as follows:

(1) Record the basic dentine shade (hue), usually at the middle third of the tooth (pre-operative, prepared abutment and after fabrication) (Figs. 4.37–4.39)
(2) Create a chromatic map showing colour variations at the cervical (chroma), incisal and interproximal sites, together with the value of the overlying enamel (value) (Fig. 4.40)
(3) Photographic documentation:
    - With different lighting to avoid metamerism and assess fluorescence and opalescence (Figs. 4.41–4.42)
    - Relative shade analysis with chosen shade tab
    - Characterisations, such as cracks, stains, mamelons and surface texture and lustre

The above are achieved either visually or digitally.

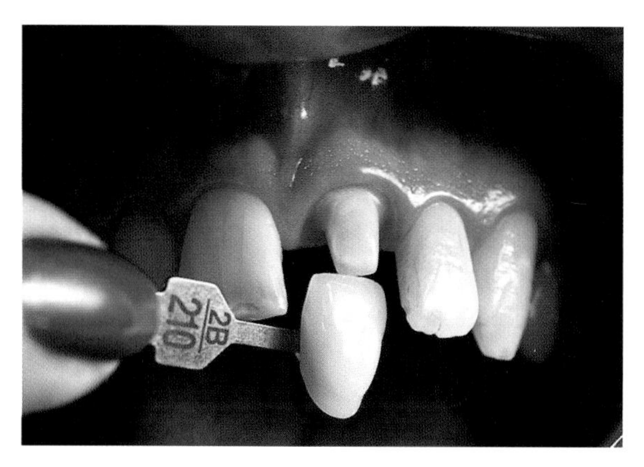

Figure 4.38 Prepared abutment shade analysis.

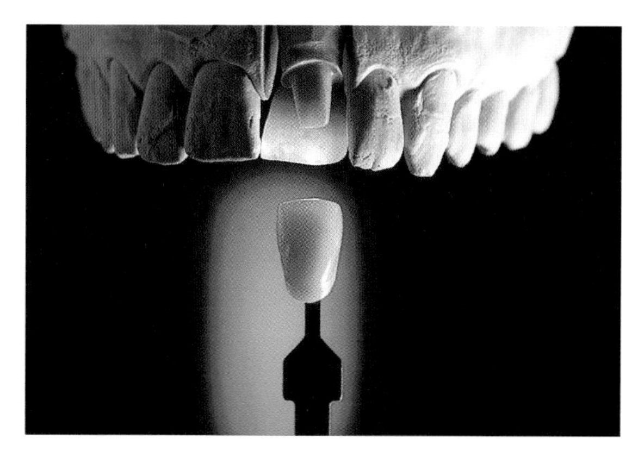

Figure 4.39 Shade verification in dental laboratory during crown fabrication.

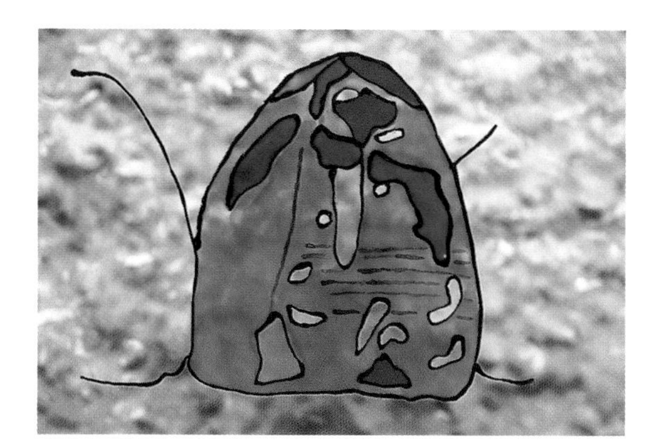

Figure 4.40 Drawing a chromatic chart for a central incisor (digital shade analysing machines automatically produce chromatic mapping charts).

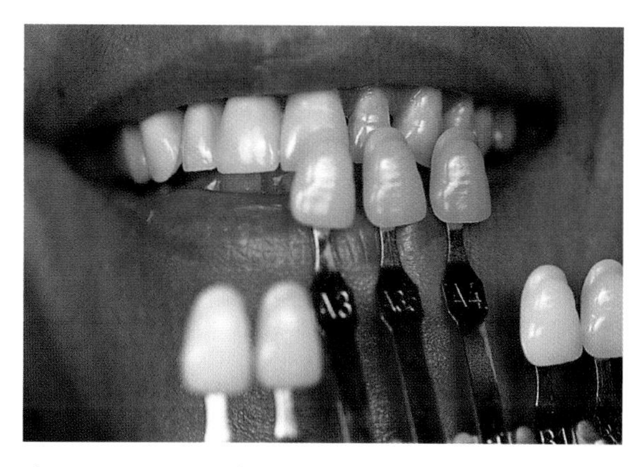

Figure 4.41 To avoid metamerism, carry out shade analysis using daylight colour corrected illumination. The colour tabs appear yellowish with electronic flash.

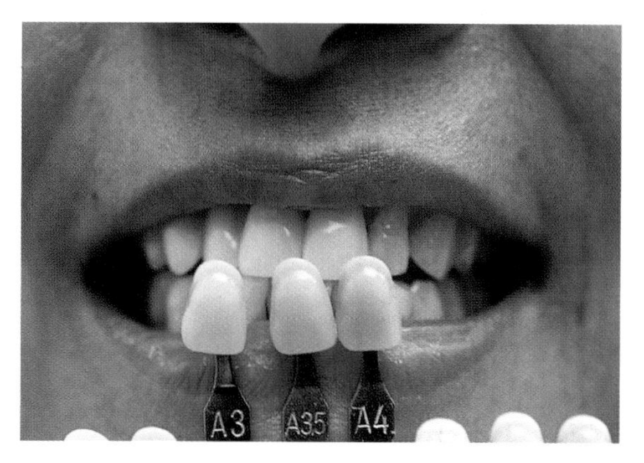

Figure 4.42 To avoid metamerism, carry out shade analysis using daylight colour corrected illumination. The same colour tabs as in Figure 4.41 now appear more realistic with daylight illumination.

Ocular shade assessment

(1) The shade analysis appointment is scheduled at the beginning of the day, when the dental team is not fatigued after a tiring day in the clinic
(2) The ideal ambience should be tranquil and serene, devoid of distractions
(3) Perform shade analysis in presence of ceramist
(4) Ensure patient is accompanied by close relatives and friends to confirm chosen shade

(5) Ensure surgery surroundings are a neutral colour or alternatively use a neutral grey card behind teeth and shade tabs
(6) Avoid lurid colour clothing and vivid cosmetics
(7) Moisten teeth, avoid dehydration of enamel or dentine
(8) Use colour-corrected daylight illumination for shade analysis
(9) To ascertain the value (brightness), look aside to activate rod cells, located peripherally to the fovea in the retina
(10) Record basic dentine shade at the middle third of the tooth (hue and chroma) in less than 5 seconds (within CAP). Use different shade guides as necessary
(11) Before repeating shade assessment, stare at blue card to avoid chromatic adaptation
(12) Create a chromatic chart of shade nuances and characterisations
(13) Photograph teeth and tabs using different lighting conditions, e.g. flash (5500 K) and natural daylight (6500 K), to mitigate metamerism, and ultraviolet and transmitted light, for fluorescence and opalescence, respectively
(14) Photograph chosen shade tab(s) adjacent to teeth for relative shade analysis
(15) Photograph teeth at a 1:1 scale for detailed characterisations
(16) Relay digitised images and chromatic map via e-mail to concerned parties (ceramist, specialist, patient).

Instrumental shade assessment

Follow steps (1)–(7) and (13)–(16). Substitute steps (8)–(12) by following instructions for the chosen type of instrument for shade analysis. Depending on the type of instrument used, photographic documentation and creating a chromatic map may not be necessary, since it may be an integral part of the accompanying software.

References

1. Myers, D.G. (1998) *Psychology.* Worth Publishers Inc., New York
2. Billmeyer, F.W. and Saltzman, M. (1981) *Principles of Colour Technology.* John Wiley & Sons Inc., New York
3. Newton, I. (1730) *Opticks.* Innys, London
4. International Commission on Illumination. (1931) *Proceedings of the English Session,* Cambridge, England. Bureau Central de la CIE
5. International Commission on Illumination. (1971) *Colorimetry: Official recommendations of the International Commission on Illumination.* Publication No. 15 (E-1.3.1) Bureau Central de la CIE
6. *Precise colour communication.* (1994) Minolta handbook, Japan
7. Munsell, A.H. (1929) *Munsell Book of Colour.* Baltimore, Maryland
8. Newhall, S.M., Nickerson, D. and Judd, D.B. (1943) First Report of the OSA Subcommittee on the Spacing of the Munsell Colours. *J Opt Soc Am,* **33**, 385–418
9. Munsell, A.H. (1961) *A colour notation.* 11th edn. Munsell Colour Co., Baltimore
10. Judd, D.B. and Wyszecki, G. (1975) Color in Business, Science and Industry. John Wiley & Sons Inc., New York
11. Marks, W.B., Dobelle W.H. and MacNicol Jr. E.F. (1964) Visual pigments of single primate cones. *Science,* **143**, 1181–1183
12. Geldard, F.A. (1972) *The human senses.* 2nd edition. p.161. Wiley, New York
13. Young, T. (1807) 'On the theory of light and colours', in: *Lecturers in Natural Philosophy, Vol. 2,* printed for Joseph Johnson, St Paul's Church Yard, by William Savage, London, p.163. 'An account of some cases of the production of colours', ibid., p. 634
14. Helmholtz, H von. (1852) Ueber die Theorie der zusammengesetzten Farben. *Müller's Arch Anat Physiol,* 461; *Poggendorff's Ann,* 87,45; *Phil Mag,* **4**, 519
15. DeValois, R.L. and DeValois, K.K. (1975) Neural coding of color. In: *Handbook of perception. Volume V: Seeing.* Ed. Carterette E.C.

and Friedman M.P. p.162. New York Press, New York
[16] Müller, G.E. (1930) Über die Farbenempfindungen. *Z Psychol Ergänzungsb,* 17 and 18
[17] Yamada K. (1993) Porcelain laminate veneers for discoloured teeth using complimentary colours. *Int J Prosthodont,* **6**(**3**), 242–247
[18] Jackendoff, R. (1987) *Consciousness and the computational mind.* MIT Press, Bradford Books, Cambridge, MA
[19] Churchland, P.S. and Sejnowski T.J. (1992) *The computational brain.* MIT Press, Bradford Books, Cambridge, MA
[20] Crick, F. and Koch, C. (1995) Are we aware of neural activity in primary visual cortex? *Nature,* **375**, 121–123
[21] Panadent Limited (1983) *Product information on Waldmann Color-i-Dent lamps*
[22] Freedman, G. (1994) Color communication. *J Cosmet Dent,* **60**(**8**), 695–699
[23] Burgt, T.P., ten Bosch J.J., Borsboom, P.C.F. and Kortsmit, W.J.P.M. (1990) A comparison of new and conventional methods for quantification of teeth colour. *J Prosthet Dent,* **63**(**2**), 155–162
[24] Photon Beard Limited, UK (1998) *Photographic lighting product catalogue*
[25] Seghi R.R. (1990) Effects of instrument-measuring geometry on colorimetric assessment of dental porcelains. *J Dent Res,* **69**(**5**), 1180–1183
[26] Knispel, G. (1991) Factors affecting the process of colour matching restorative materials to natural teeth. *Quintessence International,* **22**(**7**), 525–531
[27] Johnson, W.M. and Kao, E.C. Assessment of appearance match by visual observation and clinical colorimetry. *J Dent Res,* **68**(**5**), 819–822
[28] Goodkind, R.J., Keenan, K.M. and Schwabacher, W.B. (1985) A Comparison of Chromascan and spectrophotometric color measurements of 100 natural teeth. *J Prosthet Dent,* **53**(**1**), 105–109
[29] Judd, D.B. and Wyszecki, G. (1975) *Color in Business, Science and Industry.* John Wiley & Sons Inc., New York
[30] Kuehni, R.G. (1972) Color differences and objective acceptability evaluation. *J Color Appearance,* **1**, 3–10
[31] Douglas, R.D. and Brewer, J.D. (1998) Acceptability of shade difference in metal ceramic crowns. *J Prosthet Dent,* **79**, 254–260
[32] Warm, J.S. and Dember, W.N. (1986) Awake at the switch. *Psychology Today,* **149**, 46–53
[33] Myers, D.G. (1998) *Psychology.* Worth Publishers Inc., New York
[34] Crick, F. and Koch, C. (1997) The problem of consciousness. *Scientific American Mysteries of the Mind* (reprinted from September, 1992 issue), 19–26
[35] Glick, K.L. (1995) Color management of cosmetic restorations. *Curr Opin Cosmetic Dent,* 36–40
[36] McBurney, D.H. and Collings V.B. (1984) *Introduction to sensation and perception.* 2nd edn. p. 194. Prentice-Hall, Englewood Cliffs, NJ
[37] Goodkind, R.J. and Schwabacher, W.B. (1987) Use of a fibre-optic colorimeter for in vivo colour measurements of 2830 anterior teeth. *J Prosthet Dent,* **58**(**5**), 535–542
[38] Chu, S. and Ahmad, I. (2003) Light dynamic properties of a synthetic low-fusing quartz glass-ceramic material. *Pract Proced Aesthet Dent,* **15**(**1**), 49–56
[39] Baran, G., O'Brian, W.J. and Tien, T.Y. (1977) Colored emission of rare earth ions in potassium feldspath glass. *J Dent Res,* **56**, 1323–1329
[40] Monsenego, G., Burdairon, G. and Clerjaud, B. (1993) Fluorescence of dental porcelain. *J Prosthet Dent,* **69**, 106–113
[41] Vanini, L. (1996) Light and color in anterior composite restorations. *Practical Periodont and Aesthet Dent,* **8**(**7**), 673–682
[42] Davis, B.K., Aquilino, S.A., Lund, P.S., *et al.* (1992) Colorimetric evaluation of the effect of porcelain opacity of the resultant color of porcelain veneers. *Int J Prosthodont,* **5**(**2**), 130–136
[43] Chu, S.J., Devigus, A. and Mieleszko, A. (2004) *Fundamentals of colour: shade matching and communication in esthetic dentistry.* Quintessence Publishing Co. Inc., Chicago

5 Foundations and intra-radicular support

Introduction

Foundations (or cores) and intra-radicular supports are platforms for the eventual definitive restoration of structurally compromised teeth, either coronally mutilated vital teeth, or endodontically treated teeth requiring intra-radicular posts with a subsequent core build-up.

Before the type of foundation is chosen, it is important to remember that the strength of a tooth is directly proportional to the quantity of remaining enamel and dentine. Loss of tooth structure is attributed to caries, repeated replacement of failed restorations, fractures, endodontic access cavities and tooth preparation for extra-coronal restorations. Furthermore, endodontically treated teeth have a higher propensity to biomechanical failure because of increased loss of tooth structure,[1] increased brittleness due to a reduced moisture content,[2] and reduced proprioceptive response. The pressure threshold in root-filled teeth increases by 57%, making the tooth less sensitive to occlusal loads, and hence predisposed to fractures.[3] Preserving as much natural enamel and dentine as possible is crucial for the long-term survival of structurally compromised teeth. Any procedure reducing the amount of tooth, such as canal preparation for post placement, weakens rather than strengthens biomechanical capabilities.[4] There is also emerging debate whether or not a post is necessary,[5] and if sufficient coronal dentine is present (more than half of the coronal tooth structure); placing a post only complicates matters, jeopardising the apical seal and structural integrity. To recapitulate, the main purpose of foundations, with or without posts, is creating a platform for the definitive restoration for attaining health, function and aesthetics (see the HFA triad in Chapter 2).

VITAL TEETH – SCIENTIFIC RATIONALE

Vital teeth

As stated above, the purpose of building foundations on structurally compromised vital teeth is to support extra-coronal restorations. Repeatedly replacing failed fillings leaves the residual tooth structure incapable of supporting further intra-coronal restorations, and in order to support an extra-coronal prosthesis, a core is required for adequate resistance and retention. In addition, the tooth is further weakened by continual trauma of instrumentation, which should be minimised to prevent endodontic involvement. The essential difference between cores on vital and non-vital teeth is that, in the former, retention is solely from coronal dentine, while for the latter, additional support is gained from intra-radicular posts. A variety of methods is available for gaining retention on vital teeth including pins, cavity modifications, dentine bonding agents (DBAs) and luting cements.

Retention

Pins

Pins have been advocated for generations as a means of retaining cores on vital teeth (Fig. 5.1). The rationale is retaining as much of the remaining tooth structure as possible. However, pins have numerous disadvantages, and their use should be questioned in many clinical situations.[6] Many studies have shown that pins cause dentine crazing and tooth fracture, and are potentially perilous to the pulp and periodontium.[7] Furthermore, no difference in retention is observed with pins or other methods of supporting a core.[8]

Cavity modification

Instead of using pins, another method for retention is modifying the remaining tooth structure. This includes creating undercuts, boxes, slots or grooves for obtaining retention for the restorative material,[9] particularly in conjunction with DBAs. The advantage is that the hazardous complications of pins are obviated. Nevertheless, placing retention features into dentine also requires careful judgement. The amount of remaining tooth structure dictates whether slots are possible without encroaching into the pulp or further compromising the structural integrity of the tooth. If teeth are excessively broken down, crown lengthening or orthodontic extrusion should be considered for 'gaining' extra tooth structure. Cuspal coverage also helps retention of the final restoration, and when the cusp width is less than 1 mm, it should be reduced sufficiently to accommodate an appropriate thickness of the overlying restorative material. For porcelain onlays, a minimum thickness of 2 mm is required, together with adequate occlusal clearance (Figs. 5.2–5.4). Finally, incorporating a ferrule effect in the final restoration is another method for additional retention for absorbing functional stresses (see discussion on the ferrule effect later in this Chapter). The term ferrule means a bracelet or encompassing material. The ferrule of an extra-coronal restoration

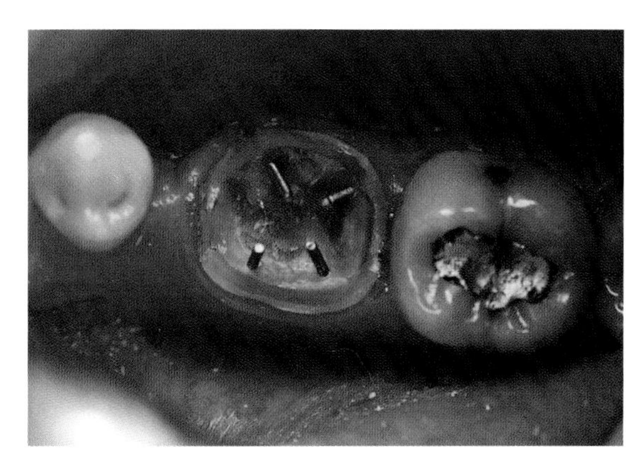

Figure 5.1 Pins are one of the oldest methods for building a foundation on structurally compromised vital teeth.

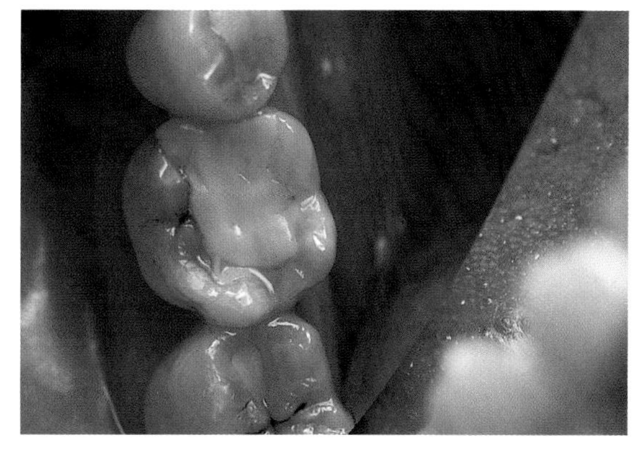

Figure 5.2 Porcelain onlay case study: pre-operative view showing failing composite filling with secondary caries in mandibular first molar.

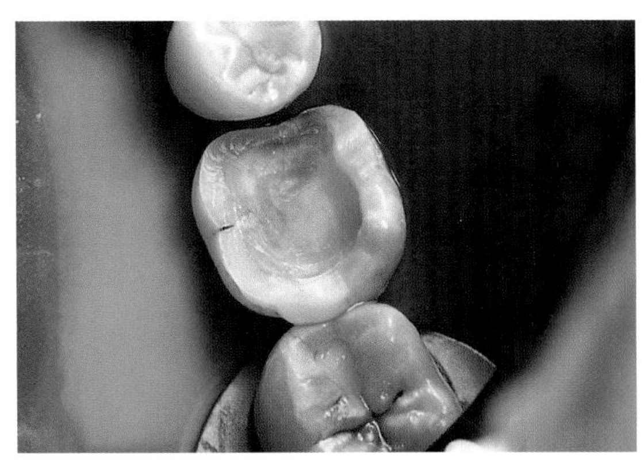

Figure 5.3 Porcelain onlay case study: preparation for indirect ceramic onlay, necessitating a minimum of 2 mm occlusal clearance to accommodate a sufficient bulk of porcelain.

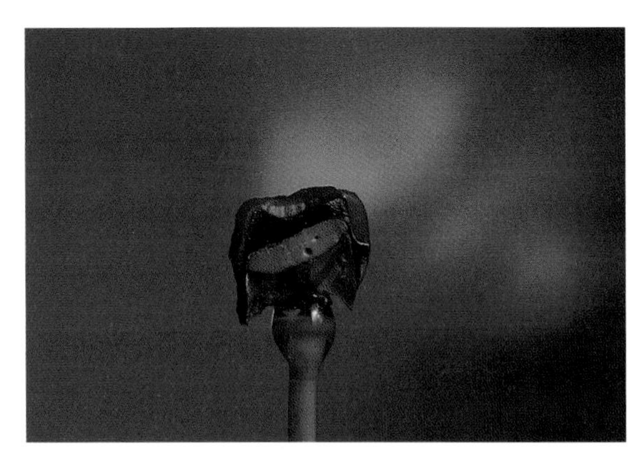

Figure 5.5 Sectioned tooth with metal–ceramic crown, which incorporates a 'bracelet' or ferrule effect (apical to veneering porcelain) encircling or bracing the tooth to provide additional strength.

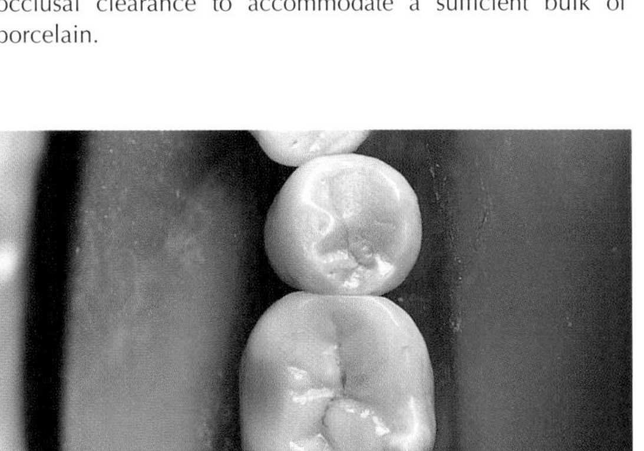

Figure 5.4 Porcelain onlay case study: post-operative view showing cemented porcelain onlay.

braces remaining dentine or the supragingival tooth. It is the restorative material of the definitive restoration (usually metal or ceramic), which covers or encompasses residual dentine. A ferrule effect is also used for a cast post/core with a built-in diaphragm or coping (Fig. 5.5).

Dentine bonding agents

Using DBAs with resin or amalgam cores increases retention by enhancing bond strength and reducing microleakage. The disadvantage is the highly technique-sensitive and protracted clinical protocol. A detailed discussion of DBAs is found in Chapter 10.

Luting cements

Following the original concept by Baldwin in 1897[10] of bonding amalgam to dentine with wet zinc phosphate cement, newer materials, such as glass ionomers (GIs) and resins, have been proposed using this method. At present, the efficacy and longevity of using GIs in a sandwich technique with composite cores is debatable.[11]

Core materials

The choice of core material will profoundly affect survival of the ultimate restoration, and is dependent on whether a fill-in or build-up is necessary. A fill-in assumes that sufficient dentine architecture is present, and that the restorative material is used purely to fill voids, without acting as a supporting platform. When minimal dentine is available, a build-up acts as the platform for supporting the extra-coronal restoration. Therefore, a build-up requires greater mechanical resilience than a fill-in material. The popular materials include amalgam, GIs, resin-modified glass ionomers (RGIs) and resin composites with DBA. Table 5.1 summarises the salient properties of fill-in and build-up restorative materials.

Table 5.1 Materials for foundations (fill-in and build-up).

Properties	Amalgam	GI	RGI	Resin composites
Strength	High (in bulk, but not thin sections)	Low	Medium	High (even in thin sections)
Seal	By corrosion products and DBA	Adhesion to tooth	Adhesion to tooth	In conjunction with DBA
Concerns	Mercury controversy, electrolysis interaction with metal prosthesis, patients with lichen planus	Hydrophilic, crack formation	Hydrophilic, crack formation	Polymerisation shrinkage, dimensional instability
Technique	Forgiving	Intermediate	Intermediate	Sensitive
Retention	Pins, cavity modifications, DBA, cements	Cavity modifications	Cavity modifications	Cavity modifications, DBA
Tooth preparation	Delayed	Delayed	Delayed or immediate	Immediate
Indications	Posterior teeth build-up	Fill-in, with adequate dentine architecture	Fill-in, with adequate dentine architecture	Anterior and posterior teeth build-up, flowable varieties for fill-in, aesthetically sensitive areas

For vital teeth, the direct technique is the method of choice, using amalgam, resin composites, GI or RGI filling materials. DBAs in conjunction with resin composites and amalgam increase retention while preserving the maximum amount of remaining tooth substrate. Amalgam has long clinical success, and using amalgam adhesives further enhances its mechanical properties (Fig. 5.6).

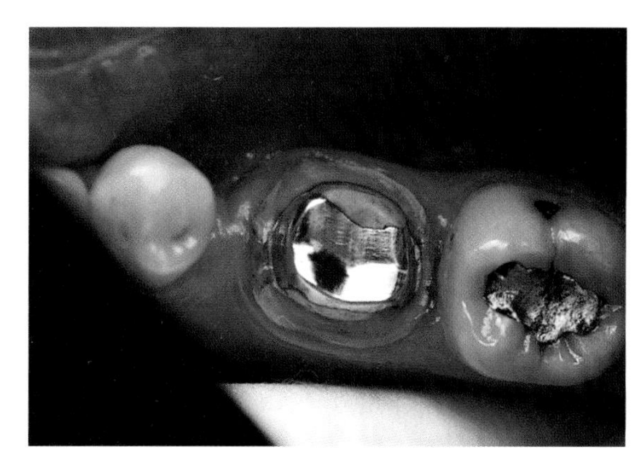

Figure 5.6 Amalgam core build-up.

GIs offer direct adhesion to dentine and are cariostatic, but due to low tensile strength and resistance to fracture, are not recommended for areas of high occlusal stresses. Composite filling materials are a better alternative, but are plagued with disadvantages of microleakage. Essentially, the linear thermal expansion of resin composites

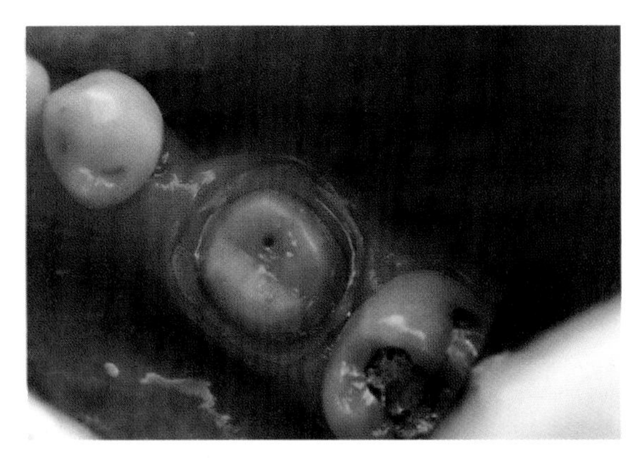

Figure 5.7 Composite resin filling core build-up.

is different from natural teeth, which causes post-operative sensitivity, pulpal pathosis and microleakage.[12] However, recent advances in resin filling materials have resulted in physical properties equalling or surpassing those of amalgam, including better handling, marginal adaptability, similar modulus of elasticity (MOE) and reduced annual rates of wear (Fig. 5.7).[13] To circumvent microleakage, flowable composites used as liners below composites offer superior accessibility and adaptability for difficult cavity recesses. The lower viscosity is beneficial for absorbing polymerisation shrinkage stresses as well as occlusal loads. A recent study assessing microleakage of teeth restored with intra-radicular posts, using different composite resin filling material with and without a flowable composite liner, concludes that microleakage is substantially reduced if a flowable composite liner is used prior to building the core with either a microhybrid or packable composite.[14]

VITAL TEETH – CLINICAL PRACTICE

Pre-assessment for cores on vital teeth

Before proceeding to build-up or fill-in structurally compromised vital teeth, the following items should be considered.

Radiographic evaluation

A radiograph will reveal the amount of residual tooth, decay, quality and extent of any existing filling, periodontal and endodontic status. In addition, appreciation of pulp and root(s) anatomy will prevent inadvertent perforation of the pulp chambers, root furcations and concavities. These findings will dictate whether the residual tooth, following removal of the offending filling and decay, is capable of supporting a core build-up with retention boxes and grooves. Vitality should also be verified, especially if the tooth has been subjected to repeated trauma of replacing defective fillings. If non-vitality is suspected, root canal therapy at this stage is prudent, rather than waiting for the inevitable after fitting the definitive restoration. Furthermore, placing an intra-radicular support will offer additional retention in cases of limited tooth substrate. In the presence of periapical or periodontal pathology, a build-up may not be feasible, without first carrying out root canal therapy or surgical crown lengthening.

Intra-oral evaluation

A careful examination, with transillumination, will reveal tooth and/or existing filling(s) fractures. Minor fractures may be salvageable, but extensive or deep vertical root fractures usually require extraction. The occlusion is also assessed, especially the inter-occlusal clearance for accommodating the build-up and final restoration. If the clinical crown height is insufficient, surgical crown lengthening or orthodontic extrusion may be considered.

Clinical sequalae for cores on vital teeth

If, following the above evaluation, a core is practical, the clinical protocol is as follows:

(1) Isolate tooth with rubber dam (Hint 5.1)
(2) Remove exiting filling(s), decay and reduce cusps that are either fractured (or display

fractures lines), or less than 1 mm in cross section

(3) Assess remaining tooth substrate for either fill-in, or build-up with retention by strategic placement of retentive boxes, grooves and pins (Hint 5.2)
(4) If necessary, place suitable matrix band and wedges for supporting the core material
(5) Select fill-in or build-up material according to Table 5.1
(6) Follow manufacturer's instructions for the chosen restorative material
(7) Remove rubber dam (Hint 5.3)
(8) Carry out immediate or delayed tooth preparation (depending on the material) for the coronal restoration (Hint 5.4)
(10) Fabricate a chairside therapeutic temporary restoration, before making an impression for the definitive restoration (see Chapter 7)

NON-VITAL TEETH – SCIENTIFIC RATIONALE

For endodontically compromised teeth, the purpose of intra-radicular anchorage is supporting a core build-up, which in turn supports the eventual coronal restoration.

Post materials

The literature is ambiguous regarding the ideal choice of post/core materials for a given clinical scenario, reporting varying survival rates depending on data derived from in vitro studies. The clinical factors, such as quantity of residual tooth structure, ferrule effect and occlusal stresses (especially non-axial), exert greater influence on the survival rate than the material from which a post is fabricated. Furthermore, the quality and precision of the definitive restoration is paramount for ultimate success of the tooth/restorative complex.[15]

Casting alloys

Custom posts are indirectly fabricated in the dental laboratory by the lost wax process using casting alloys. The existing root canal morphology dictates the length and cross-section geometry of the cast post. These passive posts are well adapted, preserving existing root canal shape, necessitating minimum shaping or modification with rotary instruments. The rationale is to fabricate a post to fit the root canal, as opposed to shaping the root canal to fit a preformed post (Fig. 5.8). The advantages include retaining residual tooth structure, unified post and core made of the same material, with long-term clinical use.[16] The disadvantages are a two-visit procedure, increased clinical time, laboratory costs, fabrication of a chairside temporary post and core, increased likelihood of bacterial contamination of post canal while awaiting cast post from the dental laboratory, and poor aesthetics if the definitive prosthesis is all-ceramic. Finally, corrosion by-products may elicit allergic reactions and cause root and soft tissue discolouration.

Prefabricated metal

Prefabricated posts are manufactured from different metals, such as stainless steel, titanium, etc., with unique serrations, surface roughness

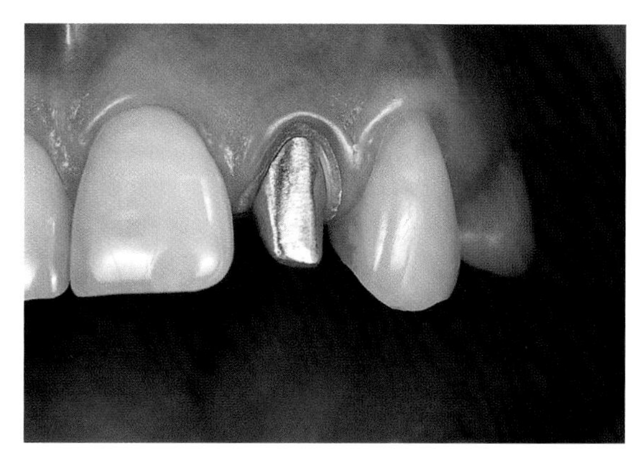

Figure 5.8 Indirectly cast gold post and core in left maxillary lateral incisor.

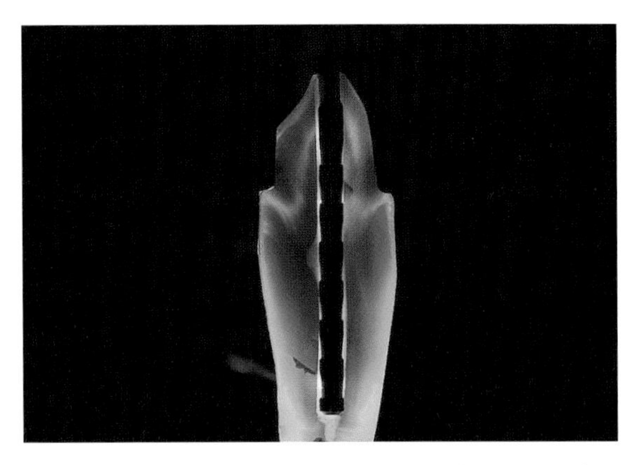

Figure 5.9 Pre-fabricated titanium post with serrations for increased retention with luting agent.

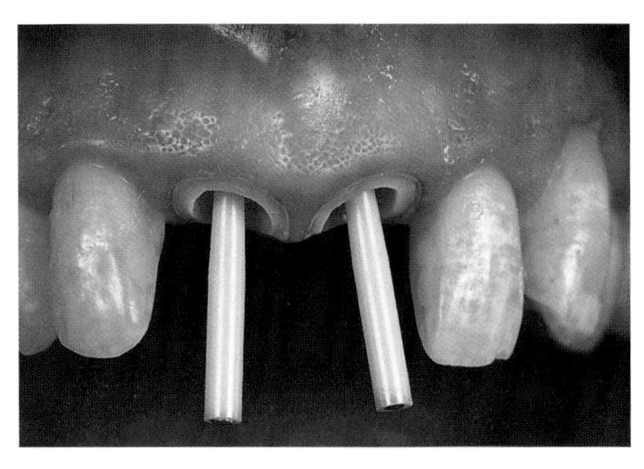

Figure 5.10 Zirconia posts in maxillary central incisors.

and cross-section geometry (tapered and/or parallel) for increasing retention (Fig. 5.9). The advantages include a single-visit procedure, less chance of contaminating the root canal with oral fluids as post placement is performed at the same time as root filling with rubber dam in situ, a core can be built using amalgam or tooth-coloured composite filling materials for improved light transmission and aesthetics. The disadvantages include dentine removal to accommodate the prefabricated shape, and conflict between ensuring a patent apical seal (minimum 4–5 mm) and sufficient post length for supporting the final restoration.

Proprietary products include ParaPost (Coltene/Whaledent, New Jersey, USA) or Dentatus Steel Posts (Dentatus, Hagersten, Sweden).

Ceramics

Ceramic varieties, such as zirconia and alumina posts, offer improved aesthetics and high fracture resistance. The prefabricated ceramic posts are either a pure ceramic, or ceramics combined with synthetic plastics. Zirconia varieties are available as smooth, tapered and parallel, or tapering at apex and parallel at the coronal aspect (Fig. 5.10). They are rounded at the apical zenith to minimise stress concentration at the root apex. Other varieties include polyester with 65% zirconium fibres, with lower MOE and stiffness compared with pure zirconia, but without compromising the advantageous light transmission properties.[17] Ceramic posts can be used with both the direct and indirect techniques, are highly biocompatible, radiopaque, and have excellent light transmission via both the root and coronal restoration. The success rates of zirconia posts are presently questionable, one study shows similar survival to cast posts[18], while another shows significantly lower survival when subjected to intermittent forces compared to carbon posts.[19] In addition, zirconia posts are stiff, with a high fracture resistance, but should the post fracture within the apical third of the canal, salvage is often challenging or impossible. The alumina varieties are indirectly fabricated, creating a unified post/core complex using a milling machine.

Proprietary products include:

- Zirconia – CosmoPost (Ivoclar-Vivadent, Schaan, Liechtenstein), ER-Cerapost (Brasseler, USA)
- Alumina – Celay (Mikrona)
- Polyester with zirconia – Snowlight (Carbotech)

Fibre

Three types of fibres are used for dental posts: carbon, quartz or glass. Either the fibres are embedded in a resin matrix, or pliable non-impregnated strands are luted with resin cements (Ribbond, Seattle, USA) (Fig. 5.11). Table 5.2 lists some common fibre posts, together with their mechanical properties.

Carbon fibre posts are biocompatible, resistant to fatigue and corrosion, have lower MOE compared with metals and are more conducive to repair. The reason for this is that fracture usually occurs at the post/core interface rather than in the root. Furthermore, numerous studies have verified that the success rate of carbon fibre posts is comparable to that of cast post and cores over a 2–3-year period.[20] The disadvantages are poor light transmission, dark colour, lack of adhesion to resin luting agents and radiolucency.[21] The dark colour of carbon fibre posts has been resolved by coating with a quartz layer to improve colour (AesthetiPost, Bisco), and if used judicially, neither the fracture resistance nor aesthetics are compromised in combination with direct composite cores.[22]

Glass and quartz fibre posts offer improved light transmission, stain resistance, superior aesthetics, and improved adhesion with resin-based luting agents compared to the carbon fibre posts (Figs. 5.12 and 5.13). The MOE is similar, but not the same as that of natural tooth structure, which minimises transmission of traumatic forces to surrounding dentine. The drawback, as with carbon fibre, is the high radiolucency.

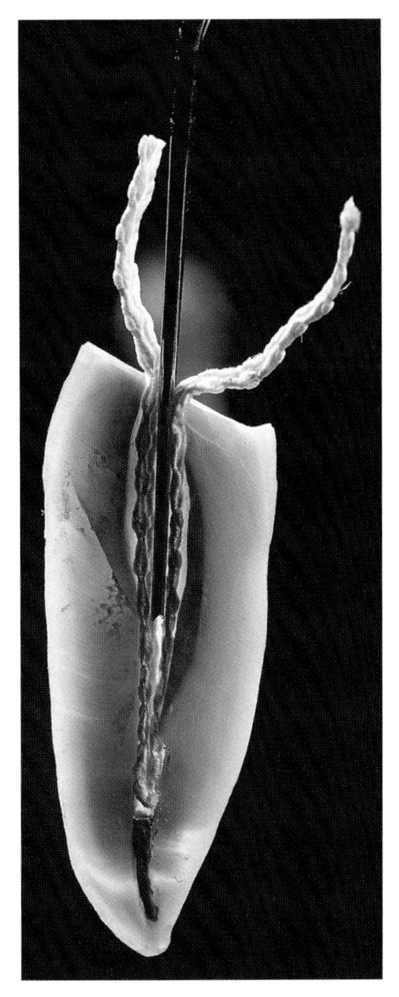

Figure 5.11 Pliable fibre (Ribbond, Seattle, USA) being used as an intra-radicular support in an eccentric shaped root canal for an eventual composite core build-up.

Table 5.2 Fibre posts.

Type of fibre	Modulus of elasticity (GPa)	Flexural strength (MPa)	Proprietary product
Carbon	145	1500	Composipost RTD, Saint-Egreve, France
Quartz	46	1400	Light-Post, RTD
Quartz	40	890	Luscent Anchors, Dentatus
Glass	45	1390	Postec, Ivoclar-Vivadent
Glass	29	990	ParaPost Fibre White, Coltene-Whaledent

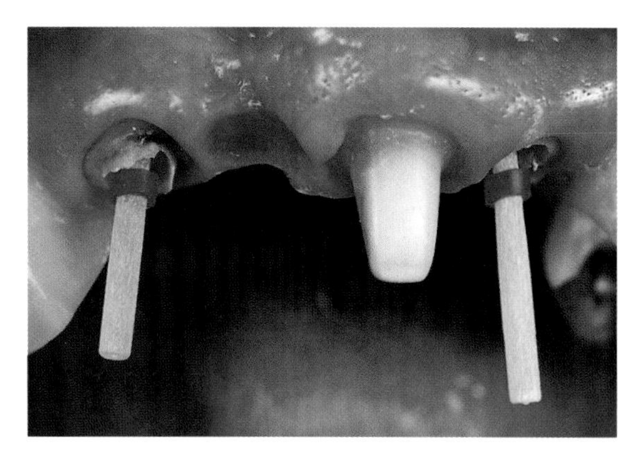

Figure 5.12 Quartz fibre posts (Luscent Anchors, Dentatus) posts for intra-radicular support in maxillary anterior teeth.

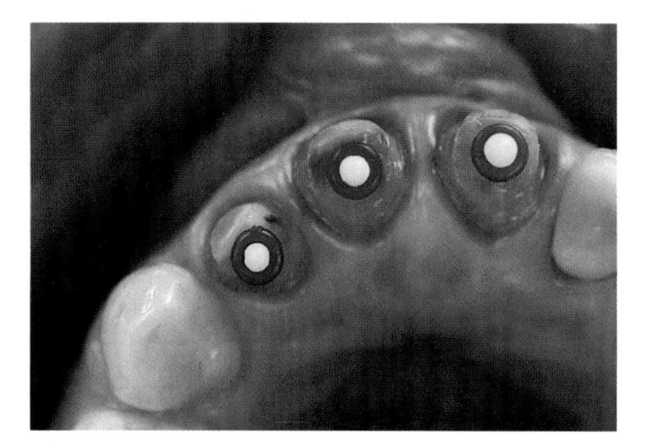

Figure 5.13 Glass fibre posts (ParaPost Fibre White, Coltene-Whaledent) with plastic rings for precise length measurements.

Criteria for intra-radicular post selection

Ideally, a post should conform to the three-dimensional shape of a root canal, without excessive pre-shaping. The physical, mechanical and optical properties should be similar to natural tooth structure, and the post should form a hermetic seal with the existing dentine for a lasting bond. In reality, none of the currently available post systems meets all these ideal criteria; a compromise is usually necessary for some beneficial properties, while sacrificing others. The ultimate success or survival rate of any post/core system is judged by its longevity. A recent study concludes that the type of post and core is irrelevant with respect to survival, the overriding factor which influences longevity is the amount of residual dentine height after preparation (ferrule effect).[23] Other studies have also reinforced the concept of retaining the maximum amount of internal and external tooth structure as the utmost important factor when restoring endodontically treated teeth.[24]

Currently, there is a lack of consensus in the dental literature for choosing an ideal post for intra-radicular support. Data and conclusions from different studies are conflicting, and choice is often dictated by prevailing clinical necessities and operator experience. However, it is important to understand the factors that influence these choices, and the discussion below endeavours to elucidate advantages and limitations for reaching an informed judgement.

Coronal dentine and the ferrule effect

According to Milot and Stein, 'if sufficient tooth structure is preserved, post selection has little or no effect on resistance to root fracture',[25] the ultimate survival of the restorative/tooth complex is dictated by the quality of the definitive restoration; an opinion which has been subsequently verified by numerous studies. However, in situations when insufficient dentine is present for the ferrule effect, or factors such as aesthetics or multiple root canals prevail, the choice of post becomes significant.[26] The ferule effect is the most significant aspect for survival of the post/core complex, and at least 1.5 mm of coronal dentine is recommended for a favourable prognosis (Fig. 5.14).[27]

Tapered vs. parallel

Tapered posts offer the advantage of conserving tooth structure near the apex due to their conical design. The disadvantages are decreased retention and pronounced wedging stresses at the apical part of the root canal, predisposing to catastrophic and unsalvageable fractures.[28] Parallel posts offer superior retention, at the expense of

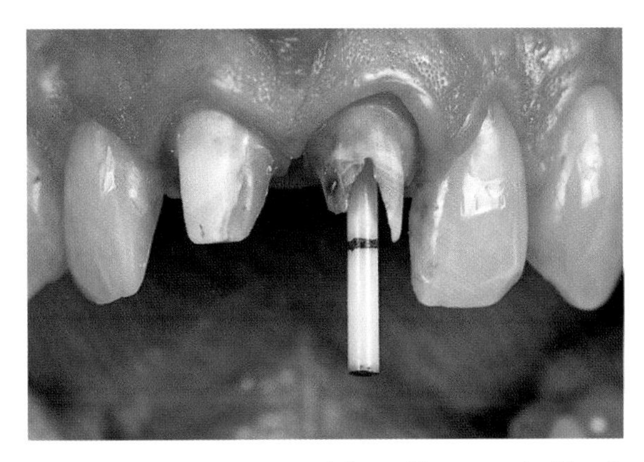

Figure 5.14 Zirconia post in left maxillary central with sufficient coronal dentine for the ferrule effect. The residual dentine should be sufficient to encircle or brace the post for support.

greater tooth removal to accommodate a cylindrical geometry. This is especially perilous with tapering root apices and thin-walled root canals. The posts should ideally mimic the canal shape, placing minimum stress on the surrounding dentine.[29] To achieve this objective, some manufacturers have a combined taper and parallel design, e.g. a taper at the apical third and parallel for the remaining coronal two-thirds.

Smooth vs. serrated

The rationale for surface roughening or serrations is to increase micromechanical retention, or locking effect, between the luting agent and radicular dentine. On the negative side, if retreatment is required, removing a highly retentive post becomes a challenge. Conversely, a smooth surface helps post retrievability, but has less retention, and increases the chance of dislodgement.

Passive vs. active

Metallic threaded posts (Dentatus Steel Posts, Dentatus, Hagersten, Sweden) are used for severely broken-down teeth with the aim of achieving maximum retention compared to passive, non-threaded varieties. The major disadvantage of threaded designs is inducing stresses, which further weaken the already fragile and reduced radicular dentine, resulting in elevated failure rates. Due to this reason, threaded posts should be used with extreme caution. Furthermore, if retention is severely compromised due to a short root, a decision regarding the long-term survival of the tooth is necessary prior to using a threaded post system.

Direct vs. indirect technique

The advantage of the direct approach is a single-visit procedure, reducing contamination of the root canal with oral fluids during post placement, ideally at the same time as root filling with a rubber dam in situ. A direct procedure also allows a wide choice of post materials; metal, ceramic and fibres. The cores can be built using either amalgam or a composite filling material. For anterior teeth, the direct technique requires a minimum 1.5 mm height and width of coronal dentine for a ferrule effect, and for posterior teeth 2 mm of coronal dentine or a deep pulp chamber. A prerequisite for ceramic posts, e.g. zirconia, is ensuring a ferrule effect of 2–3 mm to prevent root and post fracture, especially with a composite core (Fig. 5.14).[30] The ferrule effect is particularly relevant when using a resin core, which is mechanically inferior, and requires surrounding dentine for resisting occlusal loads. The canal morphology should be conducive to the preformed post, requiring minimum shaping to preserve intra-radicular dentine. The direct technique is also expedient for molar teeth with divergent roots, as a single path of insertion is not necessary as for the indirect technique.

The indications for an indirect technique are cases when there is excessive loss of coronal tooth structure and elliptical or flared canals unable to accommodate prefabricated post geometry without further canal shaping. The indirect technique is also useful if an abutment is part of the foundation for a final FPD or telescopic prosthesis, necessitating a change in the path of insertion for the final prosthesis. Additionally, a unified cast post/core complex minimises material interfaces and is beneficial for absorbing predominantly shear stresses.

There are two approaches for the indirect technique. The first is making a direct template or pattern of the canal and core build-up on the prepared abutment, using an auto- polymerising acrylic resin (Pattern Resin, GC). This pattern is either cast in metal, or milled with ceramics. A ceramic post/core complex is milled using ceramic ingots (usually alumina) in a milling machine (Mikrona). Upon delivery, the surface is sandblasted and cemented with a resin luting agent. This method produces a unified ceramic monobloc post/core complex.

The second approach is shaping of the root canal to accommodate a prefabricated post (metal or ceramic), making an impression for the ceramist to fabricate a wax pattern of the core in the dental laboratory, which is subsequently converted into either metal or ceramic. If the canal is enlarged or elliptical, it is filled with flowable composites to alter the shape for accommodating a prefabricated post (Luminex Posts, Dentatus). For the indirect ceramic core technique, leucite glass is pressed on to a zirconia post in the dental laboratory and the post/core complex cemented using an adhesive technique. Using factory-silanated zirconia posts further enhances adhesion with resin cements (Figs. 5.15–5.21). Some studies have reported

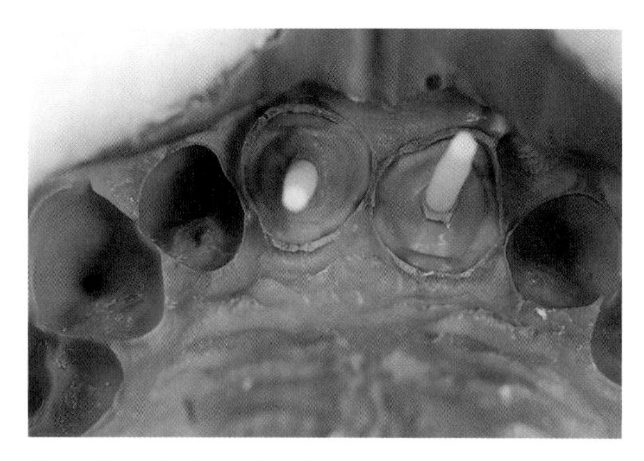

Figure 5.16 Indirect zirconia post–ceramic core case study: impressions of two zirconia posts used for intra-radicular support and to pseudo re-align maxillary centrals.

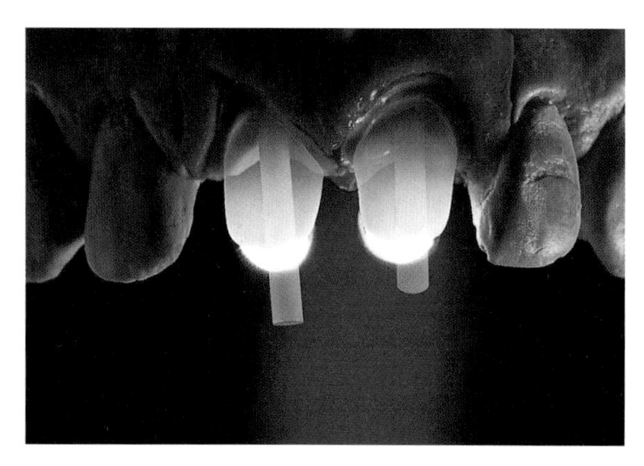

Figure 5.17 Indirect zirconia post–ceramic core case study: Empress 1 cores pressed on to zirconia Cosmoposts (Ivoclar-Vivadent, Liechtenstein) in dental laboratory.

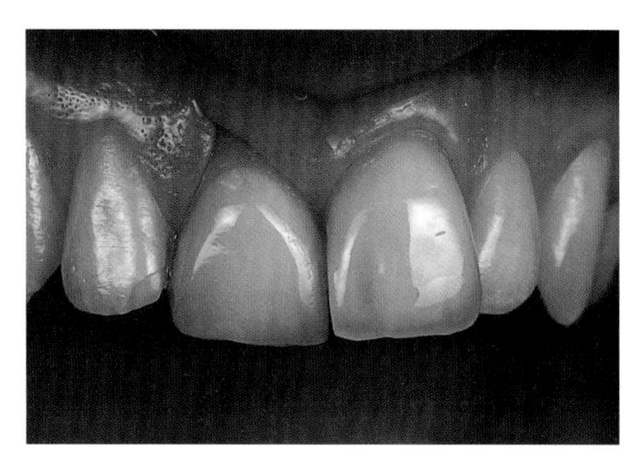

Figure 5.15 Indirect zirconia post–ceramic core case study: pre-operative status of two defective PLVs on root-filled, mis-aligned central incisors. Notice the gingival cleft on the right central, and the excessive lustre on PLVs compared to textured surfaces of natural lateral incisors.

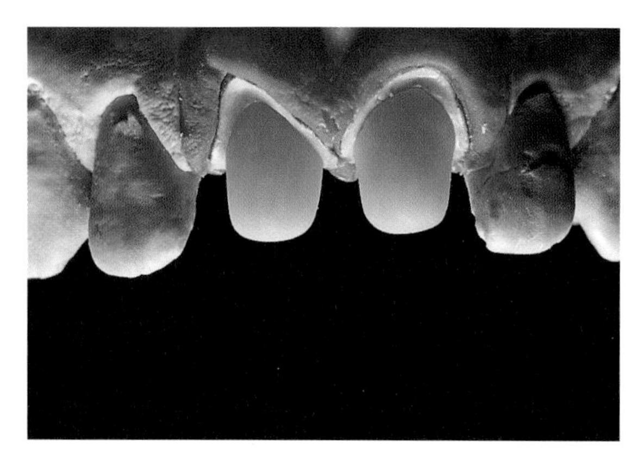

Figure 5.18 Indirect zirconia post-ceramic core case study: completed all-ceramic post/core complex.

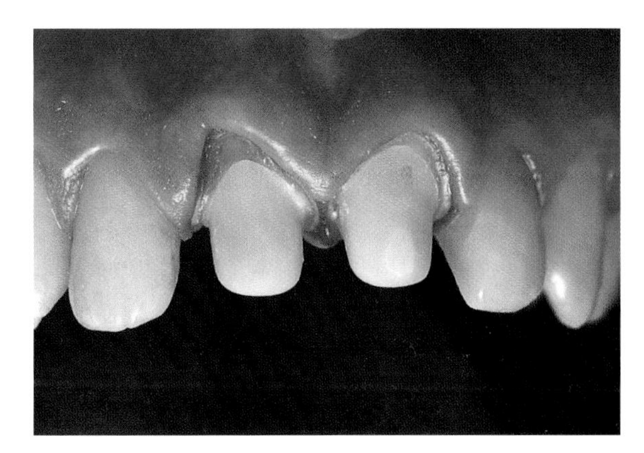

Figure 5.19 Indirect zirconia post–ceramic core case study: cemented ceramic post/core complex with clearly discernible margins for final all-ceramic crowns.

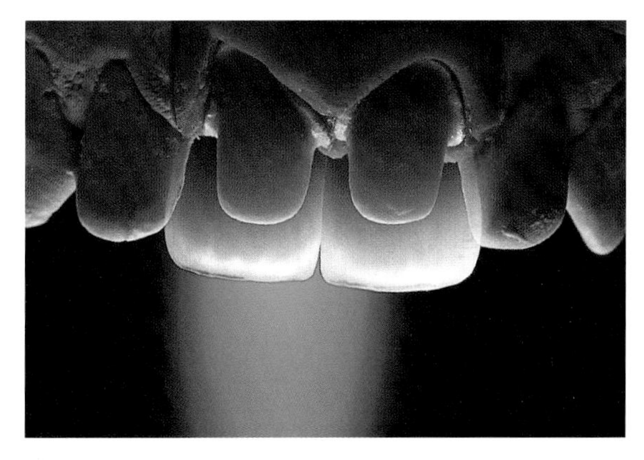

Figure 5.20 Indirect zirconia post–ceramic core case study: fabrication of two Procera alumina (Nobel Biocare, Sweden) crowns. Notice incisal translucency and incisal edge staining incorporated into veneering porcelain.

superior fracture resistance of zirconia posts with laboratory-pressed leucite cores, compared with chairside composite cores,[31] while others report little difference. This affirms the notion that using a direct technique does not compromise the biomechanical properties, while having advantages of expediency, less canal contamination and reduced number of steps compared to fabricating a direct wax pattern or impressions, temporary post, investing and casting, which all increase the chances for introducing errors.[32]

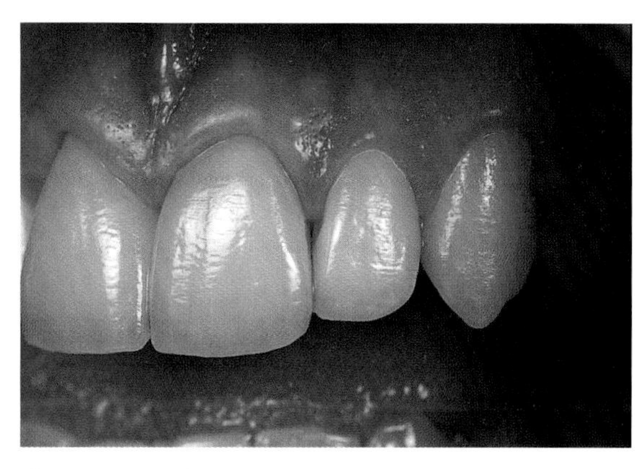

Figure 5.21 Indirect zirconia post–ceramic core case study: cemented Procera crowns showing impeccable integration with natural adjacent lateral incisors with respect to colour, texture and morphology and a healthy surrounding periodontium (laboratory work by John Hubbard, UK).

Single- vs. multi-rooted teeth

For single-rooted teeth, either a direct or an indirect technique is possible. The choice is dictated by whether the canal morphology is suitable for a prefabricated post, and the remaining coronal dentine is adequate for a ferrule effect. If the canal shape is erratic, with minimal residual dentine, an indirect approach or filling the canal with flowable composites is required. Multi-rooted teeth present difficulties for an indirect technique due to divergent roots, making a single path of insertion problematic. In these circumstances, a direct technique is favoured, assuming adequate coronal dentine and pulp chamber depth to support a chairside core.

Choice of luting agents

Similar to choosing a luting agent for crowns, the selection of cement depends on the post material (see Chapter 10). Additionally, when luting posts, the following cement properties are desirable:

- Dual or auto-cured for complete polymerisation
- Low viscosity for minimum cement thickness (this may be deleterious if prefabricated

posts are luted in flared canals, resulting in a thick cement layer prone to breakdown). For flared canals, it is prudent to shape the canal with a flowable composite prior to cementing the prefabricated post (Luminex Posts, Dentatus)
- High mechanical strength to resist stresses
- Fluoride release and cariostatic
- Radiopaque (especially when using carbon and fibre posts to delineate post on radiographs)
- Achieves a chemical bond between dentine and post material (at both cement–dentine and cement–post interfaces)

Aesthetics

If an all-ceramic restoration is chosen as the definitive final prosthesis, particularly in aesthetically sensitive areas of the mouth, masking discolouration of the underlying tooth is of crucial concern.

Tooth discolouration is categorised as superficial, extrinsic or intrinsic. Superficial discolouration is temporary stains from food dyes, tobacco and alcohol, readily removed by prophylactic measures. Extrinsic blemishes confined to the enamel layer include hypoplasia (white or brown spots, patches and surface pitting), fluorosis (mottling) and ageing (increases enamel permeability[33] with yellowish tints). In addition, erosion, abrasion and attrition also expedite discolouration. Intrinsic discolouration involves the deeper dentine layer resulting from trauma, tetracycline or sequelae of endodontic therapy. Leaching of metallic fillings (e.g. amalgam) or corrosion by-products of casting alloys of previous intra-radicular posts or prostheses also causes intrinsic staining.

There are four basic ways to obscure tooth discolouration:

- Alter the colour of the tooth substrate
- Mask or neutralise staining by a luting agent
- Mask or neutralise staining, either with a ceramic core or a definitive all-ceramic restoration by using porcelain opaquers or complementary coloured porcelains to neutralise underlying discoloured dentine
- Using all-ceramic prostheses with a dense ceramic core, e.g. Empress 2, Procera or zirconia substructures

The above methods can be used either alone, or in combination, depending on the clinical scenario and prevailing profundity of the discolouration. It must be emphasised at the outset that all these methods are unquantifiable. Each case is assessed individually according to the degree and extent of discolouration, clinician and patient expectations, and using a trial and error protocol until the desired result is achieved.

The present discussion is limited to altering the colour of the tooth substrate, methods for which include microabrasion, bleaching and light-transmitting intra-radicular posts. Microabrasion is limited to superficial, isolated stains, while bleaching is for extrinsic and intrinsic discolourations, and useful for both vital as well as non-vital teeth. The drawbacks of bleaching are its ephemeral nature, and possible root resorption for endodontically treated teeth.[34] For root-filled teeth, light transmitting white fibre, ceramic or zirconia posts[35,36] brighten the root and tooth core,[37] while metallic posts, if used with highly translucent ceramics (feldspathic and leucite glass), may be visible and detrimental to aesthetics (Figs. 5.22 & 5.23). Whilst metal posts offer excellent mechanical properties, they lack

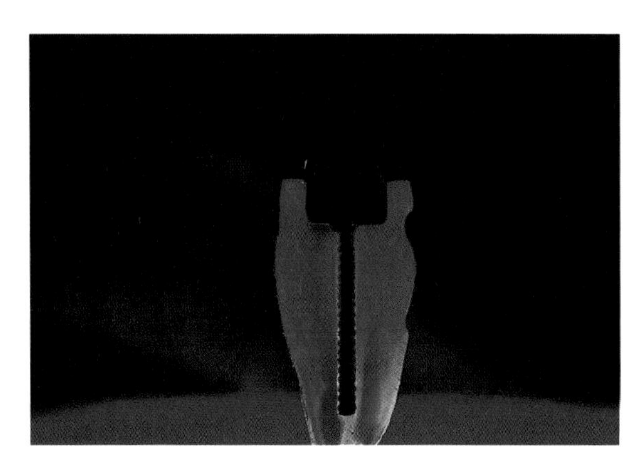

Figure 5.22 Sectioned incisor with a cast metal post and core showing that the latter impedes light transmission to the surrounding root.

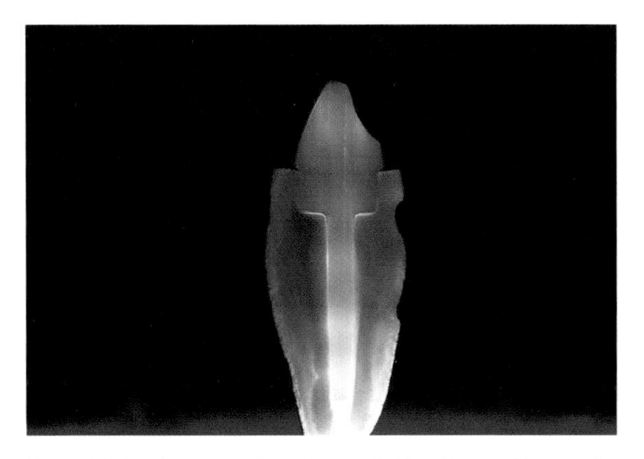

Figure 5.23 Same tooth as Figure 5.22 with an all-ceramic post/core complex, which brightens the root by allowing light transmission.

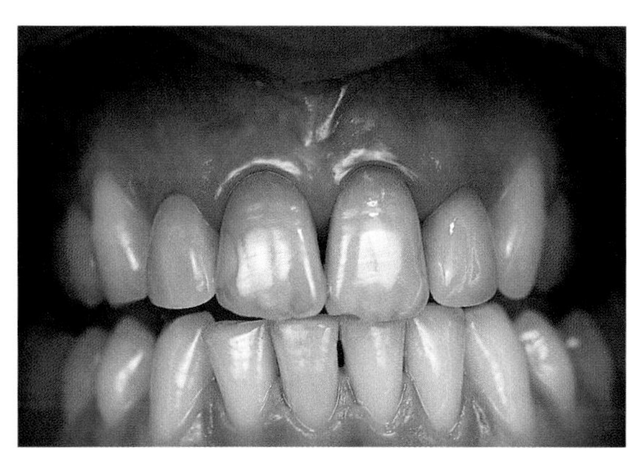

Figure 5.24 Case study, masking discolouration with light-transmitting posts and all-ceramic crowns: pre-operative status showing discoloured centrals with defective ceramic restorations on lateral incisors. All incisors were root filled following a bicycle accident.

light transmission and diffusion, often resulting in gingival shadowing at the cervical margins.

The optical behaviour of all-ceramic restorations depends on three factors:

- Relative degree of translucency or opacity of the all-ceramic system. Feldspathic or leucite ceramics (Empress I) are highly translucent, necessitating that the tooth substrate is an acceptable colour for optimal aesthetics. Alumina and zirconia ceramics are optically dense, offering increased masking capabilities but with reduced translucency
- The luting agent. Many studies have stated that the colour of an all-ceramic restoration is due to the intrinsic porcelain layering, and less dependent on the shade of the luting agent.[38] However, high chroma satins or bleach shades can alter shade with highly translucent ceramics
- Colour of tooth abutment or core. Veneering a cast gold post/core with opaque and dentine porcelains masks the metal, and approximates the colour of the core to the natural abutment. While the core colour may be acceptable, this method poses two problems. Firstly, the opaque porcelain is highly reflective, rarely seen in the natural dentition, resulting in a high value and artificial appearance. Secondly, the metallic substructure prevents light transmission via the root, and therefore compromises aesthetics of an all-ceramic crown

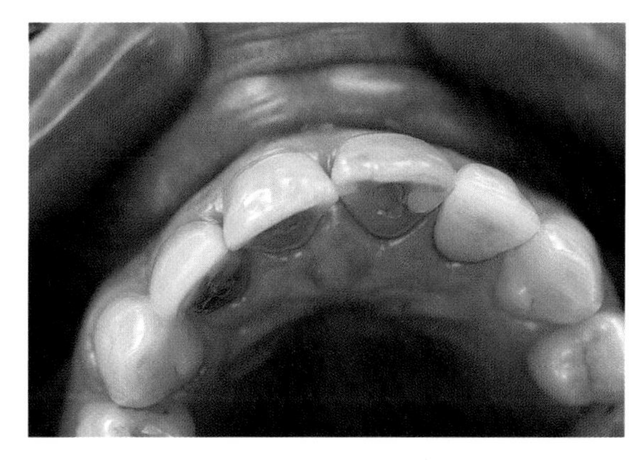

Figure 5.25 Case study, masking discolouration with light-transmitting posts and all-ceramic crowns: pre-operative status showing discoloured centrals with defective ceramic restorations on lateral incisors. All incisors were root filled following a bicycle accident.

Figures 5.24–5.36 show a case study using all three above methods to mask heavily discoloured maxillary incisors. Table 5.3 summarises post materials and criteria for selection.

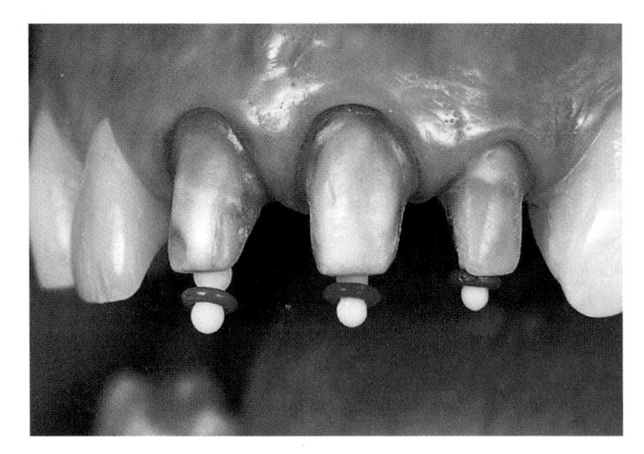

Figure 5.26 Case study, masking discolouration with light-transmitting posts and all-ceramic crowns: glass fibre posts for intra-radicular support and light transmission to brighten roots.

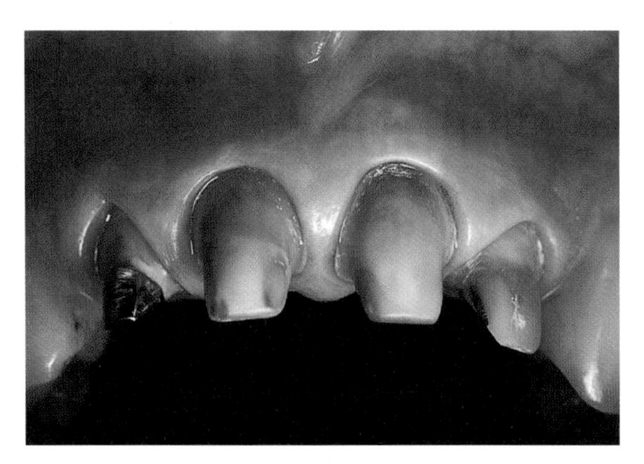

Figure 5.27 Case study, masking discolouration with light-transmitting posts and all-ceramic crowns: completed tooth preparations after cementing and trimming posts.

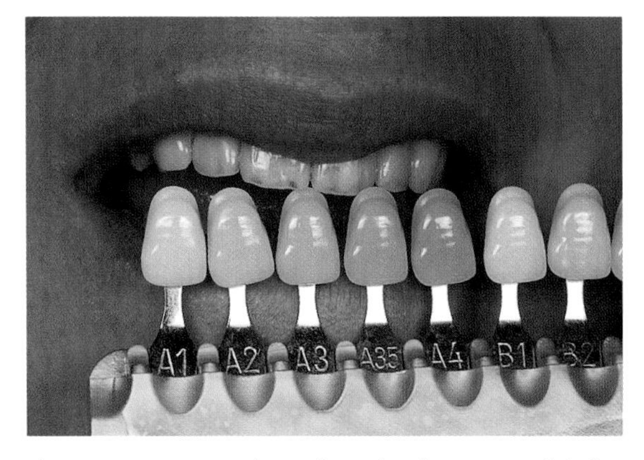

Figure 5.28 Case study, masking discolouration with light-transmitting posts and all-ceramic crowns: shade analysis with 5500 K illumination (flash) with Vita Classic shade guide.

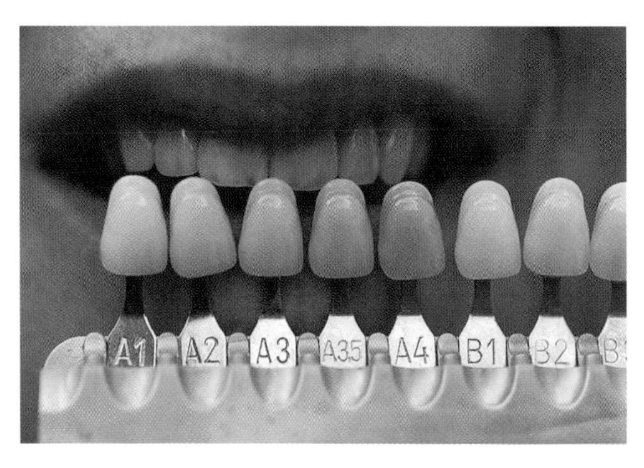

Figure 5.29 Case study, masking discolouration with light-transmitting posts and all-ceramic crowns: shade analysis with 6500 K illumination (daylight) with Vita Classic shade guide.

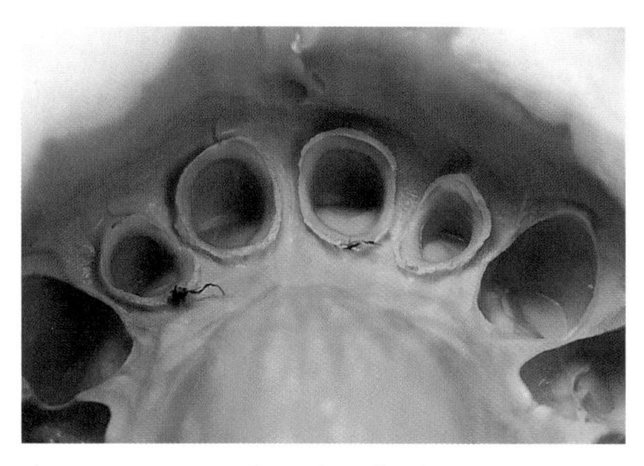

Figure 5.30 Case study, masking discolouration with light-transmitting posts and all-ceramic crowns: definitive impression with additional silicone material.

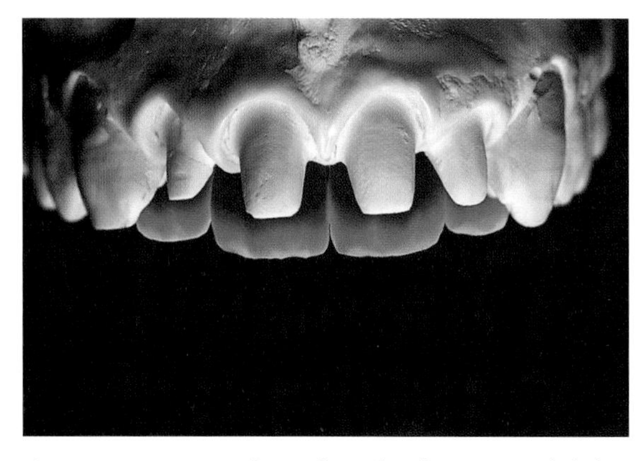

Figure 5.31 Case study, masking discolouration with light-transmitting posts and all-ceramic crowns: definitive crowns-to-tooth preparations relationship.

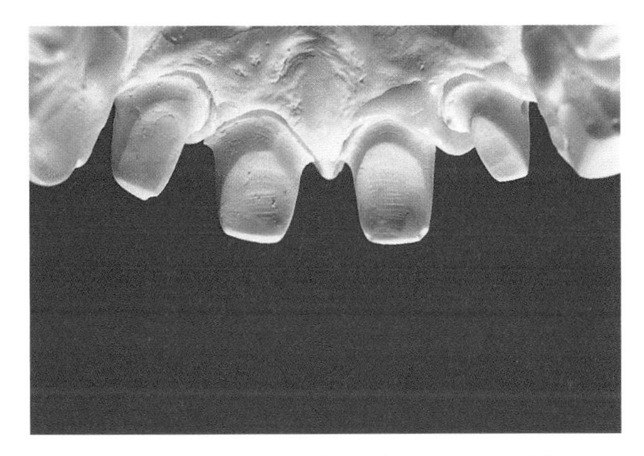

Figure 5.32 Case study, masking discolouration with light-transmitting posts and all-ceramic crowns: palatal aspect of tooth preparation showing adequate cingulum reduction to accommodate sufficient porcelain bulk.

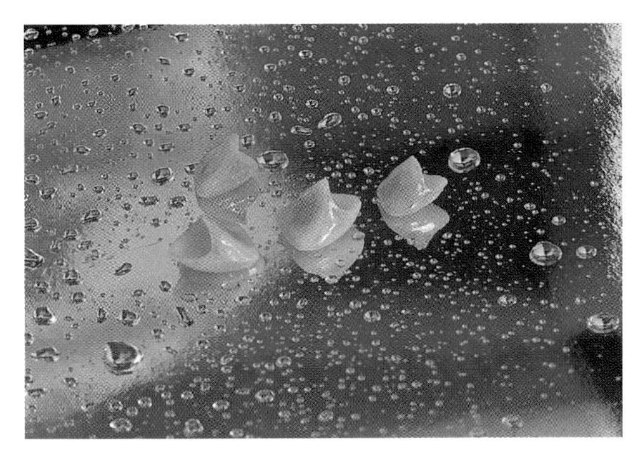

Figure 5.33 Case study, masking discolouration with light-transmitting posts and all-ceramic crowns: four completed Empress 2 crowns with dense ceramic core to mask tooth discolouration.

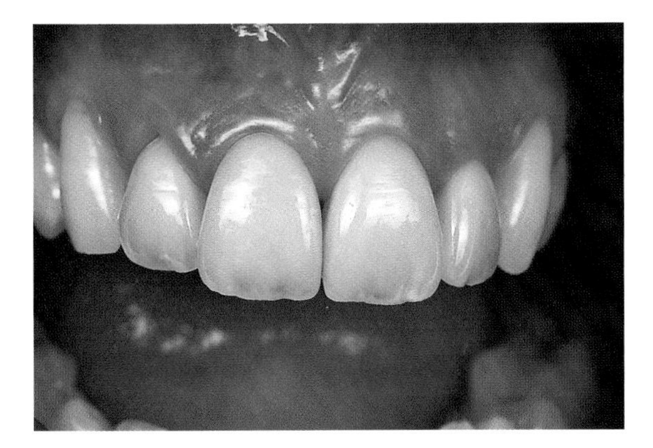

Figure 5.34 Case study, masking discolouration with light-transmitting posts and all-ceramic crowns: post-operative status showing crowns cemented with a bleach shade resin luting agent to improve colour, and further mask underlying tooth discolouration.

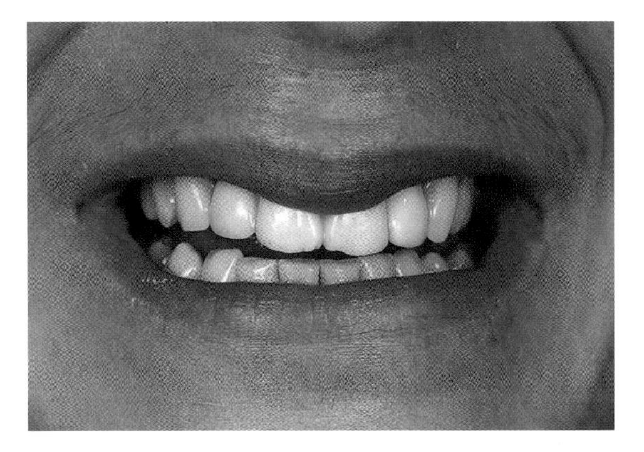

Figure 5.35 Case study, masking discolouration with light-transmitting posts and all-ceramic crowns: pre-operative dentofacial view of uneven incisal plane.

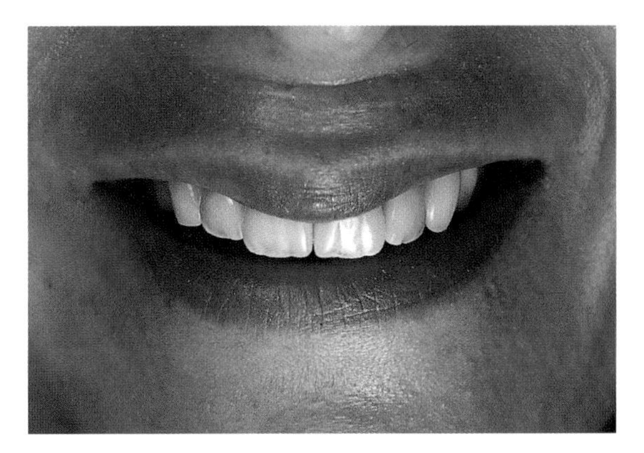

Figure 5.36 Case study, masking discolouration with light-transmitting posts and all-ceramic crowns: post-operative dentofacial view with incisal plane parallel to curvature of mandibular lip.

Types of cores

When choosing the material for the core, the fundamental principle is minimising material interfaces. This means that the fewer materials used in the post/core complex, the superior the final biomechanical properties. Similar material will cause less stress than disparate materials, reduce microleakage and increase the potential to withstand intra-oral loads. This is the rationale for using an indirect technique, because the post/core complex is a single material entity. This principle is also applicable to all components of the post/core/definitive restoration complex, by forming a monobloc structure, which is

Table 5.3 Criteria for post selection.

Selection criteria	Casting alloys	Metals	Ceramic	Fibre
Shape	Bespoke	Tapered, parallel	Tapered, parallel	Tapered, parallel
Surface roughness	Sandblasted	Unique geometry/ threaded	Smooth/sandblasted/ silanised	Smooth, unique geometry
Passive/active	Passive	Both	Passive	Passive
Technique	Indirect	Direct and indirect	Direct and indirect	Direct
Root configuration	Single, possibly multiple	Single/multiple	Single	Single/multiple
Ferrule effect	Desirable	Desirable	Essential for direct technique	Essential
Luting agent	ZP[1], GI, RGI, DR[2] with DBA, SAAR[3]	ZP[1], GI, RGI, DR[2] with DBA, SAAR[3]	DR[2] with DBA, SAAR[3]	GI, RGI, DR[2] with DBA
Aesthetics	Poor/average	Average	Excellent	Average/excellent
Clinical time	Protracted	Expedient/protracted	Expedient/protracted	Expedient
Tooth preparation	Delayed	Delayed or Immediate	Delayed or Immediate	Immediate

[1] zinc phosphate.
[2] dual-polymerisation resins.
[3] self-adhesive auto-polymerisation resins.

conducive for resisting stresses. With a direct technique, the material interfaces are increased, e.g. a prefabricated post, bonding agent and the core build-up material.

Numerous materials are available for core build-ups, which have been previously discussed for building vital teeth. When building cores on non-vital, endodontically treated teeth, two further aspects require consideration. Firstly it must be ensured that the root canal filling is not compromised during post placement. This is particularly significant since periapical pathology is more frequent with post-treated than with root-filled teeth.[39] Microleakage can potentially occur at all stages of post placement, including canal preparation, temporarisation and cementation. Secondly, the intra-radicular support further complicates matters. Ideally, a chemical bond is desirable between the post and dentine for preventing microbial ingress into the post canal. Using contemporary dental cements, a chemical bond is achievable at the cement–post interface, but the weakest link is the cement–dentine interface (see Chapter 10). The failure of the cement–dentine interface causes microleakage, leading to saliva and bacterial contamination, loss of retention (dislodgement) or ultimately root fracture.

Modes of failure

Most prosthodontic failures are caused by fatigue fractures of one or more components of the restorative/tooth complex, including the restoration, abutment, core, post and luting cement. Each component is subjected to non-axial occlusal function stresses causing fatigue fractures at the weakest point either of the restorative/tooth complex, or at the point of maximum stress. The fundamental principle for reconstructive procedures, especially of structurally compromised teeth, is to minimise non-axial (horizontal) stresses on the final prosthesis.[40] For intra-radicular supported teeth, the three main factors predisposing to failure are:

- The thin, weakened root dentine walls surrounding the post that are incapable of withstanding stresses
- Compromised retention due to a reduced surface area, leading to cement failure
- Fracture of the post itself[41]

To summarise, the three modes of failures[42] in order of increasing severity are:

- Loss of retention (most frequent) – salvageable
- Post fracture (less frequent) – possibly salvageable
- Root fracture – rarely salvageable

The above three can occur concurrently, but are discussed separately to elucidate the causative factors.

Loss of retention

Dislodgement of a post is due to loss of retention, and may be salvageable in isolation, but rarely in conjunction with root fractures. The objective is therefore to achieve maximum post retention, while mitigating risk of root fractures. Retention depends on numerous factors, such as post surface texture (and serrations), length, diameter, geometric design, timing of core preparation for the final crown and choice of luting agent. Active threaded posts offer the greatest retention, albeit at a price. Indenting the dentine with grooves obviously enhances retention, but also causes stresses that predispose to root fracture. Threaded posts should be used with caution, and if retention is severely compromised, placing a post should be questioned for the long-term survival of the tooth.

Any surface roughening, such as serrations or other unique surface topography, increases retention, irrespective of the post material or luting cement.[43] This is also true for cast posts without serrations, which exhibit less retention than serrated prefabricated posts.[44] Due to this fact, and when canal morphology is satisfactory, passive serrated prefabricated posts are an ideal choice for maximum retention. Conversely, zirconia ceramic posts offer less retention because of their smooth surface texture.

The type of cement also influences the retention of posts. Conventional cements, such as zinc phosphate, rely on mechanically interlocking surface irregularities of the root canal and post texture, while GIs and resins adhere by both mechanical and chemical bonds. The highest bond strength is achieved with resin cements, especially when pre-treatment of the post canal and post is incorporated with an adhesive cementation protocol (see Chapter 10). The positive points of resins are higher retention and resistance to fracture, reinforcing thin dentine canal walls and a MOE similar to natural tooth structure. However, the negative factors are unwanted polymerisation shrinkage stresses, microleakage from lateral canals and a demanding clinical technique.

It is well documented that ultrasonic and dental handpiece vibrations cause breakdown of the cement film between the post and surrounding dentine. Indeed, ultrasonic instrumentation is a method advocated for failed post removal.[45] This is particularly relevant to cast post and cores cemented with zinc phosphate cement, whose core should be shaped during fabrication, minimising preparation once luted to prevent dissolution of the cement film. Preparation of the core for the eventual crown within one hour of cementation has detrimental effects on retention, and should be delayed at least 24 hours post-cementation.[46]

Post fractures

Post fractures may occur in isolation or concurrently with root fractures. The important point about isolated post fractures is retrievability. This depends on the location of the fracture and the material of the post. Coronal fractures may be salvageable, but deeply located fractures in the proximity of the root apex are difficult to retrieve, due to diminished accessibility and smaller root cross-section. The material from which the post is fabricated also influences whether or not a post is retrievable. Materials, in order of ease of retrievability are fibre, metal and zirconia.

Root fractures

Root fractures are probably the most serious consequence of intra-radicular support, often necessitating extraction. During function, the least stress is concentrated within the root canal while the maximum is at the circumference. The later is the reason for incorporating a ferrule design into the definitive crown to reinforce the circumference of the root. The ferrule effect, for an extra-coronal restoration, is 1–2 mm circumference embracing sound cervical tooth structure.

To mitigate root fractures, the first point to consider is whether the chosen post will prevent or predispose to fractures. If two materials of different mechanical properties are united, stress is concentrated in the weaker material. This is apparent with metal, carbon fibre and zirconia posts, which are mechanically stronger than natural tooth structure. After loading, the weaker dentine yields, resulting in root fracture. The rationale of many newer fibre posts, whose MOE approaches that of natural tooth structure, is that deflection under load is of a similar magnitude to dentine and enamel, thereby minimising root flexion (Table 5.4).[47]

Posts fabricated from titanium and zirconia have a higher MOE and are stiffer than glass or quartz fibre, which have a lower MOE, approaching that of natural tooth, and are more elastic for absorbing and dissipating occlusal forces. The material of a post influences whether or not repair is feasible. A recent study states that titanium and zirconia posts cause catastrophic fractures at the root apices, necessitating extraction. Conversely, teeth restored with glass and quartz fibre posts exhibit coronal fractures, more amenable to repair.[48]

Table 5.4 MOE of different materials.

Material	Modulus of elasticity (GPa)
Epoxy resin	4
Dentine	15
Composite resin filling	16
Glass fibre	40
Enamel	50
Type III gold alloy	85
Titanium	110
Zirconia	210
Carbon fibre	75–215
Chrome cobalt	220

There are two opposing views regarding the stiffness of posts.[49] The first is that a post should possess mechanical properties similar to dentine, so that flexion is identical, thus reducing chances of root fracture. With an elastic post (low MOE), the tooth, post and cement all deform with a similar magnitude during function. Breakdown of the weakest point, the dentine–cement–post interface, results in dislodgement due to loss of retention, microleakage and eventual fracture of the post or core. Many studies have reported less likelihood of root fractures with elastic as opposed to stiff posts. However, following cementation of the definitive crown incorporating a ferrule effect, the difference between stiff and elastic posts is negligible.[50]

The second opinion advocates a highly stiff material (high MOE), mechanically exceeding natural tooth to withstand loads, and thereby minimise fracture. The concept is that a stiff post will dissipate forces along the post into the root canal and fracture occurs after a longer period.[51] The conclusions from the two conflicting ideas are as follows:

- With elastic posts, failure occurs within a shorter period, but is salvageable
- With stiff posts failure is delayed but is catastrophic and unsalvageable

The last item concerning root fractures is the type of cement. As well as offering superior retention, resin-based cements have a MOE similar to that of natural teeth. Hence, the cyclic deformation of resins is similar to that of dentine and enamel, with better shock-absorbing capabilities compared to conventional zinc phosphate cements.[52]

Pre-post placement assessment

In a similar vain to post selection, there is also a lack of established protocol for clinical techniques for post placement. However, before placing an intra-radicular support, the following preliminary assessment is essential to eliminate factors that may compromise long-term survival.

Endodontic factors

The starting point is radiographic assessment ensuring that the tooth is symptomless with a sound apical root filling and absence of periapical pathology. Radiographs also allow evaluation of root morphology, number, shape and width of canals, iatrogenic lateral perforations or misalignment of previous posts. The post length should be as long as possible for maximum retention (at least the length of the coronal restoration), but with at least 4–5 mm of apical root filling to ensure an adequate seal (Fig. 5.37). If the crown-to-root ratio, in addition to sufficient root filling length is not feasible, crown lengthening or orthodontic extrusion should be considered. The choice between surgery and orthodontics is determined by the gingival width and contour, especially in aesthetically sensitive areas of the mouth. Both procedures are not without problems, including an eventual lower crown-to-root ratio, insufficient dentine of 1.5 mm for the ferrule effect and compromised aesthetics. The ideal diameter of a post is also debatable, but as a general guideline, the post width should be no greater than one third of the root diameter at the corresponding depth.[53] Finally, to prevent contamination of the canal(s), the time interval between the root filling and post placement should be minimal, or they should be performed concurrently.

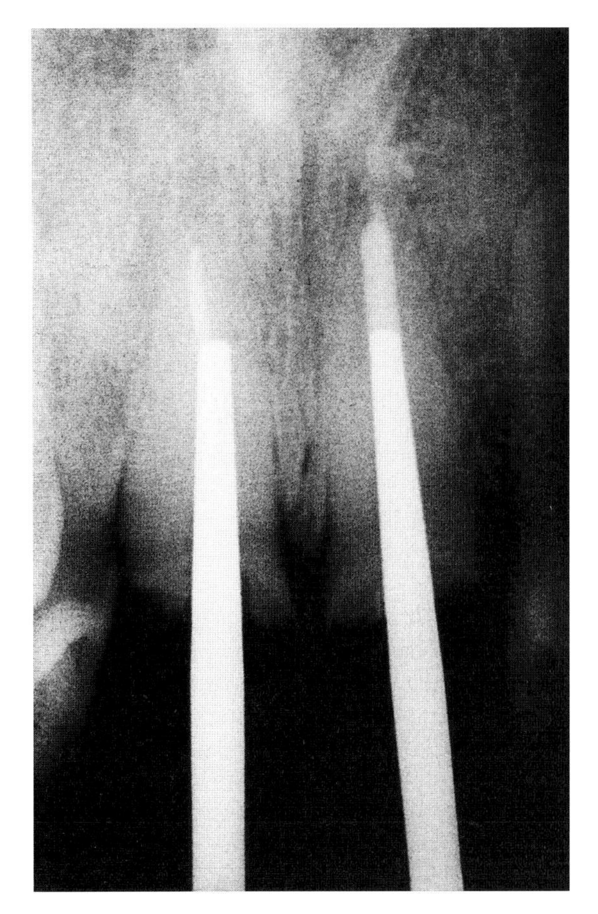

Figure 5.37 Radiograph showing two zirconia posts in central incisors with adequate (at least 4–5 mm) apical root filling.

Periodontal factors

Placing a post in an endodontically treated tooth places further stresses, and the alveolar housing should be capable of withstanding these additional forces.[54] As a generalisation, at least half of the post length should be placed in a root surrounded by crestal bone. If bone loss, following periodontal destruction, is substantial, wedging forces of the post with inadequate alveolar support may predispose to root fracture.

Choice of definitive restoration

Before deciding on intra-radicular anchorage (post/core), it is necessary to decide on the type of definitive crown. This is particularly significant if an all-ceramic prosthesis is considered, making the choice of the post and core crucial. Many all-ceramic systems are translucent (feldspathic and leucite), requiring the post/core complex to be light transmitting and of a satisfactory colour to avoid aesthetic disappointment, while others (alumina and zirconia) are optically denser with acceptable masking capabilities.

Remaining coronal dentine

If possible, the crown preparation should be carried out prior to post placement. This allows clear visualisation of the amount of residual coronal dentine (Fig. 5.38). If inadequate coronal dentine is present, an indirect post/core may be appropriate. Alternatively, if the dentine height is greater than 1.5 mm, sufficient for the ferrule effect, a direct technique is possible. For a direct composite core, especially when using zirconia posts, the ferrule effect is essential for resisting shear forces on anterior teeth. On posterior teeth, the depth and height of the pulp chamber evaluation will indicate whether a direct core is feasible.

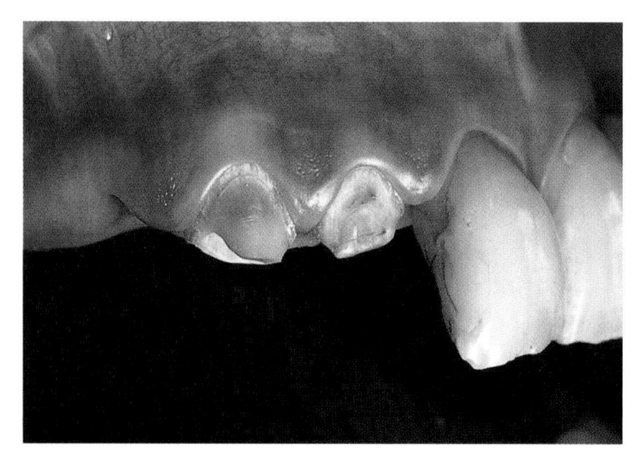

Figure 5.38 Tooth preparation on right maxillary canine and lateral incisor to assess amount of remaining residual dentine before choosing an appropriate post/core.

Tooth location

The type of tooth receiving a post/core requires two considerations, aesthetics and direction of forces. A tooth in an aesthetically sensitive area requiring an all-ceramic crown, needs a light-transmitting and tooth-coloured core. Secondly, the angle of the occlusal force is more relevant than its magnitude.[55] Anteriorly, the forces encountered are inclined, explaining the greater incidence of post-crown failures. Posteriorly, the occlusal forces are of greater magnitude but less damaging since they coincide with the long axis of the tooth, and are readily dissipated by the periodontal ligament and alveolar bone. Due to these heavier forces, cuspal coverage on posterior teeth enhances long-term success. Finally, the type of definitive restoration will also affect the amount of forces exerted, e.g. a single crown and FPD require different mechanical considerations.

Summary

Before embarking on post/core complexes, it is imperative to scrutinise the above factors, and if the clinical scenario is unsuitable, placing intra-radicular support is futile. Alternatives include accepting a poor prognosis, or extraction with subsequent or immediate implant replacement.

NON-VITAL TEETH – CLINICAL PRACTICE

Having evaluated feasibility for intra-radicular anchorage, the following is a clinical protocol for post placement and core build-up:

(1) Isolate tooth with rubber dam or non-impregnated gingival retraction cord (Hint 5.5)
(2) If possible, carry out tooth preparation for the final extra-coronal restoration to assess the amount of remaining coronal dentine for the ferrule effect
(3) If 1.5 mm height of dentine is remaining, consider a direct technique, otherwise use an indirect method

(4) Select appropriate post system according to Table 5.3 and follow manufacturer's instructions for chosen post
(5) Shape post canal: either by an additive or subtractive procedure:
   - Additive procedure (Figs. 5.39–5.44) – if canal shape is oval, elliptical, flared or with lateral iatrogenic channels or perforations, a flowable composite (with a DBA) is required to shape the canal to the geometry of a prefabricated post, or creating a suitable path of insertion/removal for an indirect technique ensuring that at least 4–5 mm of root filling is present for a patent apical seal (Hint 5.6)
   - Subtractive procedure – this involves removing radicular dentine to shape the root canal for a post. This protocol assumes that the canal is of an acceptable shape for a preformed post. The first step is removing the root filling obturation material. The choice of removal methods depend on the root filling material. The removal methods are chemical, thermal or mechanical. Chemical removal is useful for re-treating failed endodontic fillings, but has limited scope for removing gutta percha (GP) since the amount of removal is difficult to assess. In addition, some solvents, such as turpentine, cause dimensional changes in GP and increase microleakage. The thermal approach using heated instruments is ideal for GP, but unsuitable for GI and resin-based root fillings. Mechanical removal, although the most destructive, is the most widely used method for preparing root canals. Most post systems are accompanied by twist drills corresponding to post length and diameter. Initial shaping is performed with Gates–Glidden burrs of progressively increasing diameter, until the canal orifice corresponds to the twist drills of the chosen post system. Peeso drills generate excessive heat that is harmful to the periodontal cells and have a propensity to melt rather than remove GP fillers[56]
(6) If an indirect technique is used, proceed to make either a wax pattern or impression (Hint 5.7) and fabricate temporary post and crown (Hint 5.8). Forward to dental lab, and upon delivery follow from step 8 below
(7) For a direct technique, post cementation and core build-up is carried out concurrently
(8) If not already isolated, place rubber dam or retraction cord
(9) Choose core material (Table 5.1), and luting agent (Table 10.2, Chapter 10)
(10) Pre-treat post/core complex (Table 10.3, Chapter 10)
(11) Pre-treat post canal and coronal dentine with a fifth generation DBA (Hint 5.9), mix luting agent and cement post
(12) Build up direct core on to post, following manufacturer's instructions for the chosen material
(13) Remove rubber dam (Hint 5.3)
(14) Carry out immediate or delayed tooth preparation (depending on the material used) for the coronal restoration (Hint 5.4)
(15) Fabricate a chairside therapeutic temporary restoration to allow gingival healing, before making an impression for the definitive restoration (see Chapter 8).

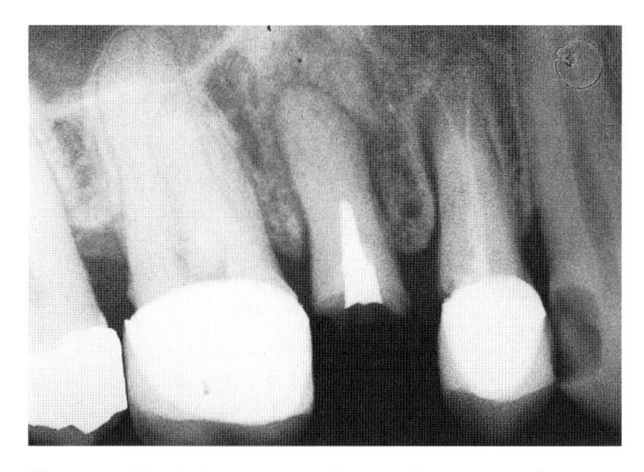

Figure 5.39 Luimex post (Dentatus) case study: pre-operative radiograph showing inadequate root filling in maxillary second premolar.

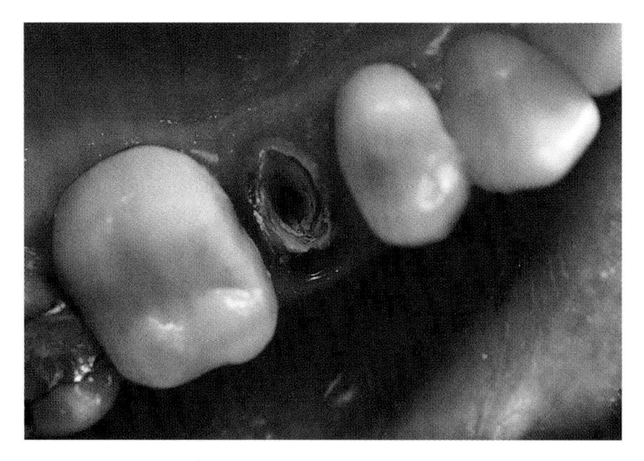

Figure 5.40 Luimex post (Dentatus) case study: following re-root canal therapy, the coronal canal orifice is flared.

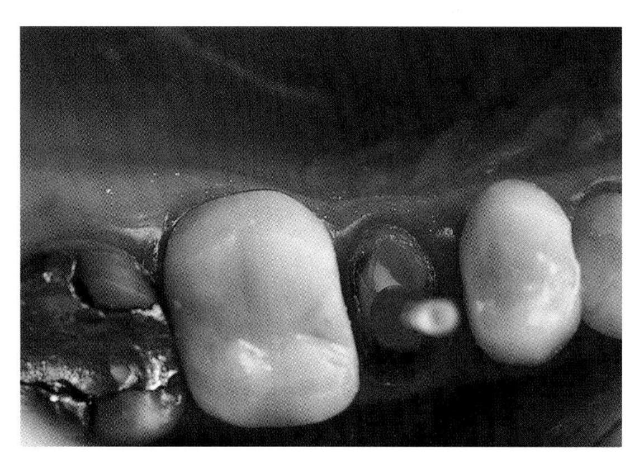

Figure 5.41 Luimex post (Dentatus) case study: flowable composite (with a dentine bonding agent) is placed in root canal and light cured with a light-transmitting post.

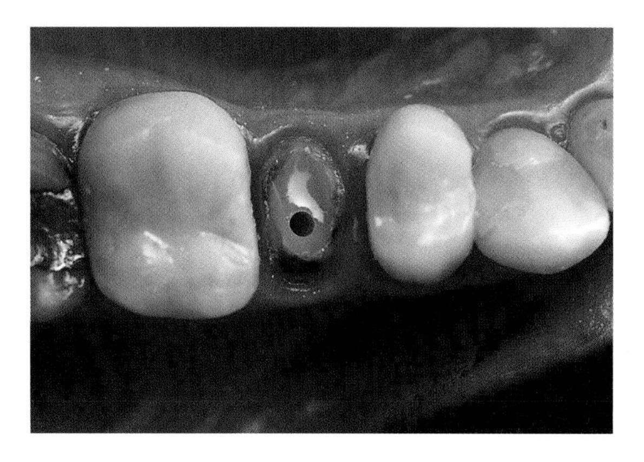

Figure 5.42 Luimex post (Dentatus) case study: the light-transmitting post is removed.

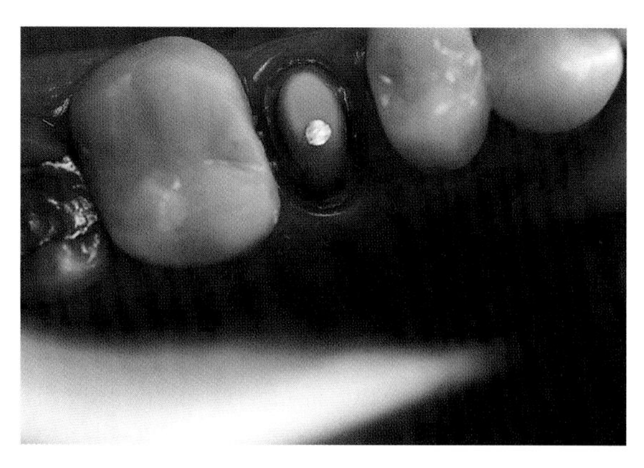

Figure 5.43 Luimex post (Dentatus) case study: a steel post, of identical diameter as the light-transmitting post, is cemented and trimmed.

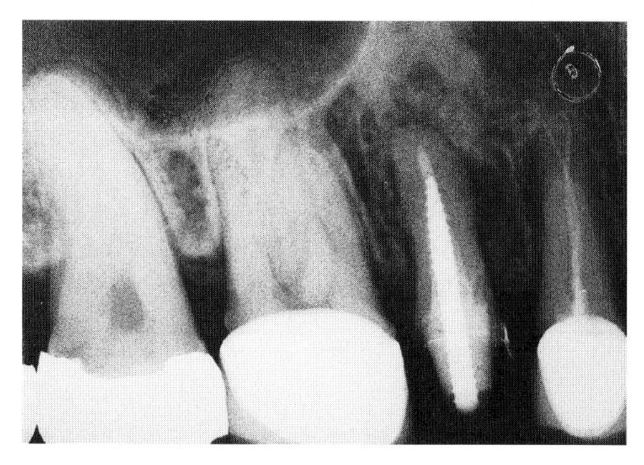

Figure 5.44 Luimex post (Dentatus) case study: post-operative radiograph showing a new root filling, shaping the flared canal with flowable composite, and a steel post with a composite core build-up.

Hints and Tips

- Hint 5.1 – If rubber dam placement is hindered by lack of tooth structure, a retraction cord provides limited isolation for protecting the periodontium, and creating an arid environment
- Hint 5.2 – Retentive boxes and grooves can be created with either a 1 mm cylindrical diamond burr or 1 mm tungsten carbide round burr. Care is necessary at the proximity to the pulp chambers and floors of cervical boxes in Class II cavities. For the latter, boxes or grooves should be at least 2–3 mm within the outer margin of the proximal box to avoid perforation of the periodontal ligament
- Hint 5.3 – If retraction cord was utilised instead of a rubber dam, and tooth preparation is immediate, the cord can be left in situ during tooth preparation and fabrication of the therapeutic temporary restoration
- Hint 5.4 – If tooth preparation is carried out immediately following fill-in or build-up, isolate the tooth and protect the soft tissues with an appropriate sized retraction cord. The cord can be impregnated with an astringent if crevicular bleeding is prevalent
- Hint 5.5 – A dry cord is ideal for absorbing crevicular fluids, visualising tooth margins and acting as an aegis for protecting biologic width integrity. If haemorrhage is anticipated, the cord can be impregnated with an astringent, or alternatively, a haemostatic agent can be applied later on to the dry cord
- Hint 5.6 – The Luminex post system is ideal for the additive procedure, which uses a light-transmitting post for complete polymerisation of the flowable composite in the root canal
- Hint 5.7 – Use appropriate lubricant or separating media to ensure post does not lock into the prepared root canal
- Hint 5.8 – Most indirect post systems have plastic posts of corresponding sizes for temporarisation
- Hint 5.9 – With chemically cured resin luting agents, avoid self-etching DBAs as the acidic inhibition layer of the latter prevents complete polymerisation of the luting agent

References

1. Sedgley, C.M. and Messer, H.H. (1992) Are endodontically teeth more brittle? *J Endod*, **18**, 332–335
2. Huang, T.J., Schilder, H. and Nathanson, D. (1992) Effect of moisture content and endodontic treatment on some mechanical properties of human dentin. *J Endod*, **18**, 209–215
3. Manning, K.E., Yu, D.C., Yu, H.C. and Kwan, E.W. (1995) Factors to consider for predictable post and core build-ups of endodontically treated teeth. Part II: Clinical application of basic theoretical concepts. *J Canad Dent Assoc*, **61(8)**, 696–701
4. Fernandes, A.S. and Dessai, G.S. (2001) Factors affecting the fracture resistance of post-core reconstructed teeth: a review. *Int J Prosthodont*, **14**, 355–363
5. Youngston, C. (2005) Posts and the root-filled tooth. *Br Dent J*, **198(6)**, 379
6. Wassell, R.W., Smart, E.R. and St. George, G. (2002) Crowns and other extra-coronal restorations: cores for teeth with vital pulps. *Br Dent J*, **192**, 499–509

[7] Webb, E.L., Straka, W.F. and Phillips, C.L. (1989) Tooth crazing associated with threaded pins: a three dimensional model. *J Prosthet Dent*, **61**, 624–628
[8] Outwaite, W.C., Garman, T.A. and Pashley, D.H. (1979) Pin vs. slot retention in extensive amalgam restorations. *J Prosthet Dent*, 41, 396–400
[9] Newsome, P.R.H. (1988) Slot retention: an alternative to pins in the large amalgam restoration. *Dent Update*, **15**, 202–207
[10] Baldwin, H. (1897) Cement and amalgam fillings. *Br Dent Sci*, **XL**, 193–234
[11] Welbury, R.R. and Murry, J.J. (1990) Clinical trial of the glass-ionomer cement-composite resin 'sandwich'. *Quintessence Int*, **21**, 507–512
[12] Prati, C. (1989) Early microleakage in Class II resin composite restorations. *Dent Mater*, **5**, 392–398
[13] Nash, R.W., Lowe, R.A. and Leinfelder, K. (2001) Using packable composites for direct posterior placement. *J Am Dent Assoc*, **132**, 1099–1104
[14] Demirel, F., Saygili, G. and Sahmali, S. (2005) Microleakage of endodontically treated teeth restored with prefabricated posts and tooth-colored restorative materials. *Int J Periodontics Restorative Dent*, **25(1)**, 72–79
[15] Torbjorner, A. and Fransson, B. (2004) A literature review on the prosthetic treatment of structurally compromised teeth. *Int J Prosthodont*, **17**, 369–376
[16] Weine, F.S., Wax, A.H. and Wenckus, C.S. (1991) Retrospective study of tapered, smooth post systems in place for 10 years or more. *J Endod*, **17**, 293–297
[17] Michalakis, K.X., Hirayama, H., Sfolkos, J. and Sfolks, K. (2004) Light transmission of posts and cores used for the anterior esthetic region. *Int J Periodontics Restorative Dent*, **24**, 462–469
[18] Strub, J.R., Pontius, O. and Koutayas, S. (2001) Survival rate and fracture strength of incisors restored with different post and core systems after exposure in the artificial mouth. *J Oral Rehabil*, **28**, 120–124
[19] Mannocci, F., Ferrari, M. and Watson, T.F. (1999) Intermittent loading of teeth restored using quartz fibre, carbon-quartz fibre, and zirconium dioxide ceramic root canal posts. *J Adhes Dent*, **1**, 153–158
[20] Hedlund, S.-O., Johansson, N.G. and Sjogren, G. (2003) A retrospective study of pre-fabricated carbon fibre root canal posts. *J Oral Rehabilitation*, **30**, 1036–1040
[21] Marinez-Insua, A., Da Silva, L., Rilo, B. and Santana, U. (1998) Comparison of the fracture resistance of pulpless teeth restored with a cast post and core or carbon-fibre post with a composite core. *J Prosthet Dent*, **80**, 527–532
[22] Hu, Y.-H., Pang, I.-C., Hsu, C.-C. and Lau, Y.-H. (2003) Fracture resistance of endodontically treated anterior teeth restored with post-and-core systems. *Quintessence Int*, **34**, 349–353
[23] Creugers, N.H., Mentink, A.G., Fokkinga, W.A. and Kreulen, C.M. (2005) 5-year follow-up of a prospective clinical study on various types of core restorations. *Int J Prosthodont*, **18(1)**, 34–39
[24] Pontius, O. and Hutter, J.W. (2002) Survival rate and fracture strength of incisors restored with different post and core systems and endodontically treated incisors without coronoradicular reinforcement. *J Endod*, **28(10)**, 710–715
[25] Milot, P. and Stien, S. (1992) Root fracture in endodontically treated teeth related to post selection and crown design. *J Prosthet Dent*, **68(3)**, 428–435
[26] Quintas, A.F., Dinato, J.C. and Bottino, M.A. (2000) Aesthetic post and cores for metal free restoration of endodontically treated teeth. *Pract Periodont Aesthet Dent*, **12(9)**, 875–884
[27] Libman, W.J. and Nicholls, J.I. (1995) Load fatigue of teeth restored with cast posts and cores and complete crowns. *Int J Prosthodont*, **81**, 155–161
[28] Cooney, J.P., Caputo, A.A. and Trabert, K.C. (1986) Retention and stress distribution of tapered-end endodontic posts. *J Prosthet Dent*, **55**, 540–546
[29] Burgess, J.O., Summitt, J.B. and Robbins, J.W. (1992) Resistance to tensile, compression, and torsional forces provided by four post systems. *J Prosthet Dent*, **68**, 899–903

[30] Meyenberg, K.H., Luthy, H. and Scharer, P. (1995) Zirconia posts: a new all-ceramic concept for nonvital abutment teeth. *J Esthet Dent*, 7(**2**), 73–80

[31] Butz, F., Lennon, A.M., Heydecke, G. and Strub, J.R. (2001) Survival rate and fracture strength of endodontically treated maxillary incisors with moderate defects restored with different post-and-core systems: an in vitro study. *Int J Prosthodont*, **14**, 58–64

[32] Mitsui, F.H.O., Marchi, G.M., Pimenta, L.A.F. and Ferraresi, P.M. (2004) In vitro study of fracture resistance of bovine roots using different intra-radicular post systems. *Quintessence Int*, **35**, 612–616

[33] Buonocore, M.G. (1975) *The nature of tooth structure in the use of adhesives in dentistry.* Charles Thomas Publishers, Springfield

[34] Javaheri, D. (2003) Techniques for nonvital bleaching. *Pract Proced Aesthet Dent*, **15**(**6**), 483–485

[35] Ahmad, I. (1998) Yttrium-partially-stabilised zirconium dioxide (YPSZ): an approach to restoring coronally compromised non-vital teeth. *Int J Periodontics Restorative Dent*, **18**(5), 455–465

[36] Ahmad, I. (1999) Zirconium oxide post and core system for the restoration of an endodontically treated incisor. *Pract Periodontics Aesthet Dent*, **11**(**2**), 197–204

[37] Gluskin, A., Ahmad, I. and Herrero, D.B. (2002) The aesthetic post and core: unifying radicular form and structure. *Pract Proced Aesthet Dent*, **14**(**4**), 313–321

[38] Paul, S.J., Pilska, P., Pietroban, N. and Scharer, P. (1996) Light transmission of composite luting resins. *Int J Periodontics Restorative Dent*, **16**, 165–173

[39] Eckerbom, M., Magnusson, T. and Martinsson, T. (1991) Prevalence of apical periodontitis, crowned teeth and teeth with posts in a Swedish population. *Endod Dent Traumatol*, **7**, 214–220

[40] Lundgren, D. and Laurell, L. (1994) Biomechanical aspects of fixed bridgework supported by natural and endosseous implants. *Periondontol 2000*, **4**, 23–40

[41] Yang, H.S, Lang, L.A., Molina, A. and Felton, D.A. (2001) The effect of dowel design and load direction on dowel-and-core restorations. *J Prosthet Dent*, **85**, 558–567

[42] Torbjorner, A., Karlsson, S. and Odman, P.A. (1995) Survival rate and failure characteristics of two post designs. *J Prosthet Dent*, **73**, 439–444

[43] Maniatopoulos, C., Pillar, R.M. and Smith, D.C. (1988) Evaluation of strength at the cement-endontic post interface. *J Prosthet Dent*, **59**, 662–669

[44] Sorenen, J.A. and Martinoff, J.T. (1984) Clinically significant factors in dowel design. *J Prosthet Dent*, **52**, 28–35

[45] Yoshida, T., Gomyo, S., Itoh, T., Shibata, T. and Sekine, I. (1997) An experimental study of the removal of cemented double-retained cast cores by ultrasonic vibration. *J Endod*, **23**, 239–241

[46] Al-Ali, K., Talic, Y., Abduljabbar, T. and Omar, R. (2003) Influence of timing of coronal preparation on retention of cemented cast posts and cores. *Int J Prosthodont*, **16**(**3**), 290–294

[47] Craig, R.G., Powers, J.M. and Wataha, J.C. (2002) *Dental Materials.* 11th edn. Mosby, St Louis

[48] Akkayan, B. and Gulmer, T. (2002) Resistance to fracture of endodontically treated teeth restored with different post systems. *J Prosthet Dent*, **87**, 431–437

[49] Asmussen, E., Peutzfeld, A. and Heitmann, T. (1999) Stiffness, elastic limit and strength of newer types of endodontic posts. *J Dent*, **27**, 275–278

[50] Freeman, M.A., Nicholls, J.I., Kydd, W.L. and Harrington, G.W. (1988) Leakage associated with load fatigue-induced preliminary failure of full crowns placed over three different post and core systems. *J Endod*, **24**, 26–32

[51] Akkayan, B. and Gomez, T. (2002) Resistance to fracture of endodontically treated teeth restored with different post systems. *J Prosthet Dent*, **87**, 431–437

[52] Junge, T., Nicholls, J.I., Phillips, K.M. and Libman, W.K. (1998) Load fatigue of compromised teeth: a comparison of three luting cements. *Int J Prosthodont*, **11**, 558–564

[53] Goodcare, C.J. and Spolnik, K.J. (1995) The prosthodontic management of endodontically

treated teeth: a literature review. Part III. Tooth preparation considerations. *J Prosthodont*, **4**, 122–128

[54] Caputo, A.A. and Standlee, J.P. (1987) Restoration of endodontically treated teeth. In: *Biomechanics in Clinical Dentistry*, pp. 185–203. Quintessence, Chicago

[55] Loney, R.W., Moulding, M.B. and Ritsco, R.G. (1995) The effect of load angulation on fracture resistance of teeth restored with cast post and cores and crowns. *Int J Prosthodont*, **8**(3), 247–251

[56] Ricketts, D.N.J., Tait, C.M.E. and Higgins, A.J. (2005) Tooth preparation for post-retained restorations. *Br Dent J*, **198**, 463–471

6 Tooth preparation

A laboratory-fabricated prosthesis, similar to other dental restorations, is essentially a fusion of two disparate materials to form a unified structure. This combination of biological (tooth) and synthetic (restoration) components aims to repair or enhance a compromised dentition. Routinely, clinicians are faced with either treating decay or improving aesthetics, both of which initially involve damaging remaining tooth substrate for achieving a therapeutic goal. Any surgical protocol inflicts trauma for the attainment of a greater good, and tooth preparation is no exception. However, minimising surgical violation mitigates iatrogenic insult, encourages faster healing and ensures longevity of the restoration. Unfortunately, scientific principles do not always dictate tooth preparation, and instead are rationalised by a variety of spurious factors. These include recommendations by peers, advertisements in journals, endorsement by opinion leaders or simply, a penchant for a particular proprietary product. Although this may appear sardonic, this is, nevertheless, not too far from the truth.

SCIENTIFIC RATIONALE

Reasons for extra-coronal restorations

The purpose of providing extra-coronal restorations are numerous; the reasons listed below often present concurrently for remedy:

- Resolving pathology, e.g. abscess, decay or fractures (Figs. 6.1 & 6.2)
- Improving function, e.g. decrease in OVD (Figs. 6.3–6.5)
- Enhancing aesthetics, e.g. misalignment, colour, shape, texture, erratic incisal plane, etc. (Figs. 6.6 & 6.7)

Before commencing tooth preparation, it is essential to reappraise the health, function, aesthetic (HFA) triad discussed in Chapter 2. Having selected the most appropriate crown for the prevailing clinical situation (Chapter 3), the next step is to prepare the abutment tooth (teeth).

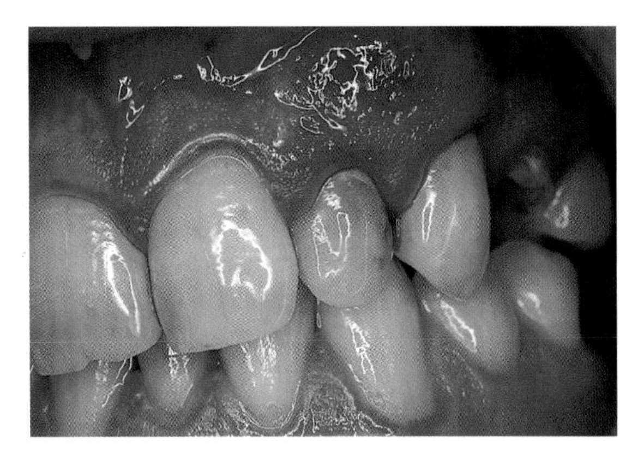

Figure 6.1 Acute abscess associated with discoloured maxillary lateral incisor.

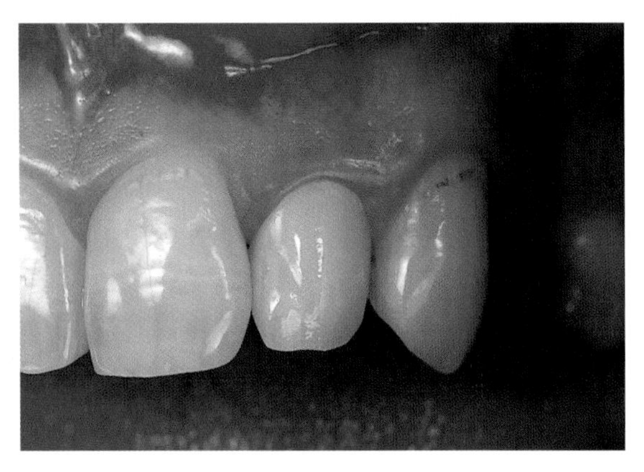

Figure 6.2 Post-operative view of patient in Figure 6.1 showing resolution of periapical pathology following root canal therapy and an all-ceramic crown.

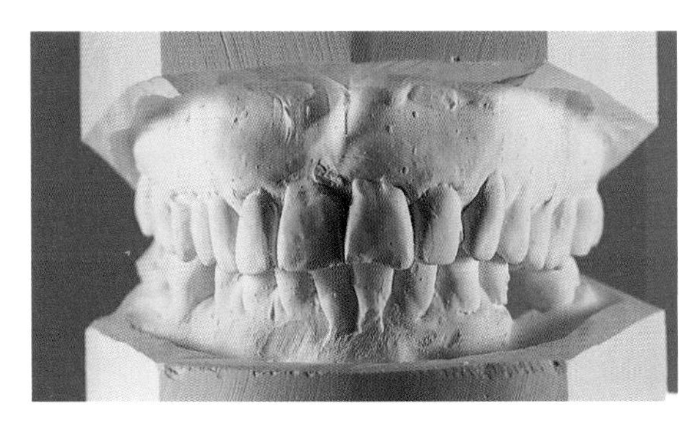

Figure 6.3 Pre-operative decrease in OVD.

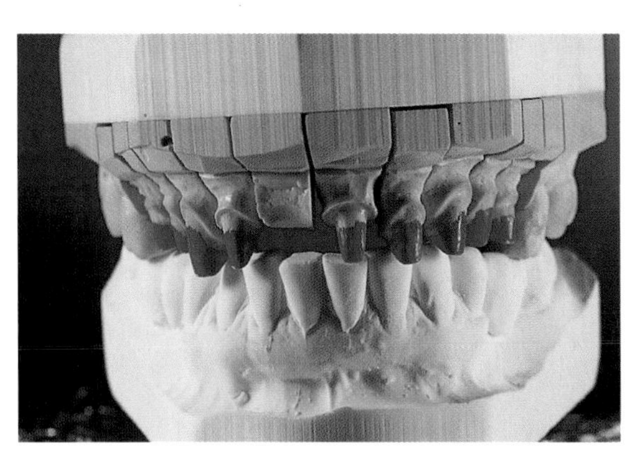

Figure 6.4 Tooth preparations for new restorations at an increased OVD.

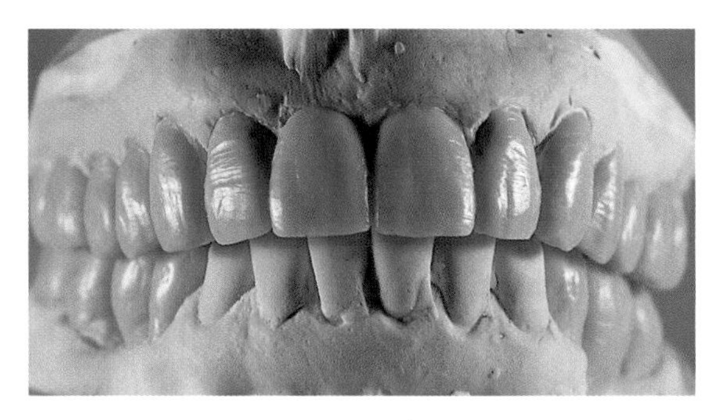

Figure 6.5 Diagnostic wax-up for proposed increase in OVD.

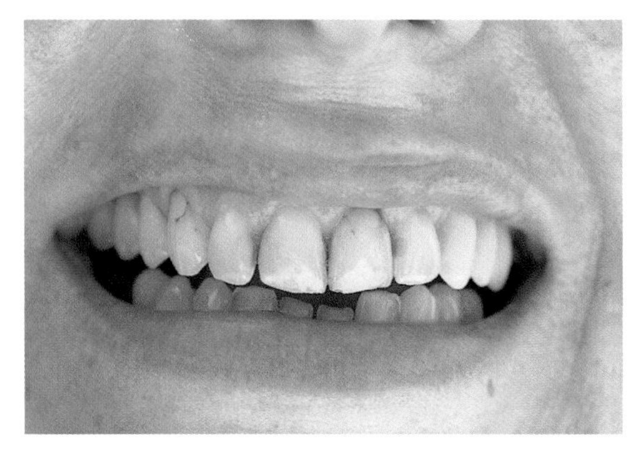

Figure 6.6 Uneven, 'rollercoaster' incisal plane.

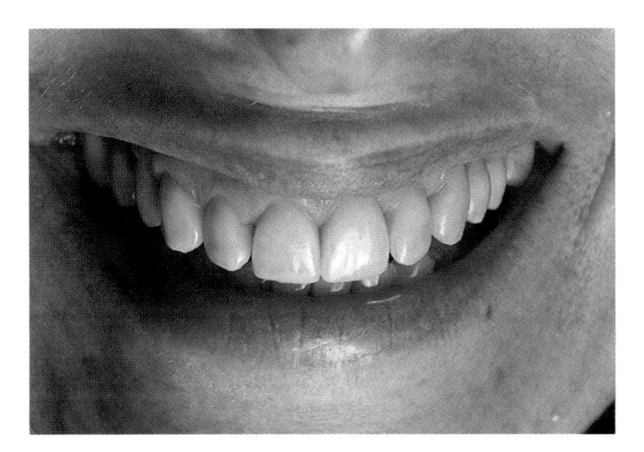

Figure 6.7 Restitution of incisal plane, coincident with curvature of mandibular lip. (Lab work by Willi Geller, Zurich, Switzerland.)

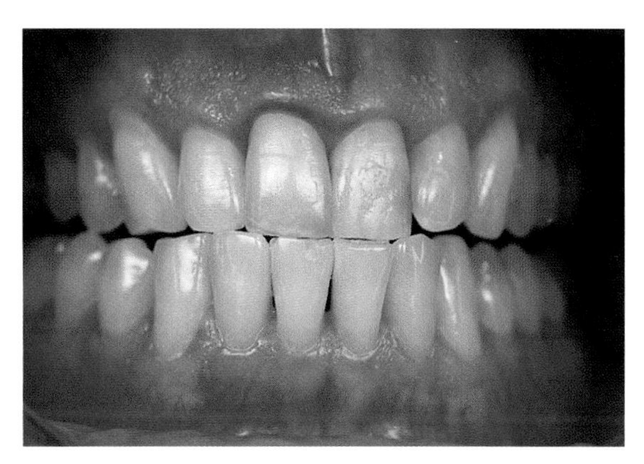

Figure 6.8 Persistent inflammation around crown on right maxillary central by crown margins impinging on the biologic width.

Biologic width

Chapter 2 emphasised the importance of preventing violation of the biologic width. The discussion also pointed out that although preset around every health tooth, the dimensions of the biologic width vary, and differential diagnosis is essential. For restorative procedures, two landmarks are used, the free gingival margins (FGMs) or the alveolar bone crest (ABC). The choice depends on clinical findings and judicious decision-making. If the survival rate of a tooth is not to be undermined, maintenance of the biologic width is imperative. This includes invasion by retraction cord placement, preparation procedures (both rotary and hand instruments), crown margin location and remnants of temporary or permanent cements. The manifestations of violating the biologic width depend on host response, all of which ultimately compromise longevity or survival of the tooth. Some examples of biologic width violation include:

- Persistent inflammation (Fig. 6.8)
- Asymmetrical gingival margins (Fig. 6.9)
- Recession (Fig. 6.10)
- Enlarged gingival embrasures (the so-called 'black triangles') (Fig. 6.11)
- Periodontal pocketing (Fig. 6.12)

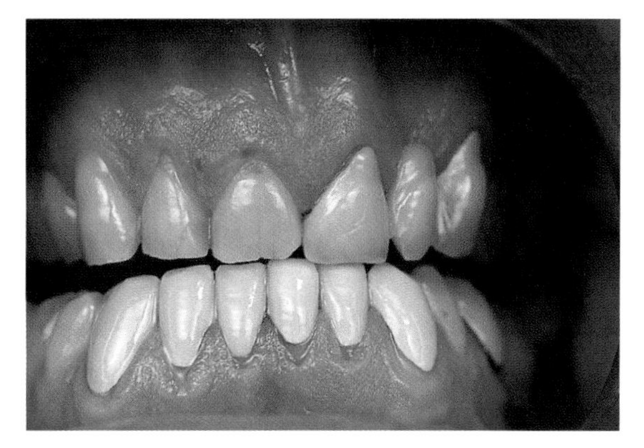

Figure 6.9 The anterior abutment (tooth #21) of a three-unit FPD shows recession (compared to the natural tooth 11) due to biologic width violation at time of cementation, resulting in unsightly, asymmetrical gingival margins.

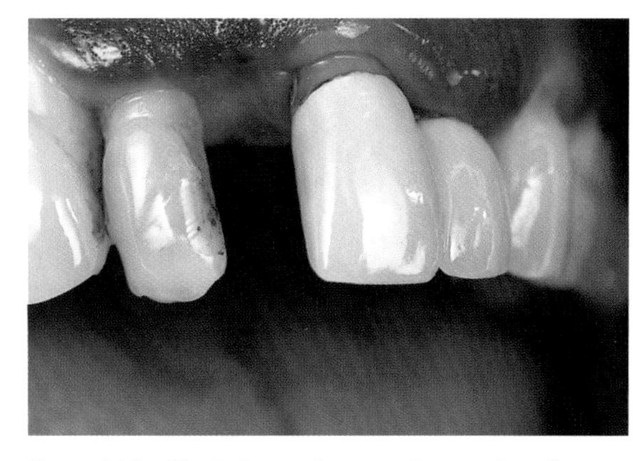

Figure 6.10 Gingival recession exposing margins of crown on left maxillary central.

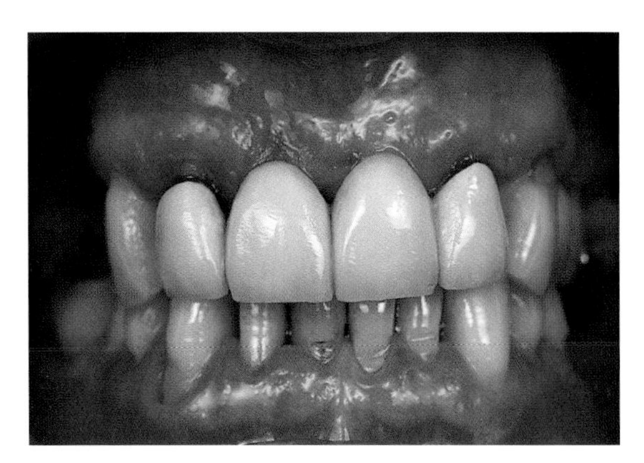

Figure 6.11 Enlarged gingival embrasures (black triangles) between crowns on maxillary incisors.

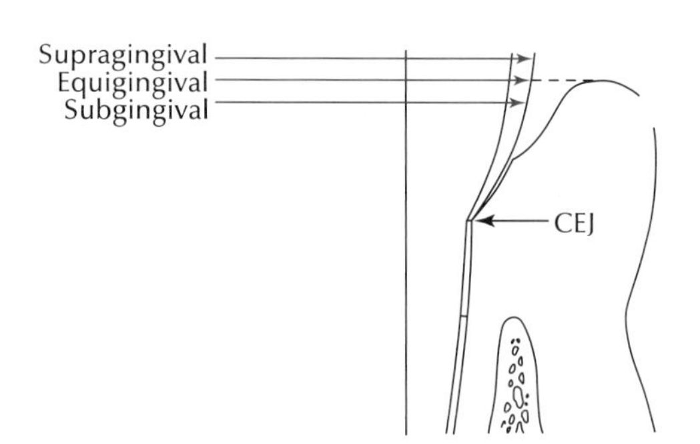

Figure 6.13 Crown margins can be supra-, equi- or subgingival.

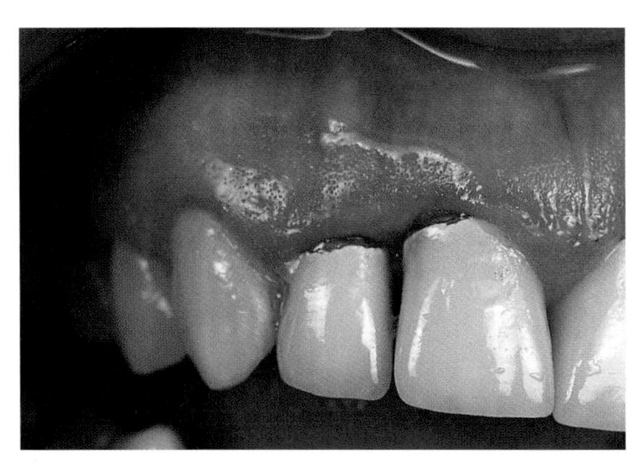

Figure 6.12 Pocket formation and periodontal abscess associated with defective crown on right maxillary lateral incisor.

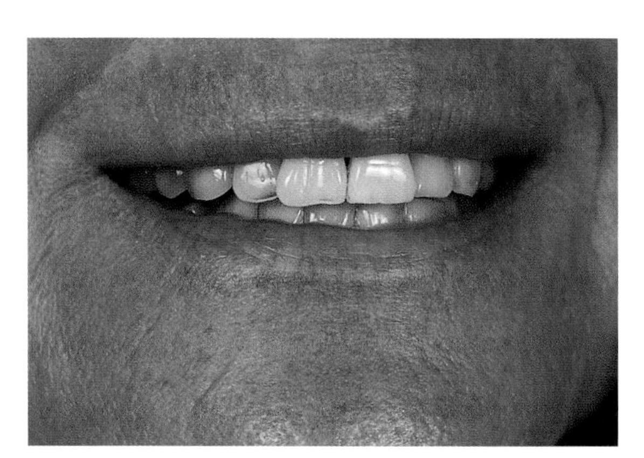

Figure 6.14 Patient with a low lip line concealing the cervical margins of the maxillary dentition.

Margin location

Crown margins can be supragingival, equigingival or subgingival (Fig. 6.13). From the aforementioned discussion, it becomes apparent that supra- and equigingival margin placement is inconsequential to the biologic width. Supragingival margins are indicated where aesthetics are of little concern, e.g. for posterior restorations, or anteriorly when the patient presents with a low lip line (Fig. 6.14). Equigingival margins are reserved for all-ceramic restorations, such as PLVs, with the proviso that the underlying tooth substrate is of an acceptable colour, avoiding an obvious cement line and colour change between the restoration and tooth (Fig. 6.15).

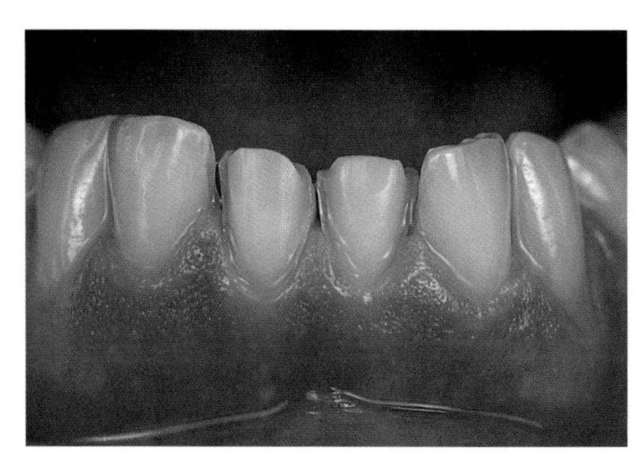

Figure 6.15 Porcelain laminate veneer preparations for the mandibular central incisors with equigingival margins (notice that the underlying tooth is of an acceptable colour).

However, subgingival margins are of paramount clinical significance. As a generalisation, if the ABC is used as a landmark for the biologic width, and sulcus depth permitting, intra-crevicular margin location should be placed at approximately half the width of the prevailing crevice. The rationale for this is that like politics, tooth preparation is an art of the possible, rarely of perfection. Hence, aiming to place a margin half the depth of the sulcus gives a degree of latitude so that, should the preparation inadvertently deviate from the ideal, the additional depth still prevents impingement into the epithelial attachment part of the biologic width. Additionally, placing margins half way in the crevice leaves sufficient space for gingival cord placement; this acts as an aegis between the epithelial attachment and the bur as well as compensating for post-preparation gingival recession, ensuring that the margins are still subgingival. On the other hand, if the FGM is used as a reference point for the biologic width, intra-crevicular margins should be placed 0.5 mm within the sulcus. Subgingival placement becomes a necessity for critical aesthetic sites, e.g. patients with a high lip line or excess gingival exposure during a relaxed smile (Figs. 6.16–6.18).

Tooth preparation should follow the circumferential FGM, which mimics the underlying alveolar bone architecture and hence ensures biologic width integrity (Fig. 6.19). Care is

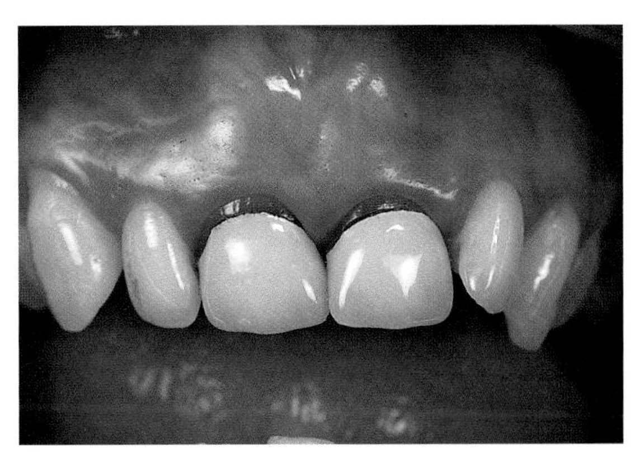

Figure 6.17 Closer view of patient in Figure 6.16 showing supragingival defective crown margins of crowns on maxillary centrals.

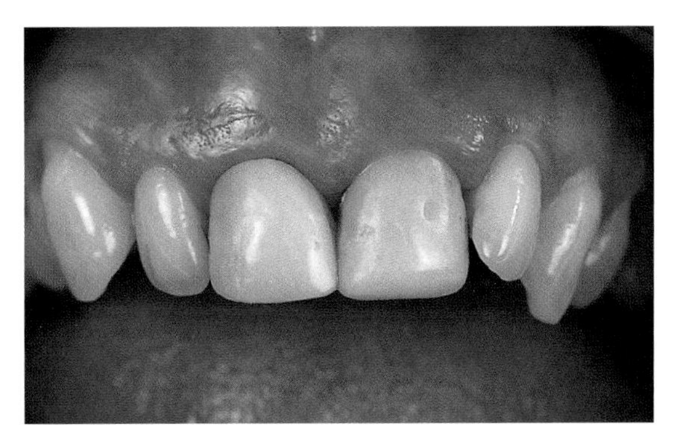

Figure 6.18 Temporary crowns with subgingival crown margins for patient in Figure 6.17.

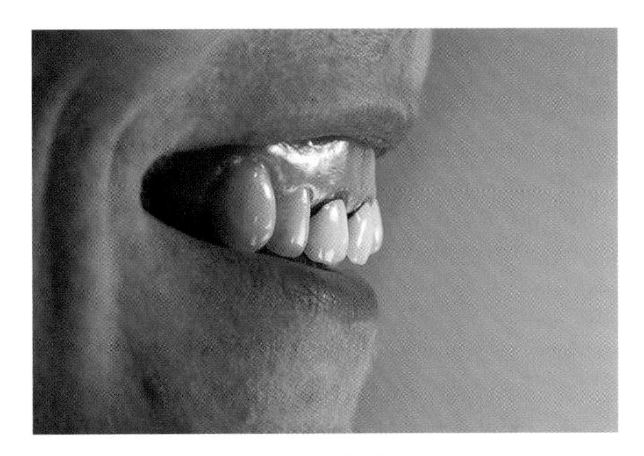

Figure 6.16 Patient with a high lip line, exposing excess gingivae during a relaxed smile, requires crowns with subgingival margin location.

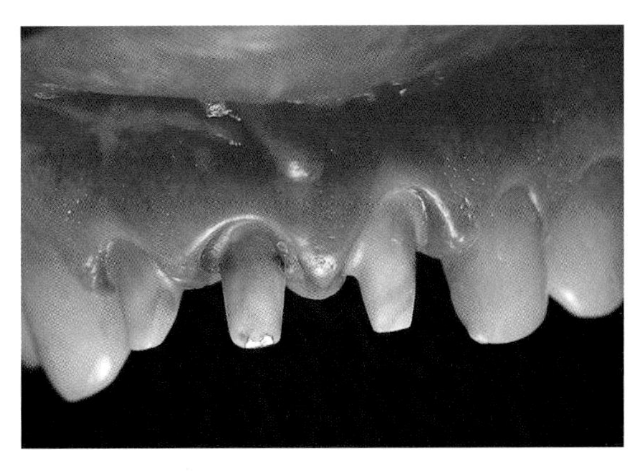

Figure 6.19 Crown preparation margins should follow the gingival margin and hence the underlying alveolar bone architecture.

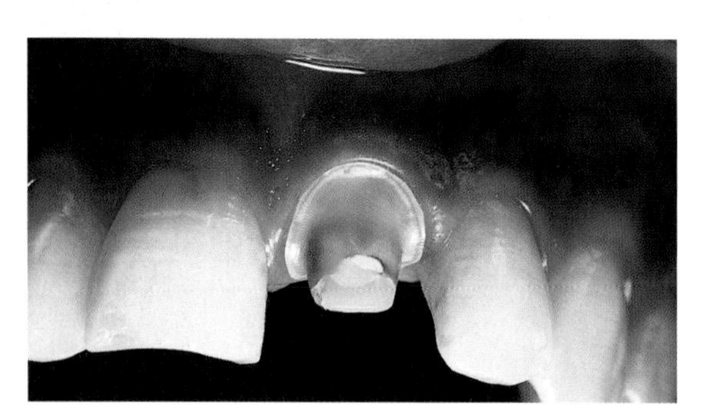

Figure 6.20 Clearly discernible crown margins mimicking the gingival scallop on maxillary left central.

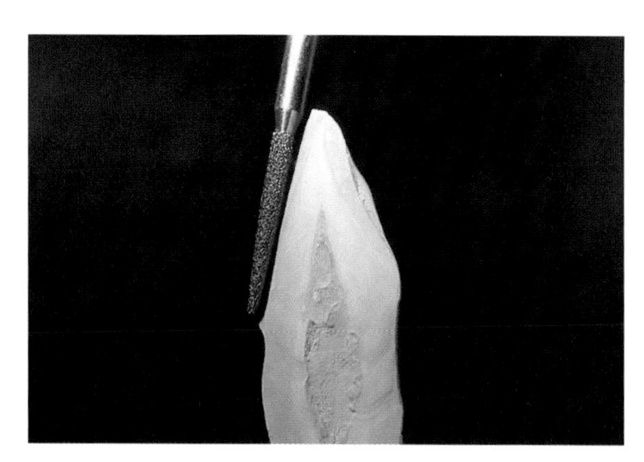

Figure 6.21 Feather or knife-edge finish line.

necessary to avoid a pitfall in the interproximal region where sulcular depth is generous (>2.5 mm). Margins could be placed deeper than the mid-facial level, but this results in 'black triangles' due to interproximal recession leading to a compromise in 'pink aesthetics'. Therefore, it is wiser to prepare a tooth mimicking the gingival scallop around its circumference, at a fixed predetermined level (Fig. 6.20).

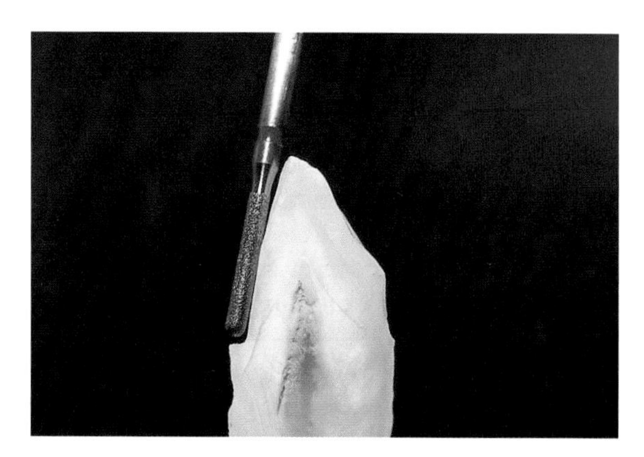

Figure 6.22 Shoulder finish line.

Margin geometry

A variety of margin designs are proposed for all-ceramic and bonded crowns. Opinions are divided depending on the factor taking precedence, i.e. aesthetic, mechanical properties of material, ease of fabrication and tooth preparation considerations.

The most popular designs include the feather or knife-edge, shoulder and chamfer. Marginal integrity, in terms of opening at the tooth/crown interface, has varying clinical acceptance with reports citing discrepancies of 120 μm, 100 μm and 50 μm.[1,2,3] The featheredge design, with an opening of 135 μm fails even the most lax acceptability of 120 μm, making its application questionable.[4] This margin design is indicated for all-metal crowns, which require minimal tooth preparation (Fig. 6.21). Furthermore, a knife-edge finish line is difficult to discern on a plaster die and can lead to poor marginal adaptability, the lack of tooth reduction results in both vertical and horizontal over-contouring of the restoration, leading to changes in the bacterial flora, with ensuing chronic inflammation and attachment loss of the surrounding periodontal ligament.[5] If knife-edge margins are used, they should be burnished and located supragingivally to avoid over-contouring or an incorrect emergence profile.

The shoulder preparation also shows diversity in geometry, with axiogingival angles ranging from 90–120° (Fig. 6.22). In a study using finite

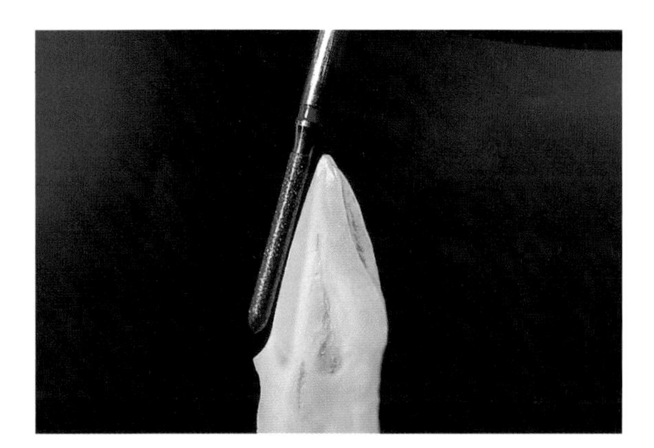

Figure 6.23 Chamfer finish line.

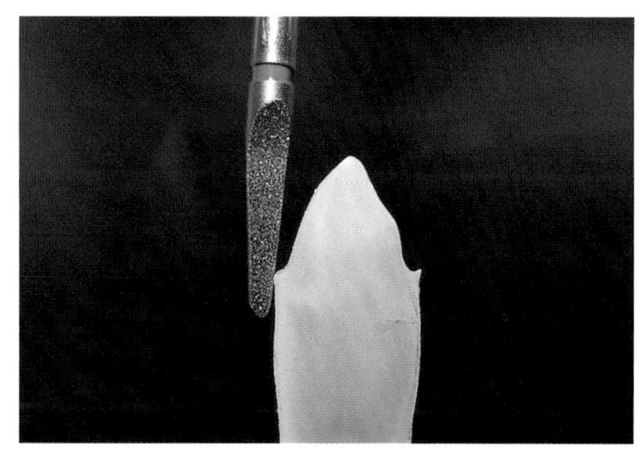

Figure 6.24 'Enamel lip' following tooth preparation (right side) is removed with diamond tips in a reciprocating handpiece (left side).

element analysis to ascertain total strain of porcelain stresses on shoulders of 90°, 120° and chamfer preparations, the chamfer showed most resilience.[6] While limited in its conclusions, this study questions conventional teaching of using shoulders when porcelain contacts the prepared tooth margin. A shoulder may be acceptable if a metal–ceramic crown is being replaced with an all-ceramic unit, and creating a chamfer would necessitate further tooth removal. Other benefits of a chamfer finish line include a marginal opening of 68 µm, facilitating scanning devices for CAD/CAM copings, expediting crown preparation,[7] and preserving more natural tooth in comparison to a 90° shoulder. Furthermore, a chamfer is aesthetically better than a shoulder since there is a gradual colour transition between the restoration and tooth substrate, avoiding an abrupt delineation between tooth and crown (Fig. 6.23).[8]

Finally, removal of serrated overhanging enamel prisms or the 'enamel lip' is needed to obtain a distinct and visible finish line. Armamentarium employed for this task includes enamel trimmers (hand instruments), rotary and reciprocating diamond tips. The smoothest finish line is obtained using diamond tips, of progressively finer grits, in a reciprocating handpiece (Fig. 6.24).[9]

Preparation design

The retention, resistance and convergence taper harmony influence tooth preparation design. Retention is resistance to displacement along the path of insertion of a restoration; i.e. the force needed to 'pull out' the prosthesis. As a general guide, at least 3 mm of natural tooth abutment is necessary for adequate retention and resistance, irrespective of the luting agent. Whilst retention has been demonstrated to have a linear relationship to preparation diameter and height, it is less representative of forces generated in the oral environment compared to resistance.[10,11] Masticatory and parafunctional force vectors encountered are lateral in nature, ranging from buccolingual, occlucogingival and linguobuccal. These non-axial forces cause fatigue, defined as cyclic loading over time. Counterbalancing fatigue, and hence improving the long-term success of a prosthesis, is dependent on the resistance, as opposed to retention form, of the prepared abutment. Resistance also demonstrates a linear relationship to height or diameter of the preparation. Additionally, resistance to fracture is also dependent on choice of cement, e.g. composite resin has three times the resistance to fracture compared with zinc phosphate.[12]

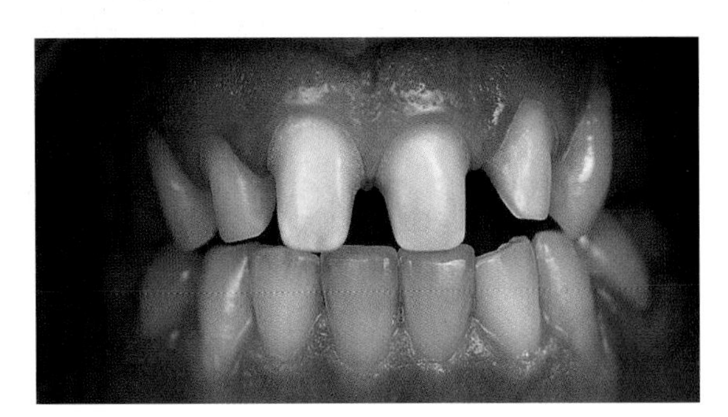

Figure 6.25 Ideal tooth preparations: 12° convergence angle.

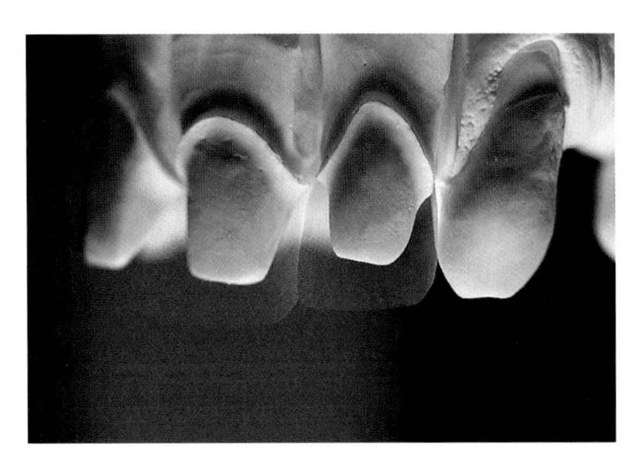

Figure 6.26 Ideal tooth preparations: plaster cast showing correctly trimmed dies with definitive crowns-to-preparation relationship.

Furthermore, using DBAs helps transfer occlusal and masticatory loads to the underlying tooth substrate for dissipation by the periodontal ligament.[13]

A 6° taper on each proximal wall, making a total convergence angle of 12°, is regarded as the standard norm (Figs. 6.25–6.27).[14] The total occlusal convergence of the preparation shows a linear, as opposed to hyperbolic, relationship to resistance to dynamic lateral loading.[15] Therefore varying the convergence angle by ±10° will increase or decrease resistance by 5–10%. Additionally, taper has a bearing on the compressive strength of the cement layer. A gradual taper exaggeration will progressively cause the cement area under compression to tend towards zero.[16]

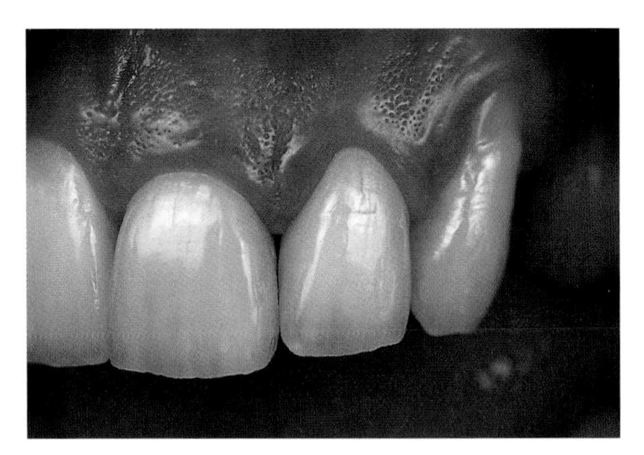

Figure 6.27 Ideal tooth preparations: definitive Procera alumina crown for patient in Figures 6.25 and 6.26.

It is important to realise that the cement compression is progressive, and does not exhibit a given cut-off point or 'limiting taper' depending on the convergence angle.[17] Therefore, although a taper increase will decrease resistance, there is no finite total convergence angle below which cement failure is inevitable.

The proverbial 1.5 mm reduction for metal–ceramic crowns is based on 0.5 mm for the metal substructure, and 1 mm for the veneering porcelain; this is purely to obtain depth of colour for achieving the desired aesthetics. Structurally, a thinner labial porcelain shoulder (less than 1 mm) is better suited to withstand tensile stresses for both labially and palatally angled loads. Other studies have further concluded that a thicker porcelain layer does not improve fracture resistance or longevity of crowns.[18] In fact, the uniformity of tooth reduction, ensuring a uniform porcelain layer, is more significant than the actual thickness of the porcelain layer.

Many clinicians assume that all-ceramic tooth preparation is more conservative than that for metal–ceramic units. This may be true for unilayer feldspathic crowns, but is untrue for most contemporary bi-layer ceramic prostheses. In order to accommodate both the dense ceramic core and veneering porcelain, tooth reduction is usually 1.3–1.6 mm, almost identical to metal–ceramic crowns. For example, if a Procera coping of 0.6 mm is required, tooth reduction is carried out with a 1.6 mm diameter bur, producing a

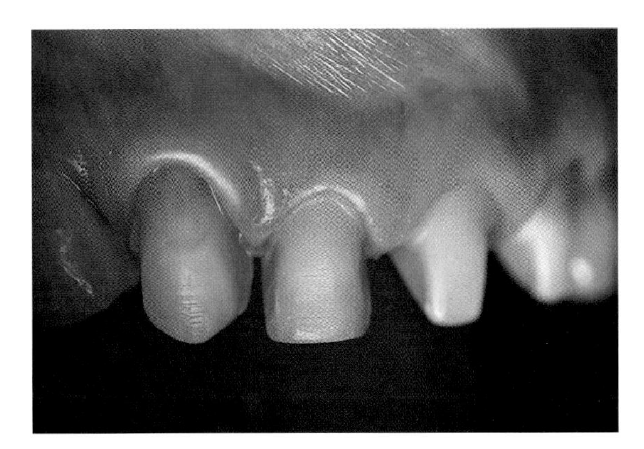

Figure 6.28 PLV tooth preparations on right maxillary canine and lateral incisor.

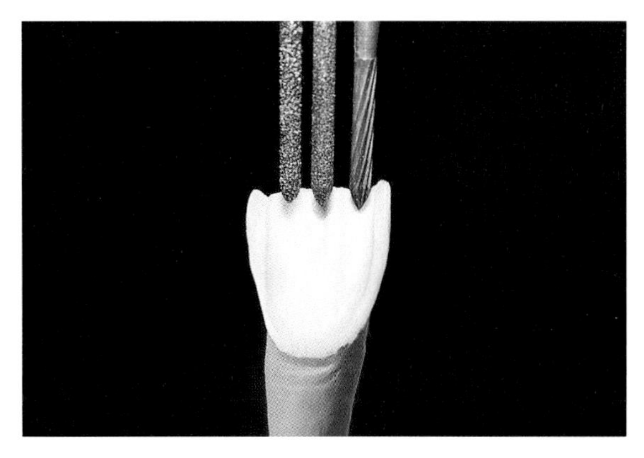

Figure 6.29 Using burs of progressively finer diamond grit (and tungsten-carbide finishing burrs) minimises pulpal temperature elevation.

reduction of 0.6 mm for the alumina coping and 1 mm for the veneering porcelain.

Tooth reduction for PLVs is usually confined to the facial aspect, and dictated by the purpose of the intended treatment (Fig. 6.28). If PLVs are used to mask discolouration, the reduction depends on the extent of discolouration and the desired final shade. However, if PLVs are used to 're-align' teeth, the reduction depends on the location of the tooth within the arch. Palatally inclined teeth requiring buccal alignment will need minimal preparation, and buccally placed teeth requiring palatal alignment will necessitate extensive tooth reduction.

Maintenance of dental hard tissue integrity

Tooth preparation, particularly for cosmetic reasons, is essentially an assault on healthy tissue to achieve a desired result. Whilst in the majority of cases the means justify the ends, precautions are necessary to mitigate damage to the triune tooth (enamel, dentine and pulp). Amount of tooth reduction is dictated by parameters such as aesthetics, obtaining a minimum thickness to avoid compromising strength of the restorative material, occlusion and pulp chamber size.

Various studies have reported non-vitality of teeth restored with artificial crowns.[19,20,21] Causes for non-vitality can be due to a dentine wound, dehydration of dentine and temperature elevation during preparation stages. Thermal shock to the pulp is dependent on pulpal dimensions and size, amount of calcified dentine and preparation techniques. The first two factors are uncontrollable but should be visualised radiographically before preparation is initiated. The last factor is primarily operator determined.

While using coarser diamond grit sized burs is procedurally expedient, it does, however, produce elevated temperatures within the pulp chamber. For example, using a 150 μm diamond grit bur raises the temperature to 40.5°C (equivalent to a temperature increase of 3.2°C), precariously close to the critical limit of 41.5°C for pulpal necrosis. On the other hand, a fine 30 μm diamond grit bur causes an intra-pulpal temperature increase of only 2.5°C. Other contributors to temperature increase are increased grinding time, relentless grinding, increased bur pressure, lack of hydraulic cooling and a cooling water temperature in excess of 32°C. Finally, as the dentine layer decreases with progressive stages of tooth preparation, its heat absorption capacity also diminishes. Therefore, in the final stages of preparation it is prudent to use burs of finer grits, as this causes less temperature elevation than coarser grits (Fig. 6.29).[22]

It should also be noted that the pulp has a 'memory' and remembers successive assaults for restorative procedures. Excluding cosmetic

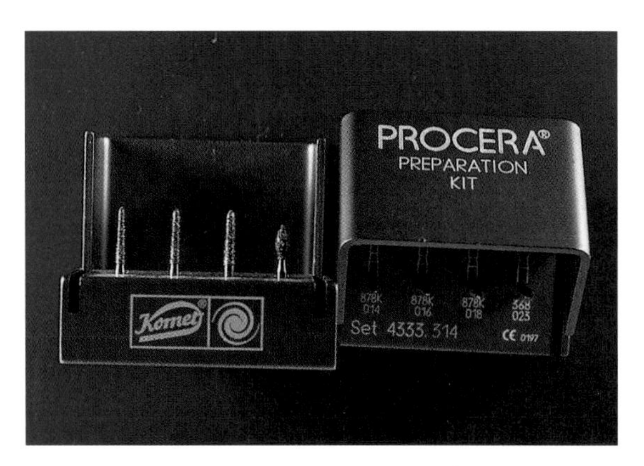

Figure 6.30 The Procera tooth preparation kits are available in medium and coarse, with diamond grit sizes of 100 μm and 150 μm, respectively. Both kits contain burs of only two shapes, the chamfers and elliptical configurations, expediting tooth preparation.

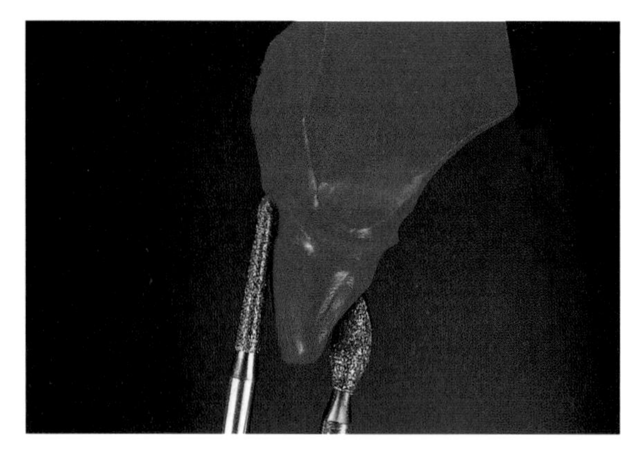

Figure 6.31 Incisors and canines are prepared with a 1.4 mm chamfer and an elliptical bur for palatal reduction.

reasons, a crown is probably the penultimate restoration, where previous fillings have failed, prior to extraction and implant placement. Considering these factors, the cumulative effect of repeated restorations eventually yields to pulpal necrosis. As a result, it is crucial to limit the time for tooth preparation to an absolute minimum, preventing damage to an already compromised pulp. Using as few burs as possible, minimal contact time with the tooth, copious irrigation and pausing to allow thermal dissipation achieves this objective.

For all-ceramic crowns, such as Procera (Nobel Biocare, Sweden), preparation is expedited by using only two types of burs. Two Procera bur kits are available, the coarse kit that contains burs of a 125 μm diamond grit, and the medium kit that has burs with a 100 μm grit, both below the critical 150 μm grit. Each kit contains burs of only two shapes (Fig. 6.30). The first is a chamfer of varying widths (1.4 mm, 1.6 mm and 1.8 mm) for circumferential reduction and an oval or elliptical shape for occlusal or palatal clearance of 1.5 to 2 mm. Using only two burs firstly simplifies preparation and ensures a calculated predetermined amount of tooth removal. Another advantage of the latter is that the diameter of chamfer bur also corresponds to the Procera copings. For example, for

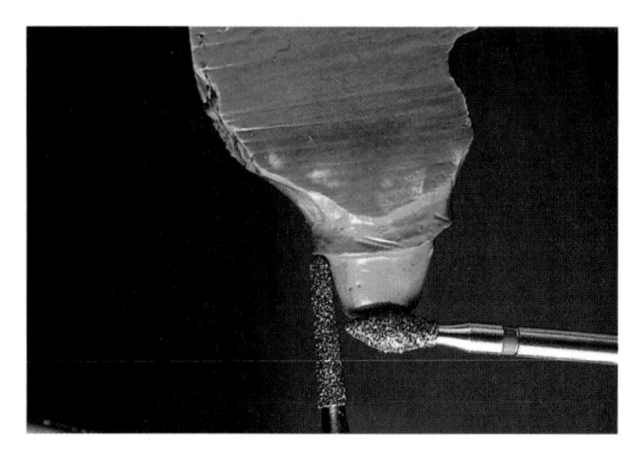

Figure 6.32 Premolars are prepared with a 1.6 mm chamfer and an elliptical bur for occlusal reduction.

anterior tooth, using a 1.4 mm bur will correspond to a 0.4 mm Procera coping, leaving 1 mm for the veneering porcelain (Fig. 6.31) and, for posterior teeth, a 1.6 mm bur will accommodate a 0.6 mm coping with 1 mm veneering porcelain (Fig. 6.32).

Another reason for sparingly using coarser diamonds is minimising enamel cracks at the preparation margins, resulting in reduced enamel toughness due to crack propagation within the enamel. To 'seal' any cracks, using diamonds of progressively finer grits removes median-type and micro-cracks between and within enamel rods. Adopting this protocol ensures the resultant preparation margins are stronger with fewer cracks.[23]

The final surface roughness of the preparation has also been a topic of debate in the dental literature. While some studies have shown little variance in retentive forces between rough and smooth preparations,[24,25,26] others have shown greater retention when a tooth surface is prepared with coarser diamond burs.[27,28] Roughness, measured in terms of Ra, of a 120 μm diamond bur is 6.8 Ra, while that for a tungsten carbide finishing bur is 1.2 Ra (Fig. 6.33). Disadvantages of a rougher surface are potential micro undercuts causing failure in complete seating of a restoration, inaccurate castings if a lost wax technique is employed and trapping air within the cement layer. Conversely, excessively smooth surfaces may cause restoration dislodgement with traditional, non-adhesive cements. Although not conclusive, but considering the above points, and the discussion relating to increased temperature and enamel subsurface damage with coarser grits, it is probably prudent to veer towards a smoother preparation surface finish.

Tooth preparation, not unlike soft tissue surgical procedure, necessitates wound closure. This includes debridement (etching with phosphoric acid to remove smear layer), disinfection and sealing to prevent bacterial invasion (application of DBA for hybridisation) and dressing with bandage (therapeutic temporary crown) to expedite healing. This protocol also reduces post-operative sensitivity, a frequent occurrence following tooth preparation, as well as improving the bond strength of the definitive restoration.[29,30]

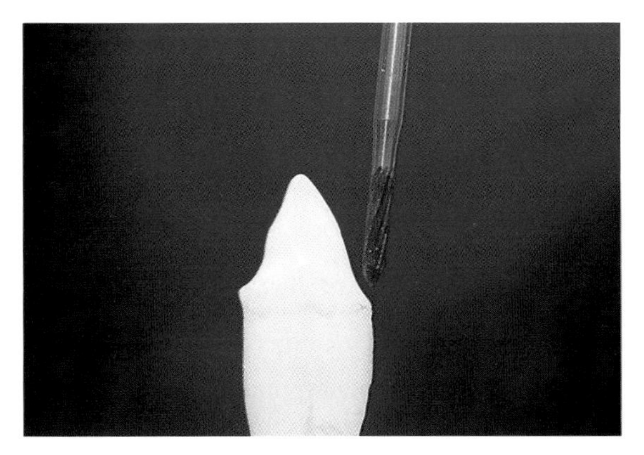

Figure 6.33 Completing preparations with a tungsten carbide finishing bur produces a smoother surface finish with enhanced enamel margin integrity.

Cutting efficiency

The cutting efficiency (CE) is dependent on a myriad of factors, including type of biological or restorative material to be cut (enamel, dentine, ceramic, cast metal or resin composite, etc.), operator kinaesthetic sense, handpiece speed and rugosity and quality of the rotary instrument. The belief that coarser grit diamond burs (>150 μm) are more efficacious is fallacious. A recent study reports that there is no increase in CE using coarser grits compared to using medium grits (100 μm).[31] The force applied on the handpiece during preparation is another point of contention. Using light pressures tends to smooth a surface, while excessive force causes pulpal damage. Furthermore, increasing the handpiece load is self-limiting, little improvement in CE is observed beyond the clinical norm range of loads between 50 g and 150 g.[32] What seems pertinent is degradation and debris accumulation of a bur, contributing to a decrease in cutting efficiency.[33] Using an ultrasonic bath to remove debris, prior to sterilisation, is therefore invaluable.

Table 6.1 summarises the salient points regarding tooth preparation.

CLINICAL PRACTICE

Anterior tooth preparation

To demonstrate the theoretical aspects, the following case study shows a sequence for tooth preparation for anterior all-ceramic crowns using the Assessment Planning Treatment (APT) acronym.

Table 6.1 Synopsis of factors determining tooth preparation.

Factor	Protocol
Crown margin placement	Depends on ABC or FGM landmark and sulcus depth: ideally placed at half prevailing sulcus depth
Margin geometry	Chamfer (unless metal–ceramic crown is being replaced with an all-ceramic unit)
Preparation design	(1) 12° total convergence angle (2) Maximise preparation height and diameter (3) Minimise tooth reduction depending on type of final crown (4) Use composite resin as luting cement (5) Mean reductions: metal–ceramic = 1.5 mm, ceramic = 1.3–1.6 mm (depending on all-ceramic system)
Dental tissue integrity	(1) Determine size and location of pulp radiographically (2) Determine degree of dentine calcification (3) Avoid using ultra-coarse burs (>150 μm) (4) Use a water cooling temperature below 32°C (5) Prepare tooth in intervals to allow heat dissipation (6) Ensure a smooth surface roughness (7) Seal with DBAs immediately after preparation
Cutting efficiency	(1) Use diamond burs of medium grit (<150 μm) (2) Avoid excessive handpiece pressure (3) Discard degraded or damaged burs (4) Clean soiled burs in ultrasonic bath

Assessment

(1) Blatant diastemae in maxillary and mandibular arches (Fig. 6.34)
(2) Maxillary median diastema of 5 mm
(3) Distal flaring of central incisors
(4) Palatal erosion due to previous episode of bulimia (Fig. 6.35)
(5) Anterior class I relationship
(6) Financial constraints limited treatment to maxillary arch. Furthermore, the mandibular lip concealed the lower anterior teeth during a relaxed smile

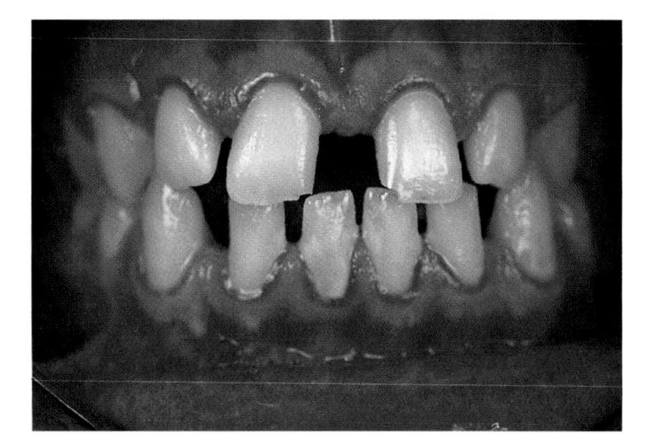

Figure 6.34 Pre-operative view showing diastemae in both arches and poor oral hygiene.

Planning

(1) Initial fixed orthodontic appliances to reduce diastemae and parallel roots to mitigate distal flaring of maxillary incisors
(2) Create a favourable width/length ratio of incisors
(3) Ensure wide contact points between incisors to prevent orthodontic relapse
(4) Provision of four full coverage Procera (alumina) crowns, for high strength and enhanced aesthetics

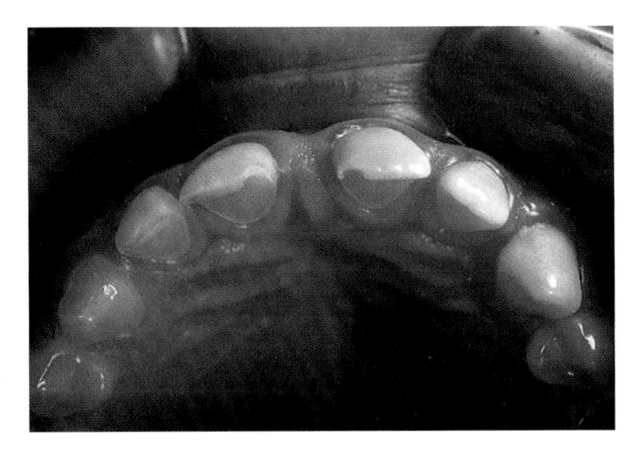

Figure 6.35 Initial maxillary median diastema of 5 mm, distal flaring and palatal erosion of the central incisors.

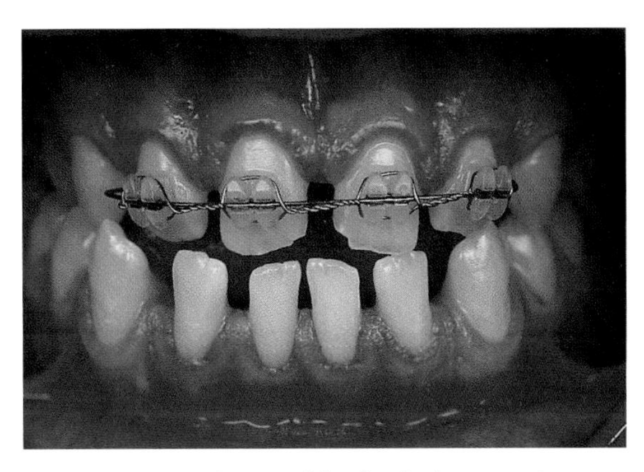

Figure 6.36 Facial view of fixed orthodontic appliance in situ to reposition maxillary anterior sextant.

Treatment

(1) Initial scaling and polishing with prophylactic and orthodontic therapy (Figs. 6.34–6.38)
(2) Decide on crown margin location position (in this case equigingival due to minimum sulcus depth). If margins are to be subgingival, use either ABC or FGM for ensuring biologic width integrity. Using ABC as a landmark, measure entire dentogingival complex from free gingival margins to alveolar crest under local anaesthesia at four sites around tooth (mesial, distal, buccal/facial and lingual/palatal), deduct 2 mm (for biologic width) to determine sulcus depth. Also, confirm location of CEJ for differential diagnosis of erratic ABC. Alternately if FGM is used as a landmark, place margins 0.5 mm within sulcus (Figs. 6.39 & 6.40)
(3) Place retraction cord, of appropriate width, within gingival sulcus to protect epithelial attachment (Figs. 6.41 & 6.42) (Hint 6.1)
(4) Use 1.4 mm chamfer burs (0.4 mm coping and 1 mm veneering porcelain), place depth cuts mesio-distally following crown contour curvature (Fig. 6.43)
(5) Repeat step (4) above for inciso-gingival and palatal aspects (in this case no palatal reduction was necessary) (Fig. 6.44)
(6) Reduce tooth according to initial depth cuts on all aspects (elliptical diamond for palatal reduction and occlusal clearance of 1.5–2 mm) (Fig. 6.45)
(7) Refine surface roughness with a 1.4 mm 12-fluted tungsten-carbide chamfer and elliptical burs (Fig. 6.46)
(8) Complete tooth preparation by removing circumferential enamel lip with diamond tip in a reciprocating handpiece
(9) Verify sinuous outline and smooth surface finish of tooth preparations
(10) Etch, blot dry and seal preparations with DBAs. Light through a glycerine gel cover to avoid interaction of oxygen inhibition layer with acrylic monomers (used for therapeutic temporary crowns) and impression materials[34]
(11) Proceed with therapeutic temporary crown fabrication
(12) At a subsequent visit, verify gingival health and stability of FGM before making impressions (Figs. 6.47–6.49)
(13) Check plaster model for clearly discernible circumferential tooth margins, and sinuous preparation outlines (Fig. 6.50)
(14) Preparations-to-definitive crowns relationship is shown in Figure 6.51.

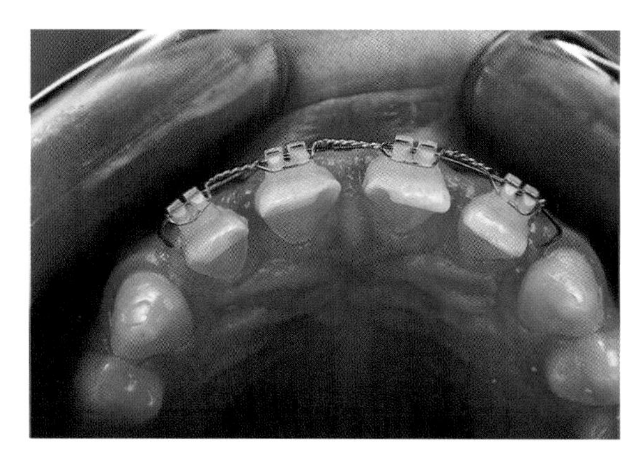

Figure 6.37 Palatal view of fixed orthodontic appliance in situ to reposition maxillary anterior sextant.

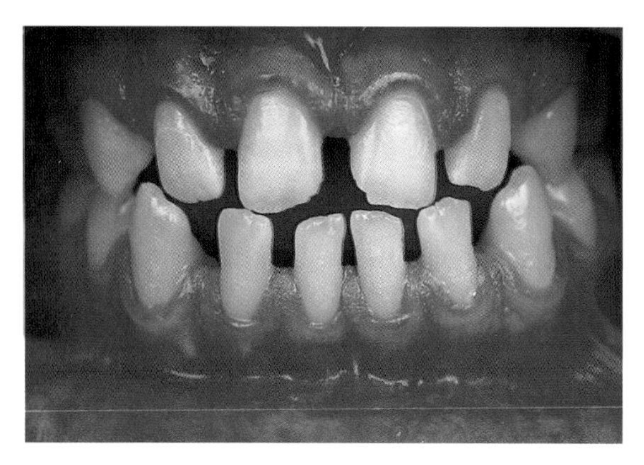

Figure 6.38 Orthodontic appliance removal, prophylaxis to improve periodontal health and reduction of median diastema to 2 mm.

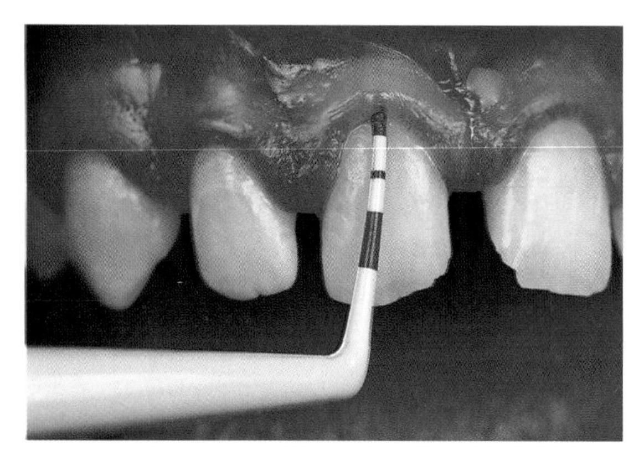

Figure 6.39 Mid-facial dentogingival complex measurement with a periodontal probe. The linear measurement is 2.0 mm indicative of a negligible sulcus depth.

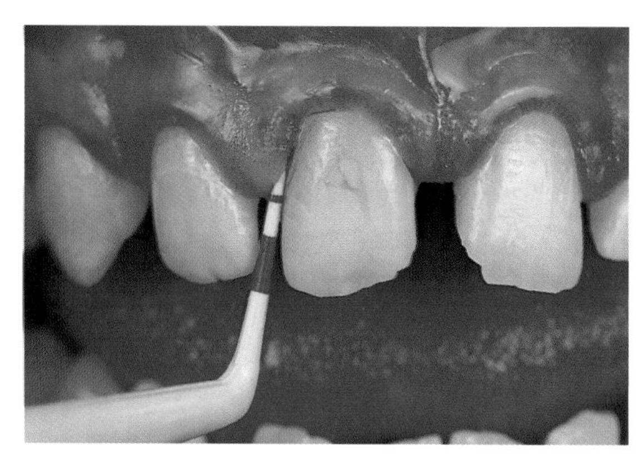

Figure 6.40 Distal dentogingival complex measurement with a periodontal probe. The linear measurement is 4.5 mm with a sulcus depth of 2.5 mm.

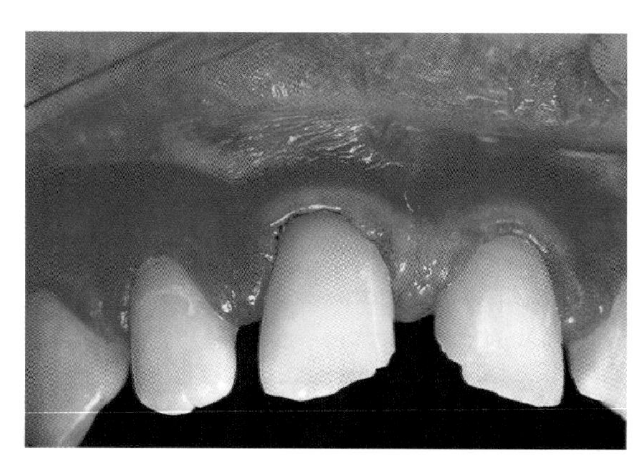

Figure 6.41 Retraction cord around tooth #11 to protect gingival margins.

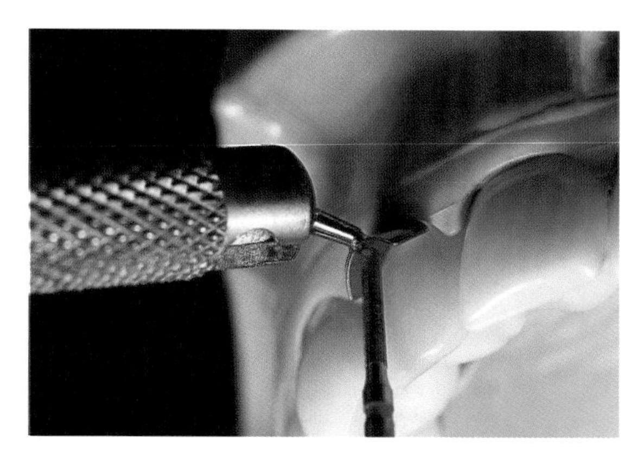

Figure 6.42 Zekrya gingival retractor to protect the FGM during crown preparation.

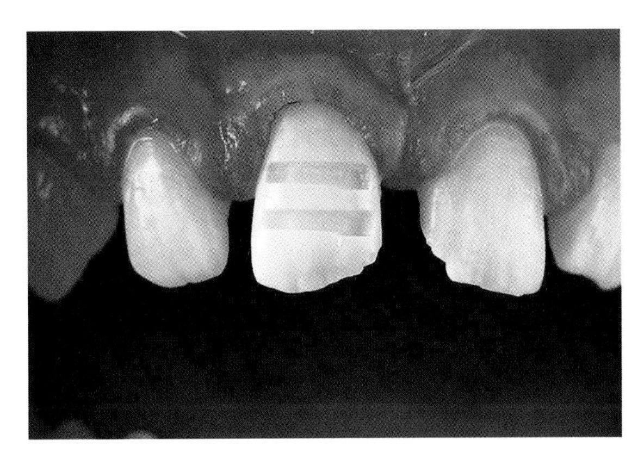

Figure 6.43 Mesio-distal depth grooves for precise tooth reduction.

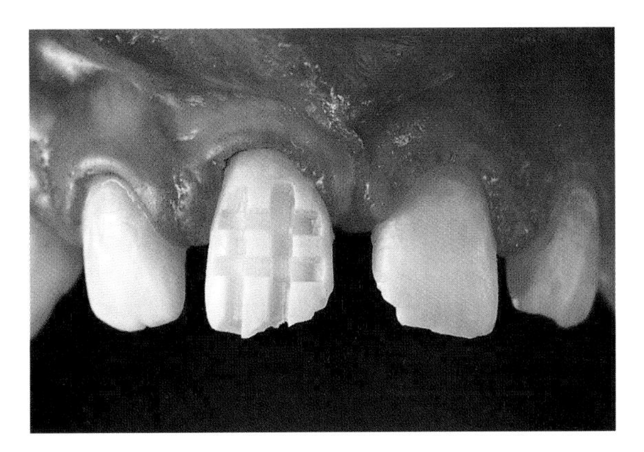

Figure 6.44 Mesio-distal and inciso-gingival depth grooves for precise tooth reduction.

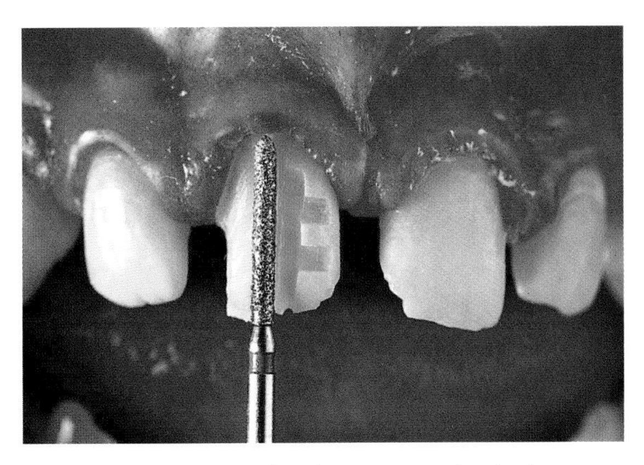

Figure 6.45 Precise tooth reduction using the depth cuts as a guide in both mesio-distal and inciso-gingival planes.

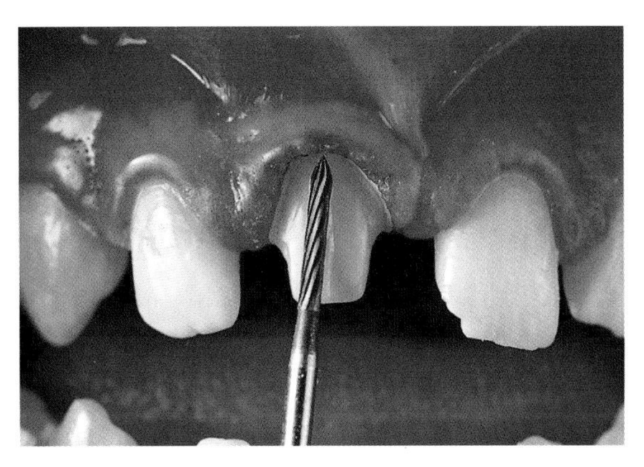

Figure 6.46 Tungsten carbide bur being used to create a smooth surface finish.

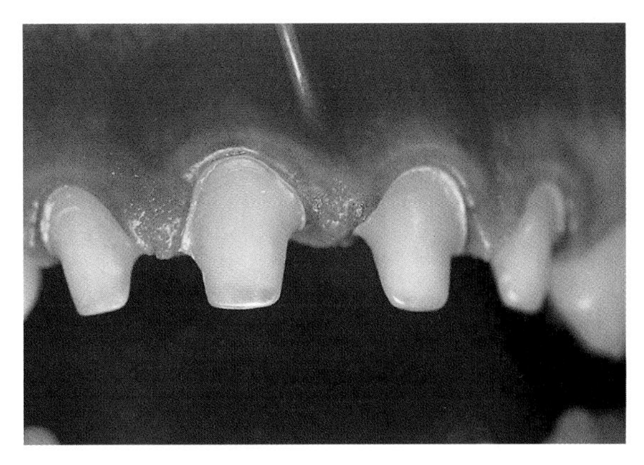

Figure 6.47 Completed tooth preparations showing distinct chamfer margins on maxillary incisors.

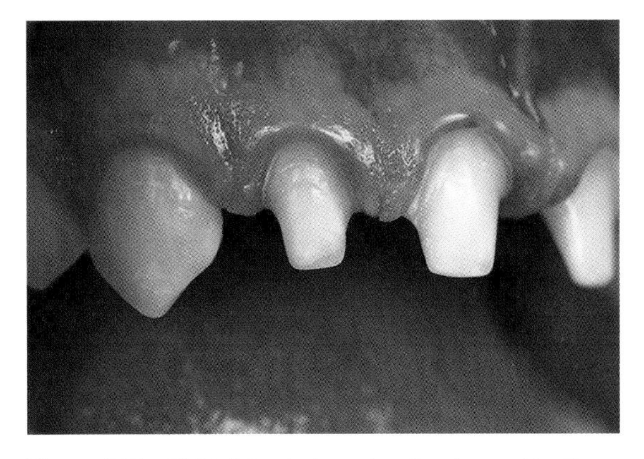

Figure 6.48 Right lateral view showing favourable tissue response following tooth preparations with sharp interdental papillae and gingival stippling.

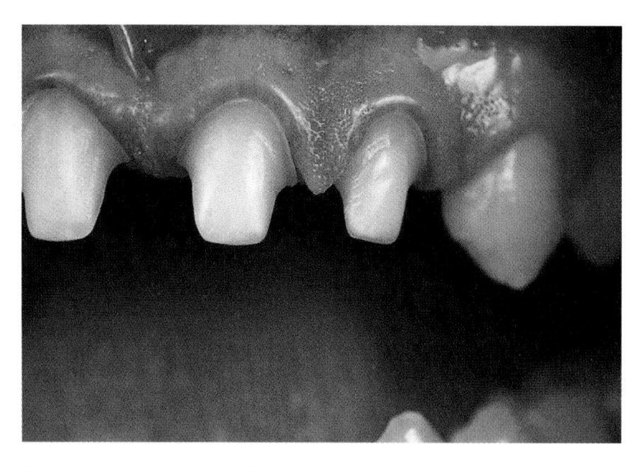

Figure 6.49 Left lateral view showing favourable tissue reaction following tooth preparations with sharp interdental papillae and gingival stippling.

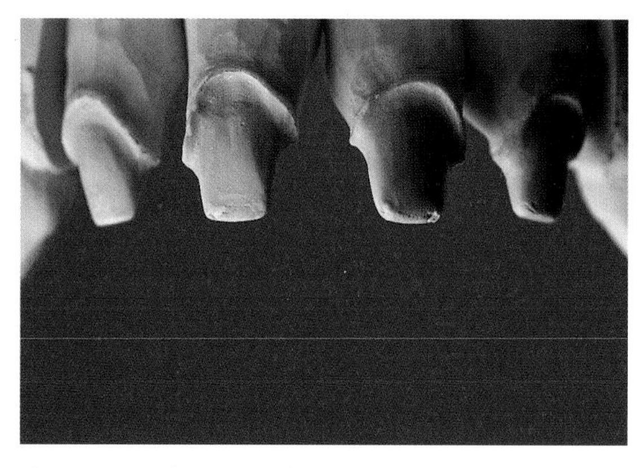

Figure 6.50 Plaster cast showing smooth preparations with sinuous outlines, devoid of undercuts.

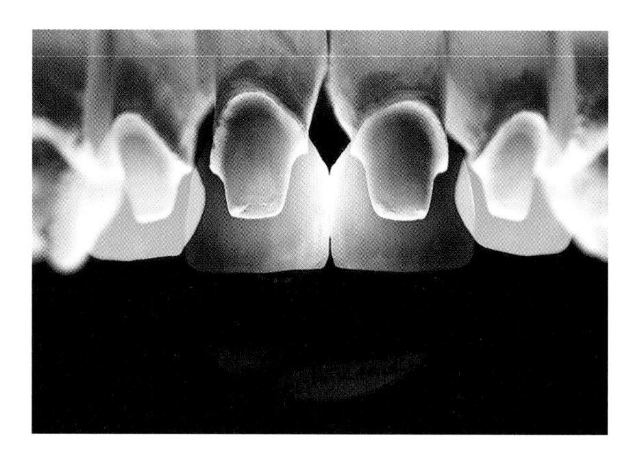

Figure 6.51 Plaster cast showing definitive crown-to-tooth preparation relationship.

Posterior tooth preparation

The following case study shows a tooth preparation sequence for an all-ceramic crown using the ATP acronym.

Assessment

(1) Heavily restored mandibular right first molar (tooth #46) (Fig. 6.52)
(2) Defective amalgam, leaky margins
(3) Sensitivity to temperature and sugary foods (vital tooth)
(4) No parafunctional habits (bruxism, etc.)
(5) No eccentric lateral or protrusive occlusal contacts.

Planning

Treatment options include:

- Replacing the amalgam – but due to decay and minimal remaining tooth structure, a direct filling would require pin retention, further weakening an already compromised tooth
- A ceramic inlay is also contra-indicated due to extensive tooth loss
- Extra-coronal restoration, e.g. metal–ceramic crown. Patient declined use of intra-oral metal
- Procera (alumina) full coverage crown for high strength (using 0.6 mm coping) and superior aesthetics.

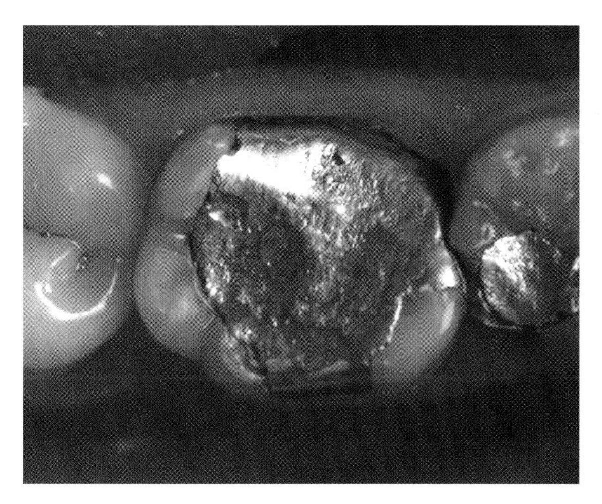

Figure 6.52 Pre-operative defective failing amalgam restoration in mandibular molar.

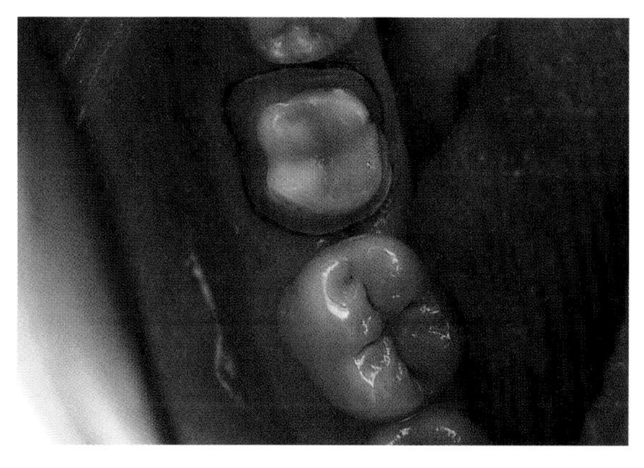

Figure 6.54 Completed tooth preparation with retraction cord in situ.

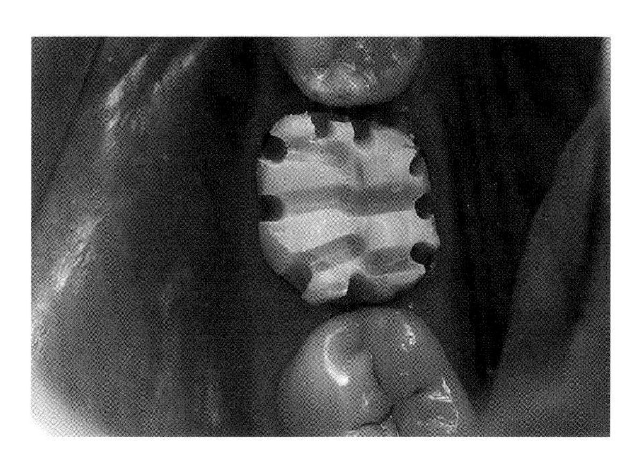

Figure 6.53 Circumferential and occlusal depth cuts in composite core build-up.

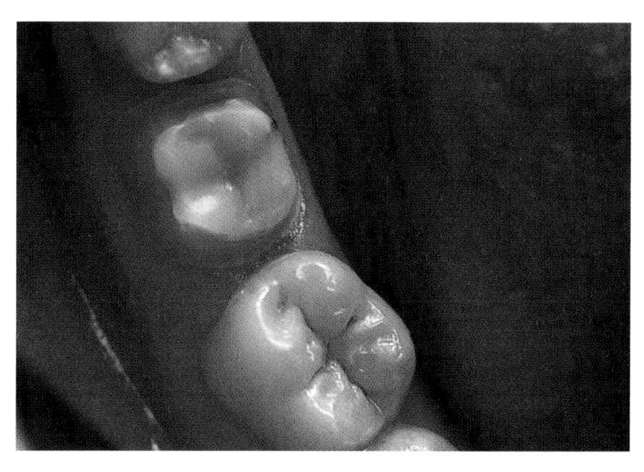

Figure 6.55 Gingival health apparent one week following tooth preparation, ready for impression making.

Treatment

(1) Remove amalgam under rubber dam isolation
(2) Build-up tooth with resin composite filling material using DBAs and intra-coronal slots and grooves for additional retention
(3) Determine sulcus depth and place retraction cord of appropriate width
(4) Use 1.6 mm chamfer bur to place depth on all aspects (Fig. 6.53)
(5) Complete tooth reduction ensuring a smooth outline, devoid of undercuts (Fig. 6.54)
(6) Protect with DBA as for anterior crowns
(7) Fabricate therapeutic temporary crown
(8) At a subsequent visit, verify gingival health before making impressions (Fig. 6.55)
(9) In the dental laboratory, using CAD/CAM Procera technology, scan die for a 0.6 mm coping
(10) Veneer coping with low fusing veneering porcelain (Fig. 6.56)
(11) At try-in bisque bake stage, check and adjust occlusal contacts (blue = working contacts, green = non-working) (Fig. 6.57)
(12) Return crown to dental laboratory for polishing and glazing
(13) Cement definitive crown (Fig. 6.58)

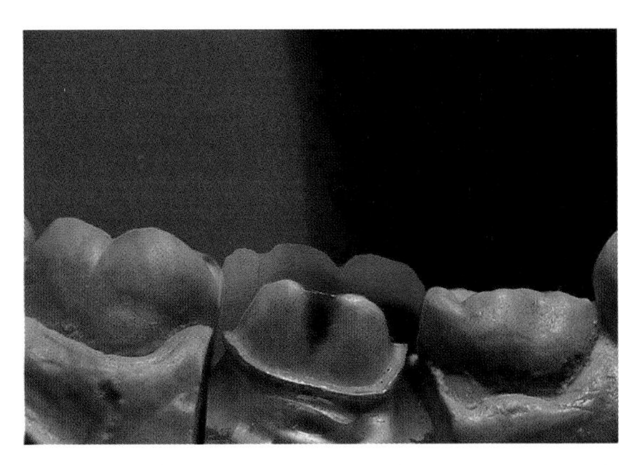

Figure 6.56 Plaster cast showing definitive crown-to-tooth preparation relationship.

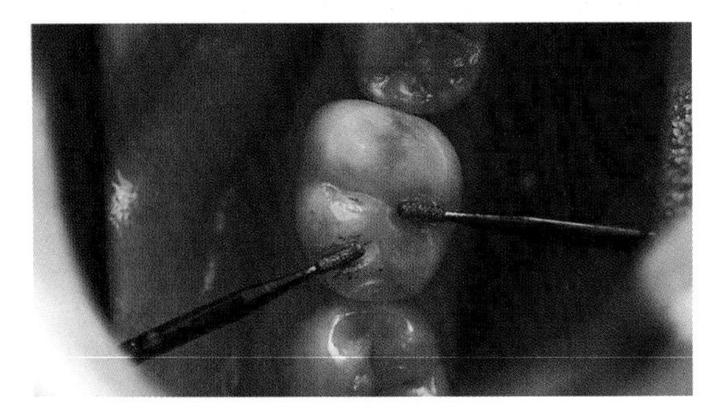

Figure 6.57 Adjusting occlusion at the bisque try-in stage.

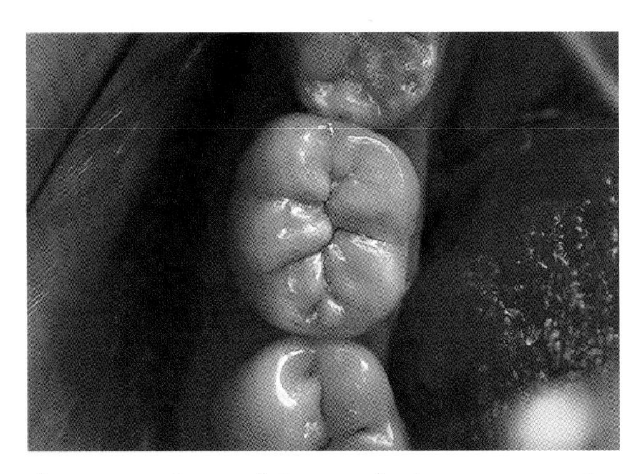

Figure 6.58 Cemented Procera alumina crown restoring health, function and aesthetics.

The final crown restores health, function and aesthetics. Furthermore, opposing tooth wear is minimised due to the low abrasive veneering porcelain.

Hints

- Hint.6.1 – If additional gingival protection and retraction are necessary, use the Zekrya gingival retractor (Dentsply) (see Fig. 6.42)

References

1. McLean, J.M. and von Frauhofer, J.A. (1971) The estimation of cement film thickness by an in vivo technique. *Br Dent J*, **131**, 107–111
2. May, K., Russel, M., Razzoog, M. and Lang, B. (1996) Precision of fit of the Procera All-Ceram crown. University of Michigan, JPD, No.4
3. West, A.J., Goodacre, C.J., Moore, B.K. and Dykema, R.W. (1985) A comparison of four techniques for fabricating collarless metal-ceramic crowns. *J Prosthet Dent*, **54**, 636–642
4. Lin, M.T., Sy-Munoz, J., Munoz, C.A., Goodacre, C.J. and Naylor, W.P. (1998) The effect of tooth preparation form on the fit of Procera copings. *Int J Prosthodont*, **11**, 580–590
5. Lang, N.P., Kiel, R.A. and Anderhalen, K. (1983) Clinical and microbiological effects of subgingival restorations with overhanging or clinically perfect margins. *J Clin Periodontol*, **10**, 563–578
6. Seymour, K.G., Taylor, M., Samarawickrama, D.Y.D. and Lynch, E. (1997) Variation in labial shoulder geometry of metal ceramic crown preparation: a finite element analysis. *Eur J Prosthodont Rest Dent*, **5**(3), 131–136
7. Bishop, K., Biggs, P. and Kelleher, M. (1996) Margin design for porcelain fused to metal restorations which extend onto root. *Br Dent J*, **180**, 177–184

[8] Burke, F.J.T. (1996) Fracture resistance of teeth restored with dentine-bonded crowns: the effect of increased tooth preparation. *Quintessence Int*, **27(2)**, 115–121

[9] Kippax, A.J., Shore, R.C. and Basker, R.M. (1996) Preparation of guide planes using a reciprocating handpiece. *Br Dent J*, **180(6)**, 216–220

[10] Kaufman, E.G., Coehlo, D.H. and Colin, L. (1961) Factors influencing the retention of cemented gold castings. *J Prosthet Dent*, **11**, 487–502

[11] Maxwell, A.W., Blank, L.W. and Pelleu, G.B. (1990) Effect of crown preparation height on the retention and resistance of gold castings. *Gen Dent*, 200–202

[12] Wiskott, H.W.A., Nicholls, J.I. and Belser, U.C. (1997) The effect of tooth preparation height and diameter on the resistance of complete crowns to fatigue loading. *Int J Prosthodont*, **10(3)**, 207–215

[13] Jensen, M.E., Sheth, J.J. and Tolliver, D. (1989) Etched-porcelain resin-bonded full-veneer crowns: in vitro fracture resistance. *Compend Contin Educ Dent*, **10**, 336–347

[14] Burke, F.J.T. and Watts, D.C. (1994) Fracture resistance of teeth restored with dentine-bonded crowns. *Quintessence Int*, **25**, 335–330

[15] Jorgensen, K.D. (1995) The relationship between retention and convergence angle in cemented veneer crowns. *Acta Odontol Scand*, **13**, 35–40

[16] Hegdahl, T. and Silness, J. (1997) Preparation areas resisting displacement of artificial crowns. *J Oral Rehabil*, **4**, 201–207

[17] Parker, M.H., Gunderson, R.B., Gardner, F.M. and Calverley, M.J. (1988) Quantitative determination of taper adequate to provide resistance form: concept of limiting taper. *J Prosthet Dent*, **59**, 281–288

[18] Malament, K.A. and Socransky, S.S. (1999) Survival of Dicor glass-ceramic dental restorations over 14 years. Part II: effect of thickness of Dicor material and design of tooth preparation. *J Prosthet Dent*, **81**, 662–667

[19] Bergenholtz, G. and Nyman, S. (1984) Endontic complications following periodontal and prosthetic treatment of patients with advanced periodontal disease. *J Periodontol*, **55**, 63–68

[20] Spiering, T.A., Peters, M.C. and Plasschaert, A.J. (1985) Thermal trauma to teeth. *Endod Dent Truamatol*, **1**, 123–129

[21] (1995) Fixed prosthodontics, avoiding pulp death. *Clin Res Assoc Newsletter*, **19(1)**, 1

[22] Ottal, P. and Lauer, H.-C. (1998) Temperature response in the pulpal chamber during ultra-high-speed tooth preparation with diamond burs of different grit. *J Prosthet Dent*, **80**, 12–19

[23] Xu, H.H.K., Kelly, J.R., Jahanmir, S., Thompson, V.P. and Rekow, E.D. (1997) Enamel subsurface damage due to tooth preparation with diamonds. *J Dent Res*, **76(10)**, 1698–1706

[24] Smith, B.G. (1970) The effect of the surface roughness of prepared dentine on the retention of castings. *J Prosthet Dent*, **23**, 187–197

[25] Ayad, M.F., Rosenstiel, S.F. and Salama, M. (1997) Influence of tooth surface roughness and type of cement on retention of complete cast crowns. *J Prosthet Dent*, **77**, 116–121

[26] Darveniza, M., Basford, K.E., Meek, J. and Stevens, L. (1987) The effect of surface roughness and surface area on the retention of crowns luted with zinc phosphate cement. *Aust Dent J*, **32**, 446–457

[27] Smyd, E.S. (1952) Dental engineering applied to inlay and fixed bridge fabrication. *J Prosthet Dent*, **2**, 536–542

[28] Tuntiprawon, M. (1999) Effect of tooth surface roughness on marginal seating and retention of complete metal crowns. *J Prosthet Dent*, **81**, 142–147

[29] Bertschinger, C., Paul, S.C., Luthy, H. and Scharer, P. (1996) Dual application of dentine bonding agents: effect on bond strength. *Am J Dent*, **9**, 115–119

[30] Paul, S.J. and Scharer, P. (1997) The dual bonding technique: a modified method to improve adhesive luting procedure. *Int J Periodontics Restorative Dent*, **17**, 536–545

[31] Siegel, S.C. and von Fraunhofer, J.A. (1996) Assessing the cutting efficiency of dental burs. *J Am Dent Assoc*, **127**, 763–772

[32] Eames, W.B. and Nale N.L. (1973) A comparison of cutting efficiency of air-driven fissure burs. *J Am Dent Assoc*, **86**, 412–415

[33] Siegel, S.C. and von Fraunhofer, J.A. (1999) Dental cutting with diamond burs: heavy-handed or light touch. *J Prosthod*, 8, 3–9

[34] Magne, P. and Belser, U. (2002) Immediate dentin bonding. In: *Bonded Porcelain Restorations in the Anterior Dentition – A Biomimetic Approach*. pp. 270–273. Quintessence, Berlin

7 Therapeutic temporary restorations

Introduction

Many synonyms are used to describe temporary restorations, including provisional, interim, prototype, non-permanent, transitional, pro-temp, short-term or disposable. The terminology is subjective, but the salient point is that a temporary restoration is not perceived as a stopgap, awaiting delivery of the final restoration or prosthesis. On the contrary, a temporary should be utilised to foresee, and correct potential problems so that aberrations are not incorporated into, or jeopardise, the permanent restoration. Consequently, a temporary, besides longevity and colour, is essentially identical to its definitive counterpart. Furthermore, an appropriate description of this restoration is *therapeutic*, since at this stage all pathology is resolved for attaining health and a stable environment prior to fitting the permanent unit(s). This implies achieving health and stability of both hard and soft tissues *before*, not *after* fitting the definitive restoration.

SCIENTIFIC RATIONALE

As discussed in Chapter 2, the requisite of a dental restoration is sequentially achieving health, function and aesthetics (HFA triad), and the therapeutic temporary restoration (TTR) is no exception. By definition, the first requirement of a TTR is retrievability, for access to the underlying prepared abutment and surrounding hard or soft tissues, for carrying out further treatment. The discussion below starts with the HFA triad, and then highlights requirements of a TTR.

Health

The primary objective of any therapy is establishing and maintaining health. In the case of a temporary restoration, its remedial role is not limited to the health of the prepared tooth substrate, but also to the surrounding periodontal

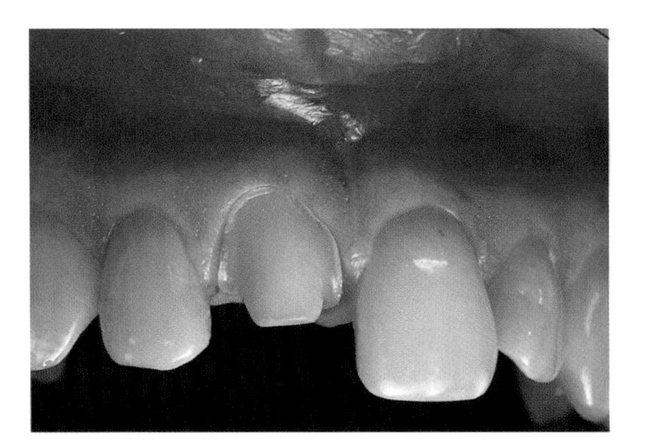

Figure 7.1 Ideal tooth preparation with adequate resistance and retention, smooth surface finish and a sinuous outline.

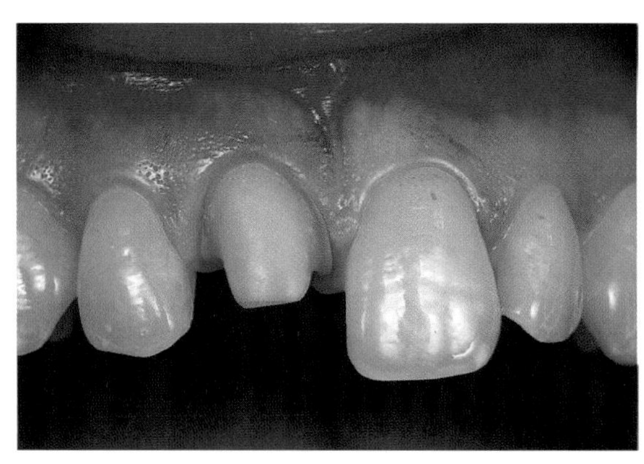

Figure 7.2 Healthy periodontal tissue around prepared tooth with knife-edge FGM and stippling of the attached gingiva.

tissues and adjacent and opposing dentition. For vital teeth, pulpal protection is essential, while for endodontically treated teeth, a coronal seal is crucial for preventing microleakage and subsequent ingress of microorganisms into the root canal and periapical regions. A hermetic seal of the temporary crown with the abutment is therefore essential.

The first item to scrutinise is tooth preparation, including retention, resistance, sinuous outline, absence of undercuts, parallelism, convergence angle and surface roughness (Fig. 7.1). Next, endodontic evaluation is carried out, which may necessitate initial or re-root canal therapy to rectify a defective root canal filling, apicectomy, intra-radicular support and subsequent core build-up, or extracting a tooth with poor prognosis with subsequent implant replacement.

Marginal integrity is also essential for achieving periodontal health; this is dependent on a correct emergence profile and appropriate crown morphology conducive for oral hygiene procedures. Modifications are carried out, and oral hygiene reinforced until inflammation is resolved resulting in a coral colour appearance of the periodontium with knife-edge free gingival margins and stippling of the attached gingiva (Fig. 7.2). Stability of the gingival architecture is essential before impressions are attempted. If gingival hypertrophy is evident, soft tissue resection and/or alterations to the temporaries are indicated. Alternatively, gingival recession requires modifications of the tooth preparation for subgingival margin concealment. This is especially relevant when crown lengthening or tissue grafts are performed concurrently with tooth preparation. In instances where biologic width violation is suspected, the appropriate treatment should be performed, such as orthodontic extrusion or osseous resection. In cases when an edentulous ridge requires surgical intervention for creating an ovate pontic site, healing is confirmed by epithelialisation of the area (Figs. 7.3 & 7.4), and, where necessary, periodontal plastic surgery

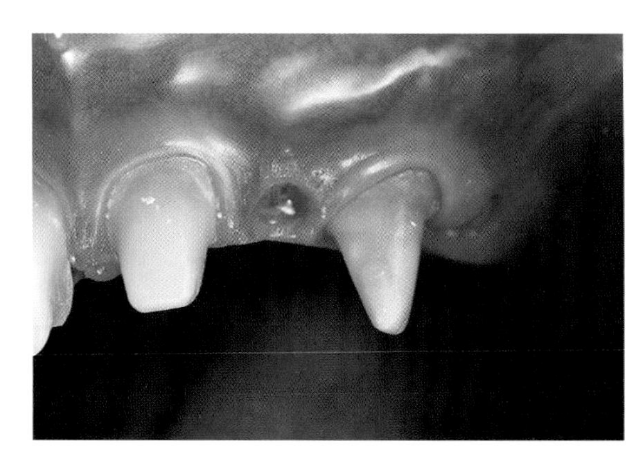

Figure 7.3 Ovate pontic created for missing lateral incisor.

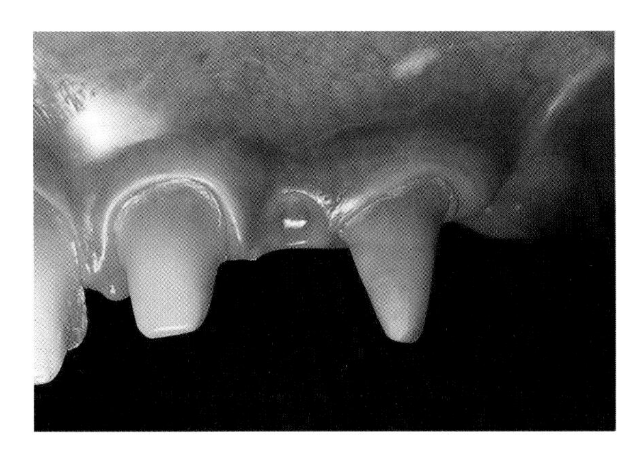

Figure 7.4 Tissue sculpturing with an acrylic therapeutic temporary restoration (bridge) 3 weeks later, showing epithelialisation of the ovate pontic site (compare with Figure 7.3).

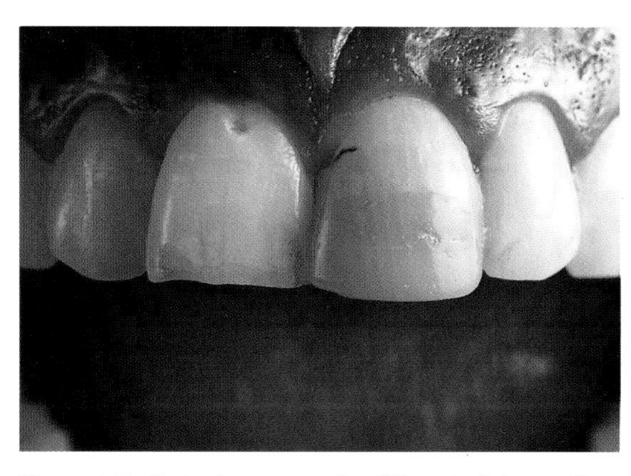

Figure 7.5 Defective composite filling in left maxillary central incisor.

and/or adjustments to the temporary pontic are made accordingly. Finally, splinting temporary crowns reduces mobility, pending periodontal therapy or extractions.

Function

A temporary restoration is an invaluable tool for assessing, maintaining or alerting occlusal and phonetic aberrations. This is particularly relevant when the abutment tooth makes initial contact in centric relation, is a guiding tooth, a working or non-working contact, when the occlusal scheme is changed or the vertical dimension is altered. Furthermore, mandibular function is verified for lateral and protrusive (anterior guidance) contacts, as well as freedom of movement and masticatory function. The temporary should not inadvertently cause pressure on adjacent or opposing teeth, causing unwanted orthodontic movement or occlusal trauma, respectively. Besides occlusion, speech impediments are also easily modified by removal or addition to the temporary, avoiding costly and time-consuming post-operative remakes. For a detailed occlusal and phonetic assessment, see Chapter 2.

Aesthetics

Many clinicians advocate, and expend enormous clinical time, creating nuances in colour and characterisations for a temporary prosthesis. The underlying premise of this onerous task is gaining instant patient gratification, and indirectly marketing the practice to the patients' family, friends and colleagues. Whilst matching the basic shade of the temporary restoration so that it is inconspicuous is essential, spending enormous clinical time creating nuances in colour and characterisation should be resisted. The reasons are as follows. Firstly, colour and characterisations are almost impossible to determine accurately with temporary restorations because the optical properties of the materials used for temporary and definitive restorations are dissimilar. Secondly, the physical properties of acrylics and porcelains vary enormously with respect to wear, staining, plaque accumulation, surface texture and roughness, which affect light interactions and hence appearance. Therefore, the time spent refining colour can be better utilised for aesthetic items that can be incorporated into the definitive restorations, such as form and shape (Figs. 7.5–7.8).

Morphological variations are the aesthetic items, which can and should be assessed during

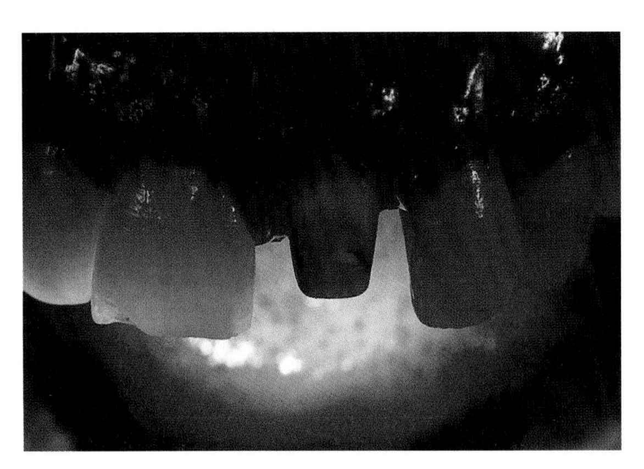

Figure 7.6 Tooth preparation for patient in Figure 7.5.

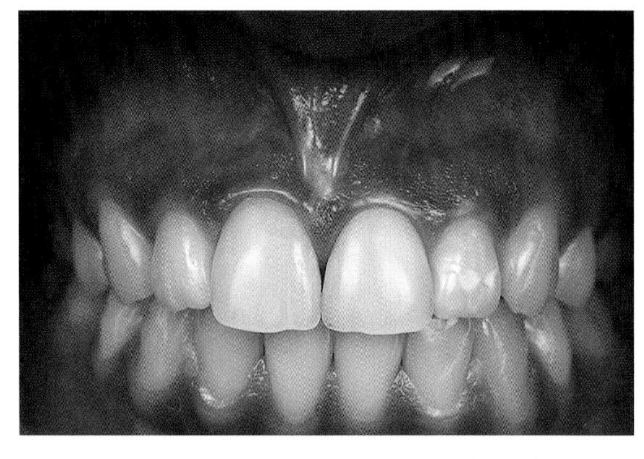

Figure 7.9 The contact point is too coronal to allow complete papilla fill between the temporary crowns on the maxillary centrals.

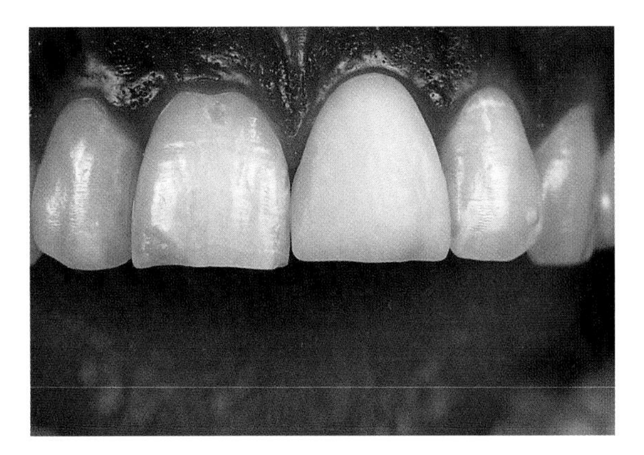

Figure 7.7 Chairside therapeutic temporary restoration on left central is shorter than contralateral central incisor.

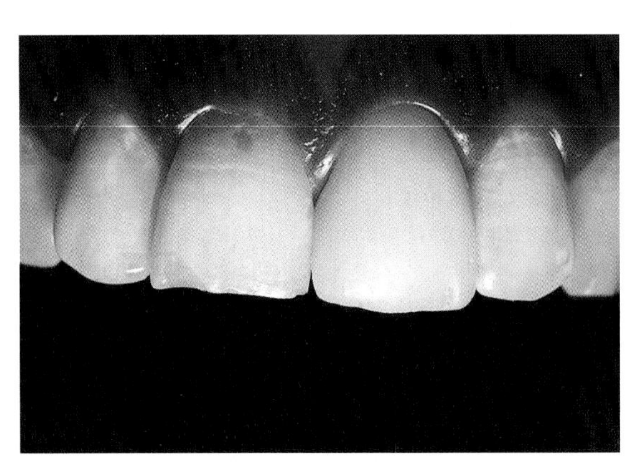

Figure 7.8 Addition of acrylic resin to finalise shape, which will act as a template for the definitive all-ceramic crown.

the temporarisation stage. These include intra-oral and extra-oral relationships. The intra-oral factors include the general shape of the tooth determined by the dental bioform or degree of gingival scallop (triangular, oval or square), contact points to ensure extent of papillary fill (Fig. 7.9), incisal embrasure angles, degree of facial and palatal contours, diastemae, imbrications, axial inclination, sagittal inclination and horizontal and vertical overbites.

The extra-oral relationships are tooth exposure (incisal edge position) during a relaxed and exaggerated smile, dental midline location, lip support and parallelism of the incisal plane to the interpupillary line and curvature of the mandibular lip (Figs. 7.10–7.12). Another issue is incorporation of patient's wishes, which are addressed at this stage (Figs. 7.13–7.17). Once these factors are finalised, an impression is made of the temporary crowns in situ, serving as a template and communication tool for liaising with the ceramist during fabrication of the definitive prosthesis.

When pre-prosthetic orthodontic movement is necessary, temporary restorations are used for assessing gingival contour and contact points for interproximal papilla fill, thus eliminating unsightly open gingival embrasures or 'black triangles'. In addition, following orthodontic movement, it is essential to confirm tooth and related gingival contour in three dimensions:

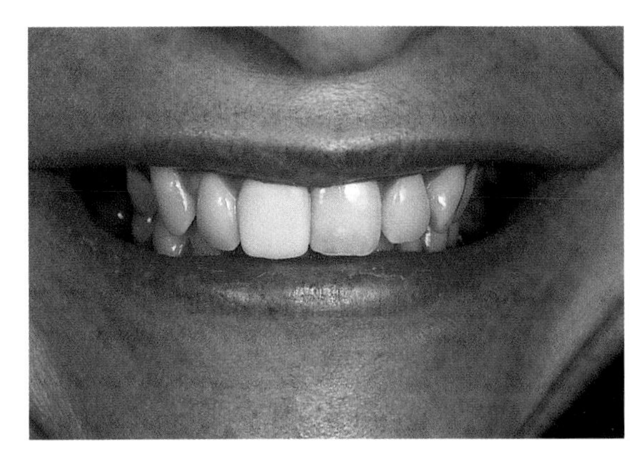

Figure 7.10 Frontal dentofacial view of temporary crown on right maxillary central to assess incisal edge position.

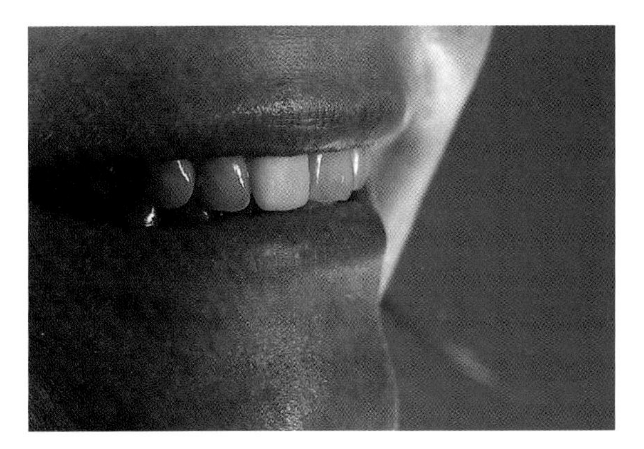

Figure 7.11 Lateral dentofacial view of temporary crown on right maxillary central to assess incisal edge position.

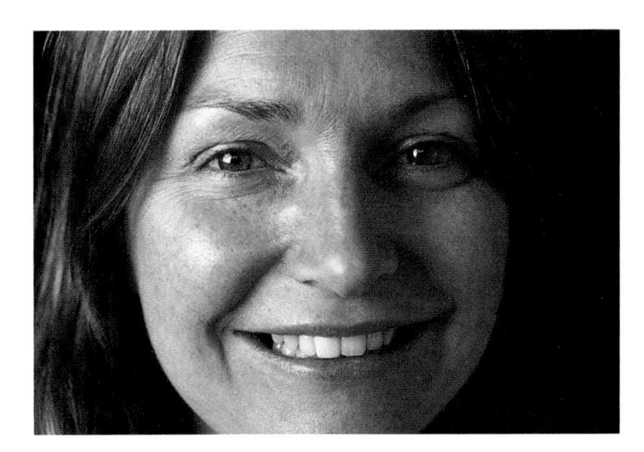

Figure 7.12 Facial view of temporary crown on right maxillary central to assess incisal edge position.

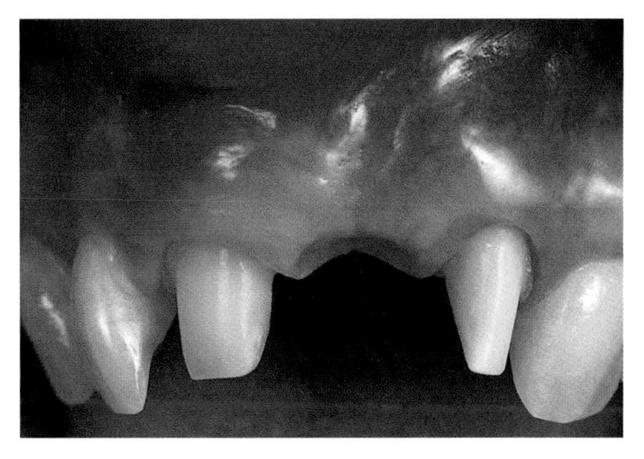

Figure 7.13 Tooth preparation for a three-unit FPD, abutments right maxillary central incisor and left lateral incisor, with ovate pontic for missing left central.

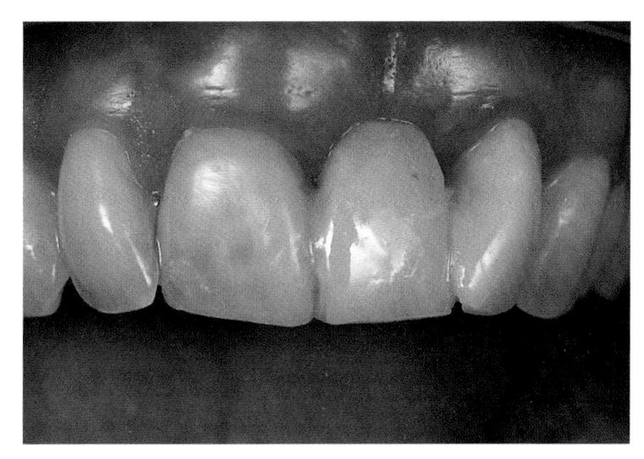

Figure 7.14 One of four sets of acrylic temporary bridges used to finalise aesthetics, before proceeding to the definitive bridge for the patient in Figure 7.13.

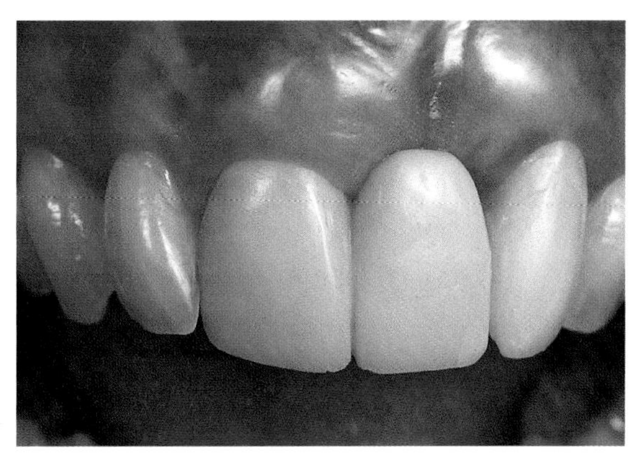

Figure 7.15 One of four sets of acrylic temporary bridges used to finalise aesthetics, before proceeding to the definitive bridge for the patient in Figure 7.13.

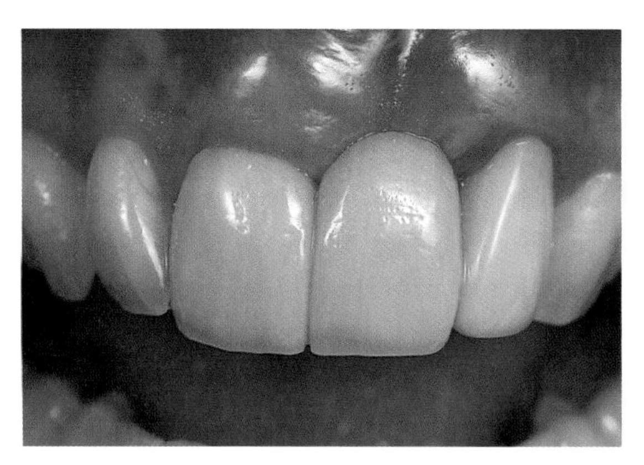

Figure 7.16 One of four sets of acrylic temporary bridges used to finalise aesthetics, before proceeding to the definitive bridge for the patient in Figure 7.13.

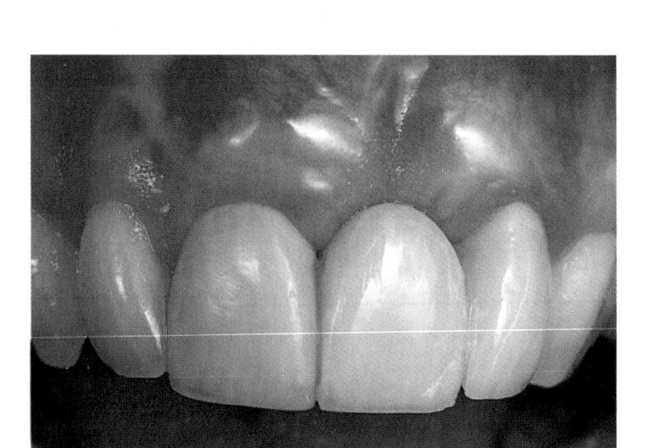

Figure 7.17 One of four sets of acrylic temporary bridges used to finalise aesthetics, before proceeding to the definitive bridge for the patient in Figure 7.13.

apico-coronal, mesio-distal and sagittal (bucco-lingual) planes.

Aesthetics is not solely limited to the prostheses. The contour, position, colour and texture of the surrounding gingival architecture are prerequisite for aesthetic appraisal. Temporary restorations, as well as achieving and maintaining periodontal health, are used to sculpture soft tissues, greatly influencing the so-called 'pink aesthetics' (Figs. 7.18–7.20).

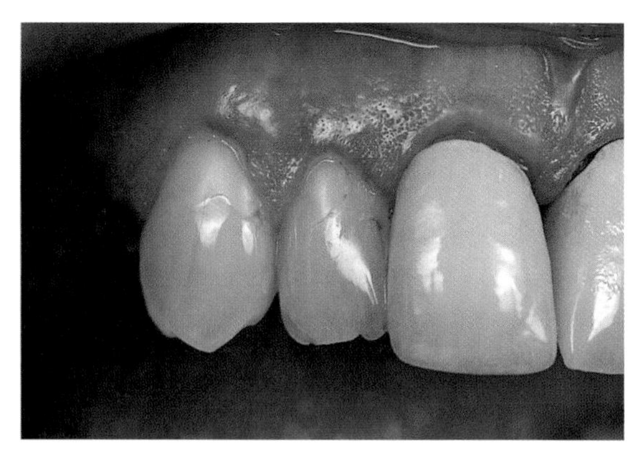

Figure 7.18 Defective metal–ceramic crowns on maxillary central incisors, with traumatised, amorphous FGMs.

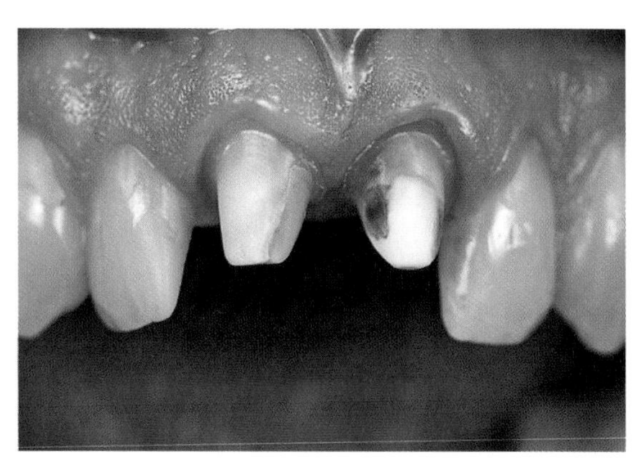

Figure 7.19 Following tooth preparations and fabricating therapeutic temporary restorations, gingival health is established, with gingival zeniths distal to the long axes of the central incisors (compare with Figure 7.18).

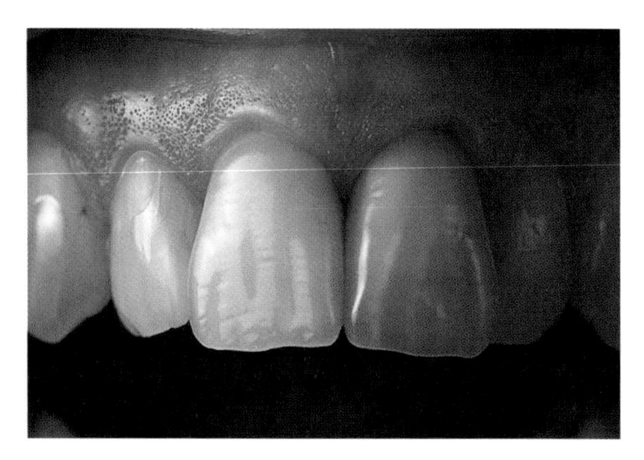

Figure 7.20 Definitive crowns for patient in Figures 7.18 and 7.19 showing impeccable aesthetics and integration of the prostheses in a harmonious co-existence with the periodontium.

Biocompatibility

Any material used in the oral cavity should be biocompatible and non-cytotoxic to vital tissues. The potentially hazardous constituent in polymer-based temporary crown and bridge materials is the unreacted free monomer, which causes pulpal and gingival irritation. Consequently, complete polymerisation is crucial to avoid traces of this residual monomer. Using heat and pressure accelerates the setting reaction and ensures it is complete.

Strength

The biomechanical properties of temporary restorations, such as adequate rigidity and resilience, are essential for resisting occlusal and masticatory forces, ensuring the restoration survives until the delivery of the definitive prosthesis. Most proprietary products display unique mechanical properties; even materials in a given generic class vary enormously, making comparisons a daunting task.[1] Hence, every product should be individually evaluated for suitability. The properties, which are discussed below include flexural strength, modulus of rupture, MOE, microhardness and fracture toughness. In order to increase the strength of temporary materials, numerous reinforcement fillers have been suggested, such as metals, glass, carbon and nylon fibres. While these increase the MOE, it is crucial that a viable bond exists between the matrix and reinforcement inclusion. If not, the filler acts as an inclusion body weakening the material. Also, when a resin is reinforced with fibres, the later should be totally immersed within the matrix. Any protruding fibres are difficult to polish, and attract food debris, encouraging bacterial colonisation. Finally, repairing a broken restoration drastically weakens the material. For example, bis-acryl materials exhibit as much as 85% reduction in strength compared with the initial intact restoration.[2]

Palliative

Palliation of the underlying tooth abutment is achieved, firstly, by protecting the exposed dentine with DBAs following tooth preparation, thereby mitigating post-operative sensitivity, and secondly, by preventing pulpal pathosis from the exothermic setting reaction of temporary crown materials.

Tooth preparation is a surgical procedure of hard dental tissues, resulting in exposed dentine tubules. If this naked dentine remains patent and unprotected, post-operative sensitivity is a common sequel causing distress and discomfort to the patient. The experienced sensitivity is explained by Brannstrom's hydrodynamic theory. This stipulates that fluid movement in the dentine tubules and the pulp chamber stimulates nerve endings which manifests as pain.[3] The situation is compounded further by bacterial invasion or toxin irritation due to microleakage. Consequently, in order to minimise these hydrodynamic changes and prevent microleakage, the dentine tubules require either sealing or blocking.

Tooth preparation with diamond burs produces a thicker smear layer compared to using steel burs. The reason is that diamonds remove enamel and dentine by a grinding action, creating more debris. Conversely, steel burs have a cutting action, which results in a thinner smear layer. The first step for dentine sealing is removing the smear layer. The most predictable method is by using a fifth generation DBA, sequentially etching with phosphoric acid, followed by priming and sealing the dentine with an adhesive resin to form the hybrid layer. Alternately the entire process, etching, priming and sealing, can be carried out using sixth or seventh generation, self-etching, all-in-one DBA (Fig. 7.21). These DBAs are relatively new, and their efficacy is unconfirmed by long-term clinical data. Which ever BDA is chosen, it is important that it contains a dentine desensitiser and disinfectant such as glutaraldehyde, e.g. Gluma (Heraeus Kulzer, Hanau, Germany). Rather than sealing, another method is blocking dentine tubules, thereby preventing hydrodynamic fluid movement. Products

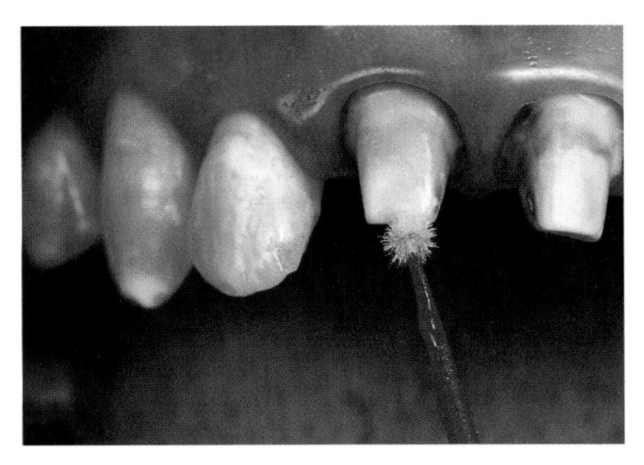

Figure 7.21 Application of a DBA immediately after tooth preparation.

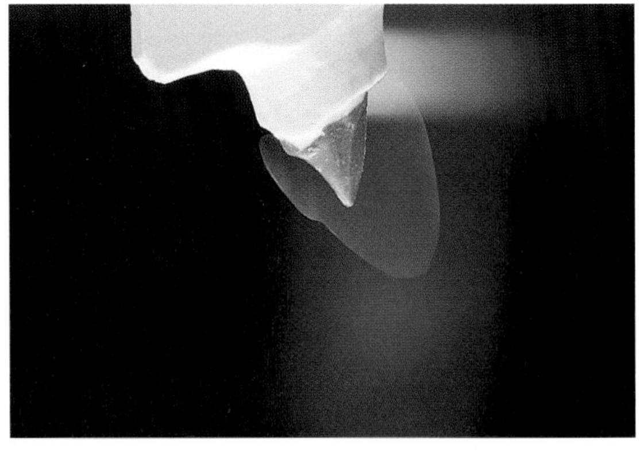

Figure 7.22 A large MO is evident at the palatal margin of this bulbous crown.

used for this technique include BisBlock (Bisco, Il, USA), which forms oxalate crystals within the tubules, halting fluid movement and alleviating post-operative sensitivity.

Most materials used for fabrication of temporary restorations polymerise by an exothermic reaction. The temperature rise during the setting reaction of different materials varies from 4.4–48°C, attributed to not only the exothermic reaction but also the energy absorbed during irradiation of light-cured resins.[4] In a seminal study on rhesus monkeys, a temperature elevation of 5.5°C resulted in 15% irreversible pulpal damage, an 11°C increase in 60% damage and a 16.6°C increase in 100% pulpal necrosis.[5] Therefore, the critical threshold for pulpal damage, which may be immediate or prolonged, is a temperature increase of 5.5°C. The temperature increase of intra-oral temporary crown materials ranges from 4–11°C, precarious to pulpal health. Consequently, it is imperative to minimise temperature rises during fabrication to safeguard pulp vitality.

The factors contributing to thermal insulation are the thickness of remaining dentine barrier,[6] the hybrid layer width, the size of DBA adhesive layer and luting or cement base.[7] The thickness of the hybrid layer (0.5–10 µm) and the overlying adhesive layer (5–10 µm) are inadequate for preventing thermal insult. Furthermore, while sealing dentine tubules with a DBA alleviates sensitivity and retards bacterial ingress, it offers little thermal protection.[8] Finally, intra-pulpal and periodontal blood supplies also dissipate temperature increases by heat convection.

To summarise, the clinically pertinent points to mitigate intra-pulpal temperature rise are material selection, material volume, type of matrix form and fabrication technique.

Marginal integrity

Obtaining a hermetic seal of the temporary restoration with the prepared teeth prevents microleakage, retards bacterial ingress that causes post-operative sensitivity, secondary caries, endodontic embarrassment, periodontal inflammation and leaching of provisional cements.

The average clinically accepted norm for marginal opening (MO) of definitive restorations is 50 µm, and a similar accuracy is desirable for a temporary crown (Fig. 7.22).[9] The MO is dependent on the intrinsic properties of the material and fabrication techniques. The major factor affecting MO is polymerisation shrinkage, apparent with most polymer-based temporary crown materials. The mean MO for temporary resin materials ranges from 24–120 µm, indicating that material selection is essential to minimise the potential restorative/tooth interface opening.[10] Polymerisation shrinkage is time and temperature dependent. The majority of shrinkage of polymer-based materials occurs in the first 5–10 minutes after mixing, a period which is crucial during fabrication of temporary restorations. Additionally, elevated ambient temperatures increase the speed, rather than the magnitude of polymerisation shrinkage-strain. The magnitude of shrinkage is dependent on factors such as filler volume (high filler equates to low shrinkage), filler particle size, amount and type of monomer, modes of polymerisation and delayed water sorption.[11] The clinical relevance is that the polymerisation should be completed within 10 minutes of mixing, and familiarity of the handling characteristics of a specific material will circumvent unwanted shrinkage.

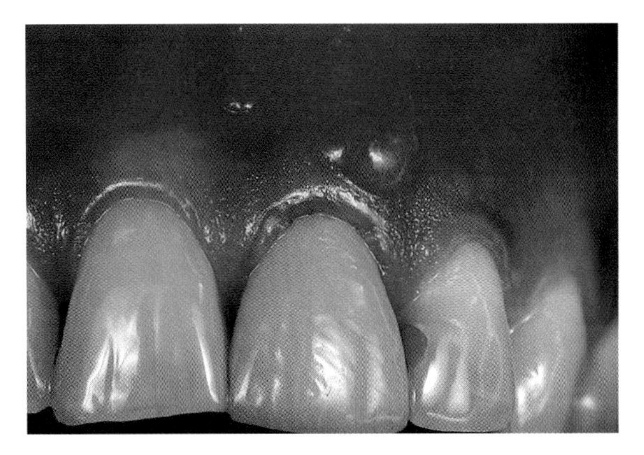

Figure 7.23 Marginal inflammation and periodontal abscess associated with defective crown margins of prosthesis on left central incisor.

Preventing plaque accumulation

The major causative factor for gingival inflammation is plaque accumulation, and this is influenced by the artificial restoration and the patient's oral hygiene regime. Combined, these two factors determine whether gingival health is possible and prolonged.[12] The criteria affecting plaque accumulation on a temporary restoration are marginal integrity, surface roughness, emergence profile and overall shape and form of the provisional, which should be conducive for deflecting food and bacteria.

Following prophylaxis, a natural tooth soon forms a biofilm composed of salivary glycoproteins. This pellicle promotes bacterial colonisation, and, if allowed to mature, becomes pathogenic. Plaque accumulation is more abundant on artificial restorations compared with enamel and dentine.[13] Consequently, the potential for periodontal inflammation with artificial prostheses is elevated. The reason for this is pronounced plaque adhesion due to rough surfaces such as defective margins, cement remnants and surface irregularities (Fig. 7.23). In addition, methods of polishing also affect the degree of accumulation. Methods of decreasing plaque accumulation are contouring with aluminum oxide discs or steel burs, pumice abrasion, polishing with silicone tips and surface sealing with an unfilled resin. For example, using a surface sealant, such as Biscover (Bisco, Il, USA), devoid of an oxygen inhibition layer, seals superficial irregularities following the finishing and polishing procedures.

The overall contour and form of a crown should be curvaceous, free of sharp line angles and free of microscopic grooves, with a smooth microtopography, helping deflect food particles and discouraging plaque adhesion. A favourable contour also facilitates cleansability and oral hygiene regimes.

Lastly, the emergence profile (EP) also influences gingival health.[14] The EP of a restoration is the cervical part, which meets the tooth apical to the preparation finish line. This tooth/restorative interface should ideally lie on a tangent (Fig. 7.24). The EP should be linear in both the vertical and horizontal planes. A vertically under-contoured margin creates a niche for bacteria, causing inflammation or caries (Figs. 7.25–7.28), whereas a vertically over-contoured margin violates the biologic width. In the horizontal plane, an under-contour results in an unsupported, flaccid FGM harbouring bacteria, inaccessible to prophylactic measures, while a horizontal over-contour causes inflammation and restricts complete temporary cement removal due to limited accessibility (Figs. 7.29–7.31).

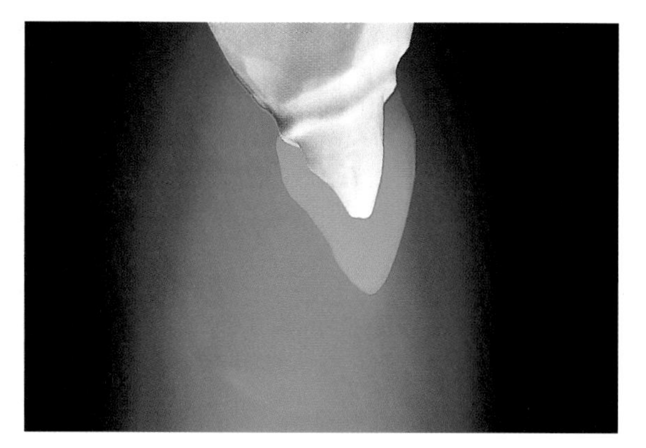

Figure 7.24 Emergence profile of crown should lie on a tangent with the root surface apical to the finish line.

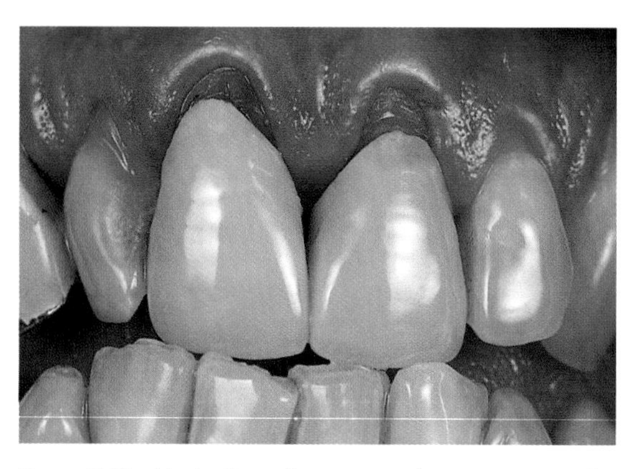

Figure 7.25 Vertically under-contoured crown case study: the vertically under-contoured crowns of the maxillary centrals are a potential niche for bacteria.

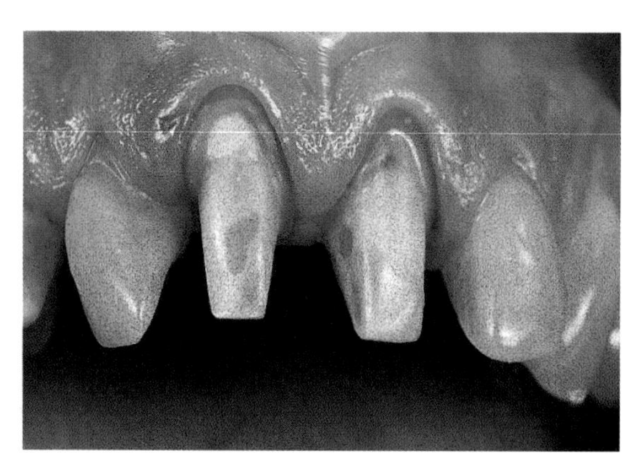

Figure 7.26 Vertically under-contoured crown case study: tooth preparations with correctly located crown margins.

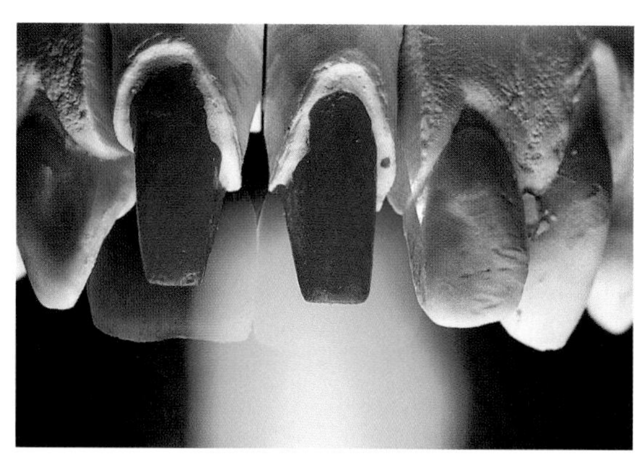

Figure 7.27 Vertically under-contoured crown case study: definitive crown-to-preparation relationship.

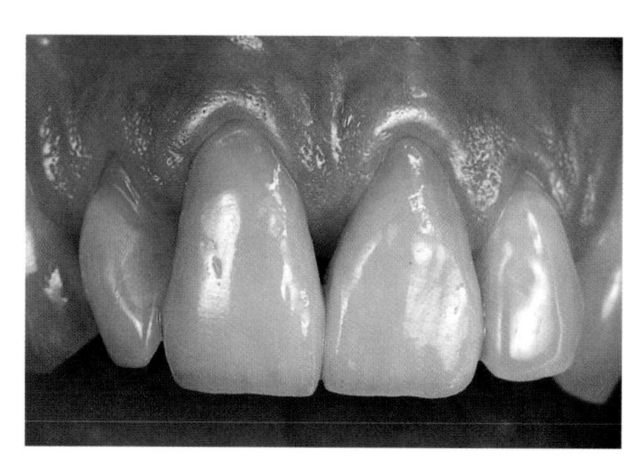

Figure 7.28 Vertically under-contoured crown case study: cemented Empress 1 crowns with correct emergence profiles (laboratory work by David Korson, UK).

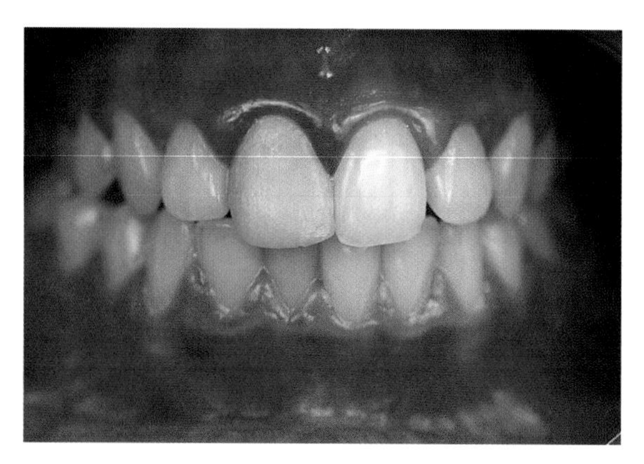

Figure 7.29 Horizontally over-contoured crown case study: gross marginal inflammation around horizontally over-contoured temporary crown on right maxillary central incisor.

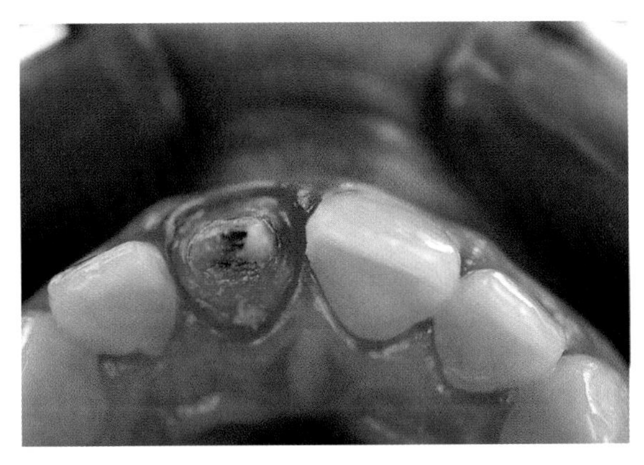

Figure 7.30 Horizontally over-contoured crown case study: crown removal shows circumferential halo indicating that crown margins are resting on marginal gingiva, not on the prepared tooth.

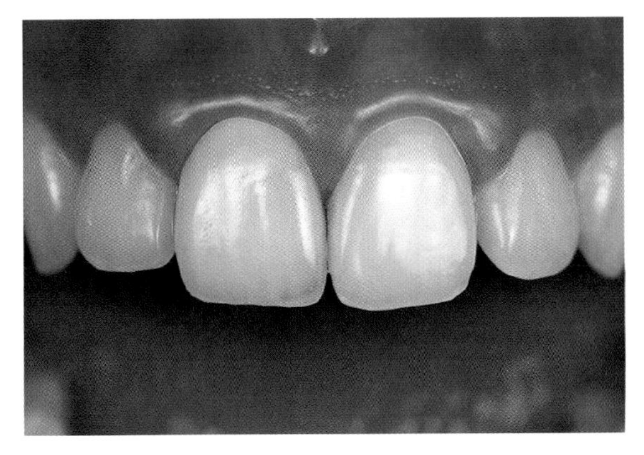

Figure 7.31 Horizontally over-contoured crown case study: replacement definitive Empress 1 crown with a correct emergence profile, allowing gingival health to be established (laboratory work by David Korson, UK).

Chromatic stability

As previously stated, it is unwise and futile attempting to ascertain the correct shade with a temporary restoration. Most temporary materials are chromatically unstable due to porosity, surface roughness, plaque accumulation, staining, incomplete polymerisation and absorption of oral fluids. Therefore, whilst it is aesthetically desirable to fabricate a provisional whose colour approximates to adjacent natural dentition, it is inadvisable to use this prototype as a guide for the shade of the final restoration (Fig. 7.32).

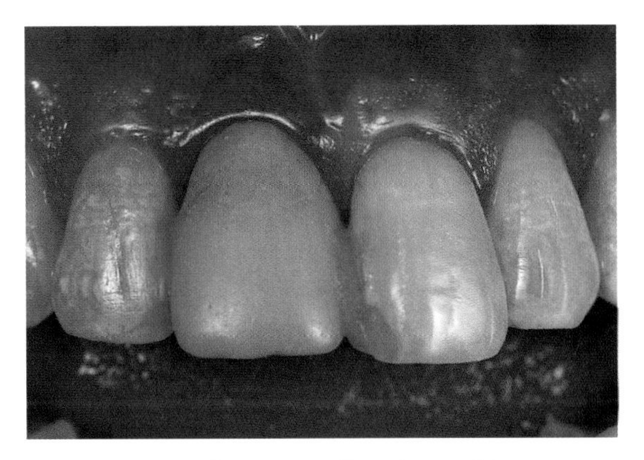

Figure 7.32 Acrylic resin readily stains, and is not appropriate for shade analysis for the definite prosthesis, as shown by the discoloured temporary crown on the right maxillary central incisor.

Handling characteristics and ease of fabrication

Clinical manipulation of a temporary restorative material is essential to expedite fabrication. Each material is unique with regard to handling characteristics and this necessitates modification of clinical techniques for optimal and consistent results. Even within a given generic class, proprietary materials often display erratic characteristics that are specific to a given product. Material selection therefore becomes essential for ensuring that the requirements discussed above are satisfied.

Material selection

Numerous factors influence the selection of materials for a temporary restoration, including the anticipated duration of the prosthesis, aesthetics, occlusal loads, repairability, ease of manipulation, number of units and whether adjunct treatment is required, e.g. orthodontic, periodontal or endodontic. No single material satisfies all criteria, and, in many instances, a compromise is necessary. Alternatively, combinations of materials can be used for fabricating temporary restorations, exploiting beneficial properties of different generic classes of products. Most materials used for making temporary crowns and bridges are resin based, which are chemical-, light- or dual-cured. For ease of handling, many are available in dispensing cartridges ensuring consistency of mix and disposability. The list below discusses some contemporary materials, citing advantages and limitations, and their suitability for specific clinical scenarios.

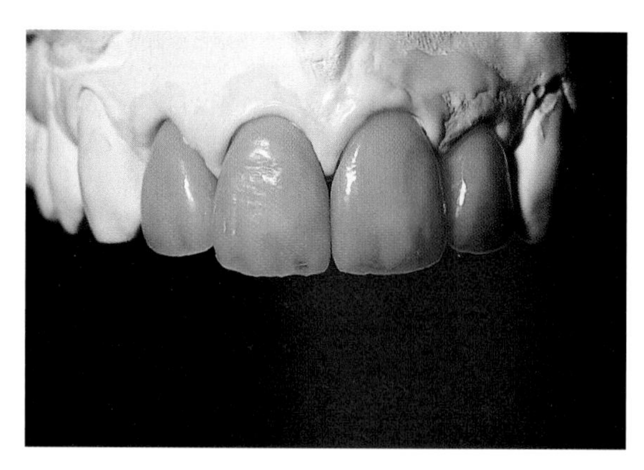

Figure 7.33 Laboratory-fabricated acrylic crowns for maxillary incisors.

Polymethyl methacrylate (PMMA)

Most indirect temporary restorations are fabricated using this generic class of materials. They are the oldest acrylics used in dentistry, and were once advocated for definitive restorations, either alone, or with a metal substructure. The laboratory process of heat and pressure curing also enhances the physical and mechanical properties. Hence, the main advantages are good mechanical properties, e.g. flexural strength and fracture toughness and excellent aesthetics.[15] The disadvantages are a highly exothermic setting reaction, making intra-oral use prohibitive. In addition, the residual monomer is a pulpal irritant, while pronounced polymerisation shrinkage compromises margin integrity. To negate these undesirable properties, PMMAs are used in small volumes to minimise shrinkage, e.g. PMMA shells made in the dental laboratory, which are subsequently filled and relined with polyvinyl ethylmethacrylates (PVEMAs) directly on the prepared tooth abutment. This procedure exploits the strength and aesthetics of PMMAs, while overcoming the shortfalls of polymerisation shrinkage for a superior marginal seal (Figs. 7.33 & 7.34).

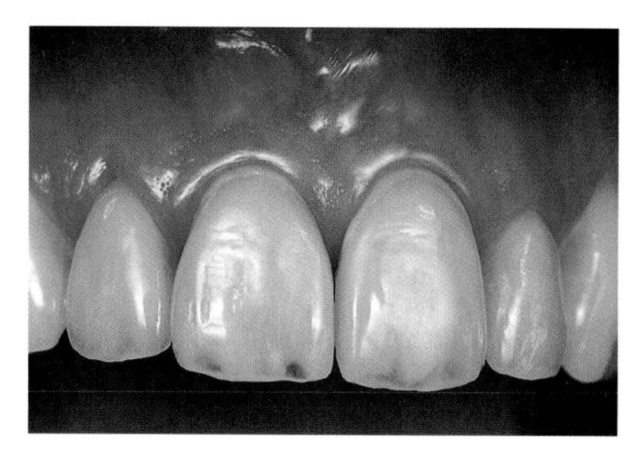

Figure 7.34 The temporaries in Figure 7.33 were relined at chairside to improve marginal fit before cementing with a provisional luting agent (notice cervical additions).

Polyvinyl ethylmethacrylate (PVEMA)

Of the acrylics, PVEMAs are an ideal choice for intra-oral use, due to a lesser exothermic reaction, e.g. Trim (HJ Bosworth Co., Il, USA) and SNAP (Parkell, NY, USA) (Figs. 7.35 & 7.36). The monomer of ethyl methacrylate has reduced toxicity compared to PMMAs. However, porosity compromises strength and aesthetics, and, if

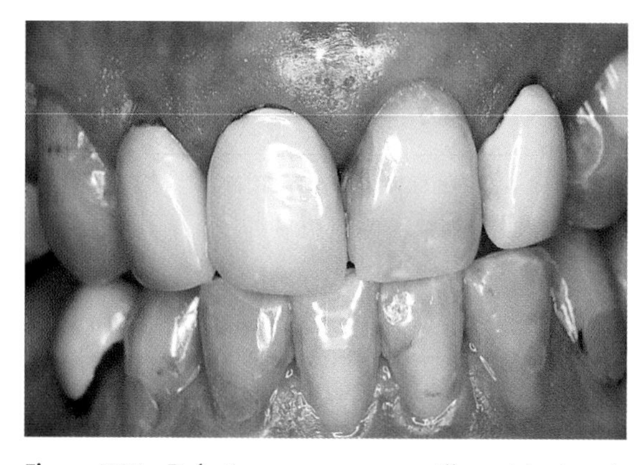

Figure 7.35 Defective crowns on maxillary right lateral, central incisors and left lateral incisor.

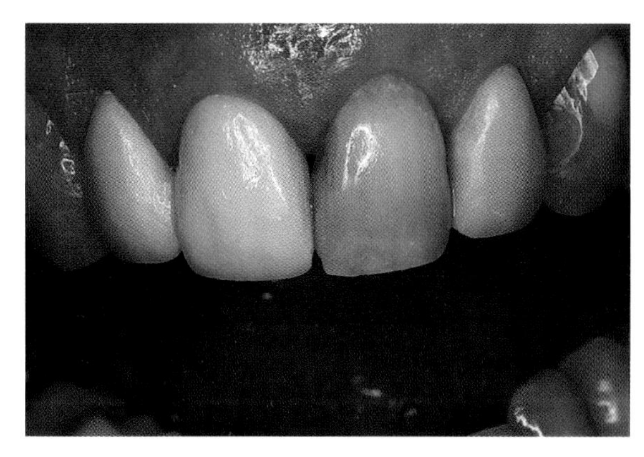

Figure 7.36 Chairside acrylic temporaries for patient in Figure 7.35 with improved marginal integrity.

worn for long periods, the surface discolours and stains are readily conspicuous. The mechanical properties are also mediocre, and the lower fracture toughness often predisposes to unwanted fractures. Repair of fractures and filling air blows or voids is relatively simple by additions of a low viscosity mix, or alternatively a flowable light-cured resin composite. Nevertheless, as stated above, a repaired restoration is significantly weaker than the original intact prosthesis.

Bis-GMA resin

The benefits of bis-GMA resins are similar to those of conventional restorative filling materials made of the same compound, including malleability, large choice of shades and ease of fabrication. They are available as light- and dual-cured varieties. The strength is intermediate compared to acrylics, with fracture toughness greater than PVEMA but lower than PMMA.[16] The main disadvantage is brittleness, causing minor or catastrophic fractures, especially if used for multiple splinted units.

Bis-acryl resin composite

The bis-acryl composite materials are probably the most popular and widely used materials for intra-oral temporary crowns, e.g. Protemp (3M-ESPE, St Paul, Minnesota, USA). Material presentations include cartridge delivery (eliminating mixing), variety of shades and various setting modes (chemical-, dual- and light-cured), which all expedite chairside fabrication. The benefits include resistance to wear due to increased micro-hardness, high modulus of rupture and MOE. There is average fracture toughness.[17] Polymerisation shrinkage is less than PMMAs, with lower temperature elevation during setting, and low pulpal irritancy. The major disadvantages are difficulty relining margins, poor polishability and, hence, compromised aesthetics. Indications include single units, or short spans for short duration.

Urethane dimethacrylate (UDMA) resin

UDMA is the ubiquitous resin matrix for many contemporary composite filling materials. The major difference between the restorative and temporary material is that the latter is not loaded with filler particles and therefore has increased flowability, e.g. Triad, (Dentsply, Germany). The UDMA resin has high fracture toughness and low exothermic reaction. The heat generated is not from the setting reaction (as with acrylics), but due to radiation absorption during curing with a visible light source. Furthermore, pulpal irritation is almost eliminated due to the absence of a monomer. The disadvantages are poor marginal integrity and polishability, resulting in inferior fit and aesthetics, respectively. However, to overcome poor aesthetics, a universal hybrid restorative material (with filler loading) can be used to veneer the temporary crown. This technique is also beneficial using PVEMA as a core and veneering with a hybrid composite.

CLINICAL PRACTICE

Fabrication

The dental literature is crammed with techniques for fabricating temporary restorations and ingenious methods are proposed depending on clinical scenarios. It is important to realise from the outset that technique is paramount, superseding the choice of a given class of temporary material or a specific proprietary product. Essentially, techniques can be categorised as direct (chairside fabrication) or indirect (constructed in a dental laboratory). The direct method is instant and economical, but time consuming, and often results in restorations with poor physical and aesthetic properties. This method is indicated for a limited number of teeth, up to three units, for short duration of wear. The indirect method offers superior aesthetics and is ideal for prolonged wear due to mechanical resilience (plus the option to reinforce with metal or fibres), but with increased costs. A combination technique is also possible, exploiting the advantages of both direct and indirect methods, while overcoming their limitations.

Successful fabrication of TTRs involves two entities: the external contours and internal contours. The factors influencing external contours are tooth morphology, which depends on dental bioform, gingival architecture, aesthetics, occlusion, contact points and phonetics. The internal contours (or adaptation) are determined by tooth preparation geometry, including retention and resistance form, surface roughness, type of margin finish line, preparation outline, and presence or absence of undercuts.

Matrices

The external contours of TTRs are achieved using matrices, categorised as:

- Existing anatomical form
- Proposed anatomical form
- Preformed anatomical form

Table 7.1 summarises the criteria for choosing a matrix.

Existing anatomical form

If the existing tooth morphology is acceptable, it can be used as a template for the TTR. An alginate or electrometric impression is made for creating the anatomical form (external contours). A silicone impression, rather than an alginate, is preferred since the former is dimensionally stable, can be stored, and is reusable if a remake is necessary.

Proposed anatomical form

In many instances the reason for providing indirect restorations is to alter aesthetics, occlusion and function, which consequently requires modification of existing tooth morphology. This is

Table 7.1 Criteria for choosing a matrix.

Criterion	Existing anatomical form	Proposed anatomical form	Preformed anatomical form
Status quo	Yes	No	No
Altering aesthetics, occlusion and OVD	No	Yes	No
Units	Up to three	Unlimited	Single
Duration of wear	Short	Long	Short
TTR material choice	Limited	Any	Limited
Expediency	Yes	No	Yes
Cost	Low	High	Medium

carried out either intra-orally or in the dental laboratory. If minor changes are necessary, hybrid/flowable composite or wax is added until the desired shape is achieved. Alternatively, for extensive changes, a diagnostic wax-up of the proposed anatomy is fabricated in the dental laboratory (Figs. 7.37 & 7.38). An impression is then made of the wax-up using a silicone material ensuring that adjacent teeth, as well as surrounding 1–2 mm of soft tissues are recorded for precise intra-oral location of the matrix. The advantage of using a silicone matrix is heat dissipation during the polymerisation of the temporary restorative materials. The disadvantage is difficulty locating the silicone impression and tray on to the prepared teeth intra-orally, due to lack of transparency.

Another method is to pour a plaster cast of the impression of the diagnostic wax-up and fabricate a vacuum-formed polypropylene matrix. The latter matrix can only be formed on a stone replica of the wax-up, since the heat generated during vacuum forming would melt the diagnostic wax-up. Since the matrix is transparent, precise location on to the prepared teeth is facilitated. Another benefit is that visible light-cured temporary resin material can be utilised. The major disadvantage is that the thin shell is not an effective heat sink for materials with exothermic reactions.

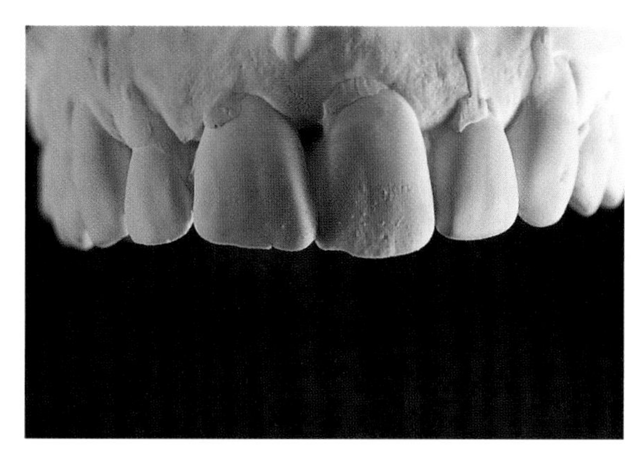

Figure 7.37 Pre-operative cast showing uneven incisal plane and poor width/length ratio of maxillary incisors.

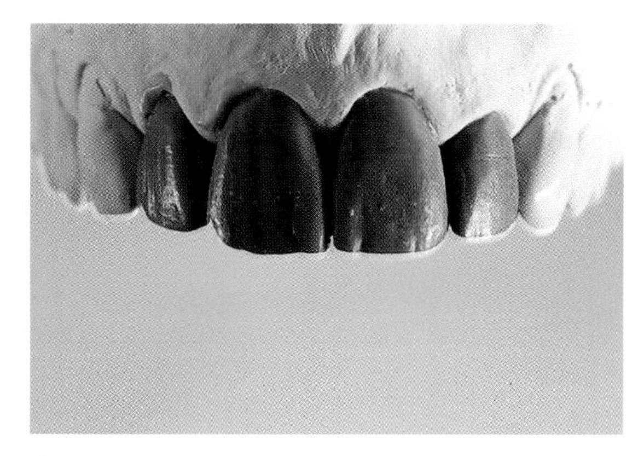

Figure 7.38 Proposed diagnostic wax-up to improve aesthetics for patient in Figure 7.37, which is used to fabricate laboratory acrylic temporaries (see Figures 7.33 and 7.34).

Preformed metal and plastic crown forms

Prefabricated crowns are available in metal (aluminum or stainless steel) or plastic (acrylic or polycarbonate). Both types require filling with a resin for internal adaptation of the prepared tooth abutment. The metal varieties offer rigidity and durability, but require extensive shaping to conform to the occlusion and to obtain accurate margins. In addition, trimmed steel margins can act as a scalpel, lacerating the soft tissues. The plastic variety offers immediate aesthetics, but also requires prolonged clinical time for shaping and verifying margin integrity and occlusion. Another advantage of the clear plastic varieties is ease of location and the ability to use light-cured temporary crown materials. As a generality, preformed crowns are indicated for single units, and are worn for short periods.

Techniques

Having chosen and fabricated the appropriate matrix for the external contours of a TTR, the next stage is forming the internal contours. This is achieved by using one or more of the abovementioned materials. Numerous factors influence the choice of material, depending on the clinical requirements of a TTR. Table 7.2 presents guidelines for making the correct choice depending on clinical requirement. However, rather than trying to master every material, it is prudent to familiarise oneself with a few products and obtain predictable and consistent results.

There are three fundamental techniques for fabricating TTRs: direct, indirect and a combination of direct–indirect. In the author's experience, the methods and materials described below for each technique produce predictable results. However, the clinician may wish to modify these steps, omitting superfluous steps or adding stages to modify procedures to tailor them for specific clinical needs.

Direct technique

(1) Refine existing anatomy and aesthetics by additions with a flowable composite (or wax) and trim with diamond burs, discs and silicone polishing tips. Alternatively, a preformed crown can be utilised for the external contours, omitting steps (2) and (3) below
(2) Block pronounced gingival embrasures with wax
(3) Fabricate a matrix using a silicone impression material, or a vacuum-formed sheet (from diagnostic wax-up) for short-span bridges
(4) Carry out tooth preparation
(5) Following tooth preparation, place matrix on to the abutment and adjacent teeth, verifying correct seating and location
(6) The prepared teeth should already be isolated with retraction cord, and any loose emanating strands are gently replaced into the gingival crevice, to allow visualisation of the circumferential preparation finish line. This ensures that the marginal integrity is not compromised by adherence of the cord to the temporary restorative material
(7) Apply phosphoric acid etchant to remove the smear layer (Hint 7.1), followed by a DBA incorporating desensitisers or alternatively use a dentine tubule blocking agent. Whilst DBAs afford little thermal protection to the underlying pulp, they do however alleviate post-operative sensitivity by sealing the tubules and preventing bacterial ingress
(8) Lubricate the abutment, surrounding and antagonist teeth liberally with petroleum jelly, to reduce thermal insult to the pulp and protect the gingival tissues. This separating medium also prevents locking of the restoration on to the abutment and in the gingival embrasures
(9) Choose material for internal contours from Table 7.2, e.g. a PVEMA such as SNAP, and mix according to manufacturer's instructions. The usual mixing time for SNAP at room temperature is 2–3 minutes, and the flowable mixture is poured into the matrix (Hint 7.2)
(10) Place the SNAP-loaded matrix on to the abutment(s) ensuring correct seating and location
(11) Flush with water for cooling and reducing temperature elevation
(12) Once the rubbery stage is reached (4 minutes from the start of mixing), remove the matrix with the temporaries, trim excess from undercuts and re-seat temporaries without the matrix on to the abutment(s), ask patient to close in centric occlusion for 30 seconds (Hint 7.3)
(13) Remove temporaries from mouth and allow extra-oral setting for another 2 minutes until rigid (Hint 7.4)
(14) Once rigid, check marginal integrity, emergence profile, occlusion, aesthetics and passive seating. Marginal discrepancies and voids are filled by additional material, mixed to a lower viscosity with a dull appearance (indicative of monomer evaporation). Unduly liquid mixes are avoided, since they contain large volumes of unreacted free monomer, which causes pulpal and gingival irritation. Alternately, voids

or alterations to the morphology can be corrected by additions with a flowable composite

(15) Carry out gross trimming with tungsten carbide acrylic burs at low speeds. Excessive high-speed diamond burs tend to melt rather than cut acrylic resin. Finer refinements to margins, anatomy and occlusion are performed with aluminum discs, silicone tips and chamois leather mops (Hint 7.5)

(16) If relining of the internal contours is necessary, use a mix that is neither thin nor liquid, to avoid irritation by any unreacted free monomer

(17) The restoration is luted with fine particle zinc oxide eugenol cement with sufficient rigidity, such as Temp Bond (Kerr, Michigan, USA). Varieties of eugenol-free and clear cements are also available, preventing interaction with bonding agents and enhancing aesthetics, respectively. For acrylic laminates, spot etching the abutment with 37% phosphoric acid, and luting with a flowable composite (without bonding agent) is an alternative method for temporary cementation

(18) Once set, remove excess cement and retraction cord with a sharp probe, and use dental tape or floss to remove interproximal remnants

(19) Finally, irrigate of the margins with 0.2% chlorhexidine liquid to flush cement fragments and encourage gingival health.

Table 7.2 Criteria for selection of material for internal contours of a TTR.

Criterion	PMMA	PVEMA	Bis-GMA	Bis-acryl	UDMA	Reinforce
Intra-oral	U	S	S	S	S	C
Extra-oral	S	C	S	C	S	S
Manipulation/handling	S	S	C	C	C	C
Aesthetics	S	C	S	C	C	C
Structural integrity/resilience	S	C	C	C	C	S
Reparability	S	S	C	C	C	C
Expediency	C	S	S	S	S	C
Cost	C	S	S	C	S	C

S – Superior.
C – Compromise.
U – Unacceptable.

Indirect technique

This technique is less laborious than it initially appears, and the benefits of superior aesthetics and physical and mechanical properties often outweigh the additional time and cost.

(1) The external contours can be either the existing teeth if the aesthetics are acceptable, or a vacuum matrix using a polypropylene sheet on a stone model of the diagnostic wax-up
(2) Carry out tooth preparations with a retraction cord in situ so that the circumferential finish line is clearly discernible. A clear vacuum matrix (placed onto the prepared teeth) is particularly useful for checking that tooth reduction is sufficient to accommodate the restorative materials of the definitive prosthesis (metal and/or porcelain)
(3) Make an impression, using a silicone impression material, of the tooth preparation following sealing the freshly cut dentine with a DBA or dentine tubule blocking agent
(4) The impression is cast using rapid setting stone by either the clinician, or an on-site dental laboratory
(5) Block interproximal gingival embrasure undercuts with wax, and liberally lubricate the preparations, adjacent and antagonist teeth and soft tissues with petroleum jelly
(6) The stone model of the preparations is coated with a silicone-separating medium
(7) If the temporaries are intended for long duration of wear, reinforcement by metals, fibres or rods is incorporated within the PMMA resin
(8) The pre-operative impression or clear vacuum matrix is filled with a PMMA resin, cured by heat and pressure in a hydro flask
(9) Once set, follow steps 15–19 in the direct technique for finishing, polishing and cementing.

Direct–indirect technique

The direct–indirect technique exploits the strength, physical and aesthetic properties of the indirect method, while ensuring a precision fit by directly relining on to the intra-oral tooth preparation. This technique for fabrication of TTRs combines both extra- and intra-oral stages, the first nine steps are performed in the dental laboratory, and the remaining in the surgery.

(1) The external contours can either be an impression of the existing anatomy, or of a proposed anatomy (diagnostic wax-up)
(2) A plaster cast is poured of the existing anatomy or the diagnostic wax-up
(3) A vacuum-formed transparent matrix is fabricated from step (2) above
(4) Tooth preparation(s) are simulated on the plaster cast. This can also be used as a guide for intra-oral tooth preparation, or a pre-operative diagnostic tool for assessing feasibility of a proposed treatment plan
(5) The stone model of the preparations is coated with a silicone-separating medium
(6) If the temporaries are intended for long duration of wear, reinforcement by metals, fibres or rods is incorporated within the PMMA resin
(7) Shells of the external contours are created either by painting the inner surface of the clear vacuum matrix with a PMMA or a composite resin, before heat and pressure curing (Hint 7.6)
(8) Once cured, the temporaries are trimmed and polished (step (15) of direct technique)
(9) The transparent matrix and shells of the external contours are returned to the surgery
(10) The clinician carries out tooth preparations, using the matrix as a guide
(11) Once completed, gingival embrasures are blocked and petroleum jelly applied to teeth and soft tissues
(12) The shells are seated, ensuring correct location and filled with a PVEMA to create the internal contours. The next stages are the same as for the direct technique, steps (9)–(19). Constant irrigation with water is imperative to allow heat dissipation, since the thin shell(s) offer little heat convection compared to a silicone impression matrix.

Hints and tips

- Hint 7.1 – Avoid desiccating the dentine following etchant removal, which may elicit pulpal inflammation
- Hint 7.2 – Allow the mixture to reach a dull appearance, ensuring evaporation of the free monomer, and minimising its associated toxicity
- Hint 7.3 – To dissipate heat, some authorities advocate the repeated 'on-off' technique until the material is rigid. Whilst this rationale is sound, repeated seating results in a poor marginal fit, often necessitating relines. Furthermore, if the measures outlined above for heat insulation are followed (silicone matrix, water cooling, isolation with petroleum jelly), undue damage to the pulp and soft tissues is avoided
- Hint 7.4 – Placing the temporaries in boiling water or a stream of hot air accelerates the polymerisation reaction, i.e. the speed, rather than the magnitude of shrinkage. The total setting reaction should be completed within 10 minutes of the start of mixing
- Hint 7.5 – Sealing with a surface sealant such as Biscover, which is devoid of the oxygen inhibition layer, emulates a glaze and seals surface discrepancies following the polishing procedures
- Hint 7.6 – The advantage of using a composite resin is a vast shade range

References

[1] Haselton, D.R., Diaz-Arnold, A.M. and Vargas, M.A. (2002) Flexural strength of provisional crown and fixed partial denture resins. *J Prosthet Dent*, **87**, 225–228

[2] Koumjian, J.H. and Nimmo, A. (1990) Evaluation of fracture resistance of resins used for provisional restorations. *J Prosthet Dent*, **64**, 654–657

[3] Camps, J., Pizant, S., Dejou, J. and Franquin, J.C. (1998) Effects of desensitizing agents on human dentine permeability. *Am J Dent*, **11**, 289–290

[4] Lloyd, C.H., Joshi, A. and Mcglynn, E. (1986) Temperature rises produced by light sources and composites during curing. *Dent Mater*, **2**, 170–174

[5] Zach, L. and Cohen, C. (1965) Pulp response to externally applied heat. *Oral Surg Oral Med Oral Pathol*, **19**, 515–529

[6] Tjan, A.H.L. and Dunn, J.R. (1988) Temperature rise produced by various visible light generators through dentinal barriers. *J Prosthet Dent*, **59**, 433–438

[7] Voth, E.D., Phillips, R.W. and Swartz, M.L. (1966) Thermal diffusion through amalgam and various liners. *J Dent Res*, **45**, 1184–1190

[8] Usumez, A., Ozturk, A.N. and Aykent, F. (2004) The effect of dentine desensitizers on thermal changes in the pulp chamber during fabrication of provisional restorations. *J Oral Rehab*, **31**, 579–584

[9] LaMar, F.R. (2004) Guest editorial. Microgap or macrogap: significance of the marginal discrepancy between implant crown and abutment. *Int J Periodontics Restorative Dent*, **24(3)**, 207

[10] Tjan, A.H.L., Tjan, A.H. and Grant, B.E. (1987) Marginal accuracy of temporary composite crowns. *J Prosthet Dent*, **58(4)**, 417–421

[11] Kim, S.H. and Watts, D.C. (2004) Polymerisation shrinkage-strain kinetics of temporary crown and bridge materials. *Dental Mat*, **20**, 88–95

[12] Sorensen, J. (1989) A rationale for comparison of plaque-retaining properties of crown systems. *J Prosthet Dent*, **62(3)**, 264–269

[13] Glantz, P.O. (1969) On wettability and adhesiveness. A study of enamel, dentine, some dental restorative dental materials and dental plaque. *Odontol Rev*, **17**(Suppl 20), 1–124

[14] Martignoni, M. and Schonenberger, A. (1990) *Precision Fixed Prosthodontics: Clinical and Laboratory Aspects*. Quintessence Publishing Co. Inc., Chicago

[15] Moore, B., Goodcare, C., Swartz, M. and Andres, C. (1989) A comparison of resins for fabricating provisional fixed restorations. *Int J Prosthodont*, 2, 173–184
[16] Gegauff, A.G. and Pryor, H.G. (1987) Fracture toughness of provisional resins for fixed prosthodontics. *J Prosthet Dent*, 58, 23–29
[17] Ireland, M.F., Dixon, D.L., Breeding, L.C. and Ramp, M.H. (1998) In vitro mechanical property comparison of four resins used for fabrication of provisional fixed restorations. *J Prosthet Dent*, 80, 158–162

8 Biological impressions

Introduction

Shavell coined the phrase 'biological impressions', to signify impressions that capture, with fidelity, healthy tissues in their natural habitat.[1] Most indirect dental restorations are made with only an impression as the unifying element linking the three protagonists, ceramist, patient and dentist (or CPD) (Fig. 8.1). The intrinsic qualities of an impression are to record as much and as accurate detail as possible. This necessitates faithfully recording the prepared, adjacent and opposing dentition, together with the surrounding soft tissues. Whether an impression is for a laminate, inlay, crown, bridge, denture or implant, the objective is to reproduce accurately a facsimile of anatomical structures as a morphological platform for fabricating the proposed restoration. This implies that the tissues are neither escharotic nor necrotic.

Two types of biological impressions are required: dental and gingival. The dental biological impression is one that replicates abutment teeth following preparation. By definition, this requires deflecting the gingival crevice to accommodate an impression material that will reproduce the preparation margins for obtaining a correct emergence profile. The gingival biological impression records the periodontium in a non-deflected state. The latter is made after fabricating the definitive restoration, at the try-in stage, when the gingival tissues have recoiled to their normal position. By locating the restoration on an untrimmed plaster model, the rendezvous of a restoration with the surrounding soft tissues is visualised. This allows assessment of the cervical transmucosal soft tissue support and contact points. Following modifications, a non-violent coexistence between the two entities, restoration and soft tissues, is achieved.[2]

SCIENTIFIC RATIONALE

Making precise impressions depends on two variables, the primary and secondary determinants. While there is only one primary determinant, without which an accurate impression is unattainable, there are numerous secondary determinants, which are discussed initially,

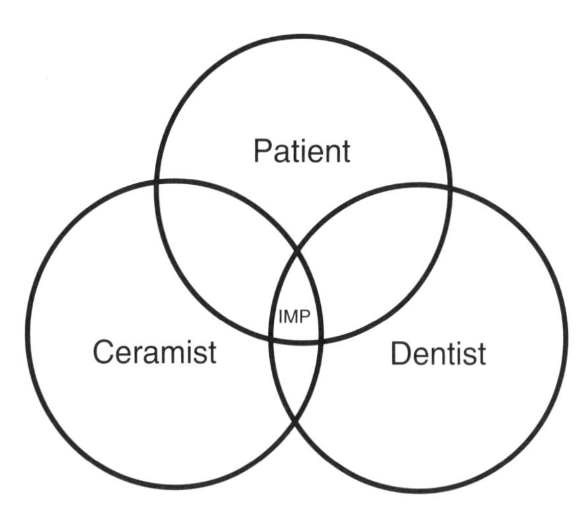

Figure 8.1 The impression is the key element linking ceramist, patient and dentist.

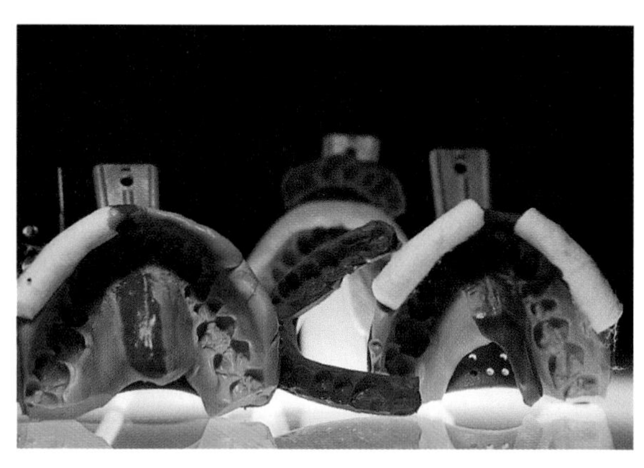

Figure 8.2 Rigid plastic stock trays are satisfactory for making impressions for up to three units.

before considering the crucial primary determinant.

Secondary determinants

The following list is not exhaustive, but emphasises pertinent points of the secondary determinants.

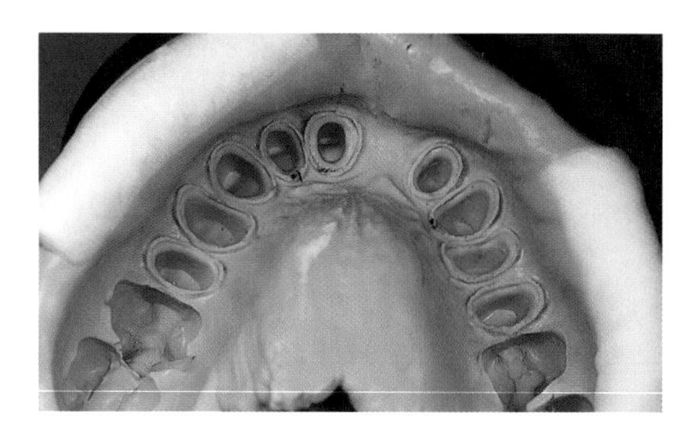

Figure 8.3 Full maxillary intra-arch impression.

Stock vs. custom trays

The rationale for using custom or special trays is to control dimensional stability, and hence minimise polymerisation shrinkage. This was particularly significant with earlier elastomeric materials, but is less relevant with contemporary formulations. The newer materials are relatively stable, exhibiting sufficient stiffness and rigidity. The advantages of custom trays are ease of location and seating in the oral cavity, patient comfort by avoiding sharp tray flanges impinging into the sulci, and capturing posterior teeth without the need to modify stock trays with wax or compound materials. As a general guideline, stock trays are acceptable for one to three units in conjunction with a heavy-bodied or putty base (Fig. 8.2).

Inter- vs. intra-arch

Intra-arch impressions record an entire arch including contralateral teeth (Figs. 8.3–8.6), while inter-arch impressions record the antagonist dentition. The latter is carried out using 'triple trays' and benefits include eliminating an opposing arch impression and bite registration. While the resulting impression records both the prepared teeth and occlusal registration, the technique is trying for both the clinician and ceramist. Furthermore, inter-arch impressions

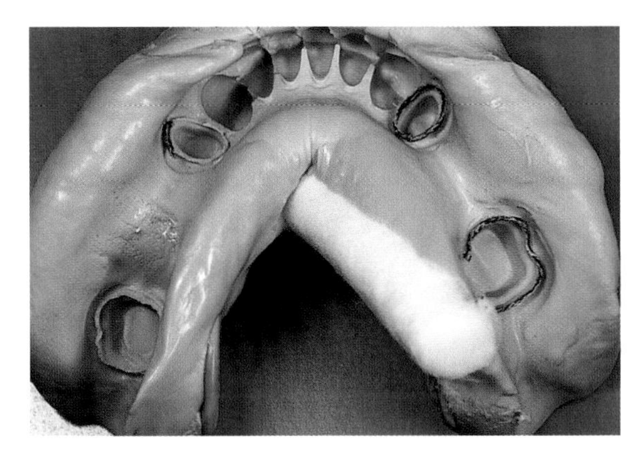

Figure 8.4 Full mandibular intra-arch impression.

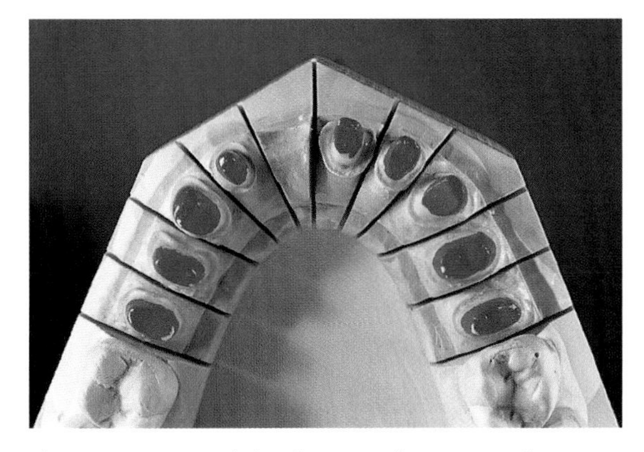

Figure 8.5 Trimmed dies from maxillary intra-arch impression in Figure 8.3.

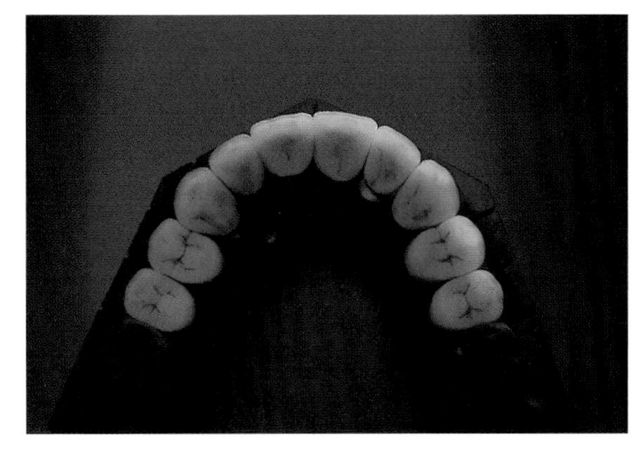

Figure 8.6 Completed crowns for patient in Figure 8.5.

are limited to one or two units. Further disadvantages include distortion of tray when the patient occludes,[3] verifying whether the teeth are in centric occlusion, and ensuring that at least two teeth either side of the prepared abutment are included.

If, however, the tooth to be restored has interferences (working or non-working side), or is the initial contact in CR or a guiding tooth, interarch impressions are essential to allow mounting on a semi-adjustable articulator.

Closed vs. open tray

The rationale for an open tray is that drilled holes in the impression tray act as vents for excess material and air to escape. In theory, this is valid, but clinically there is little improvement of the resulting impression. Furthermore, since excess material has to be rapidly mopped after tray insertion, there is increased patient discomfort, often eliciting a reflex gagging response.

One vs. two stages

The basis of a two-stage impression is ensuring a solid platform for the subsequent wash stage. The procedure involves taking an initial impression with putty (using a rigid metal or stock tray), usually separated by an acetate or polypropylene sheet, in effect, to form a custom tray. The second stage is injecting a light-bodied wash over the prepared teeth and reseating the tray. The obvious disadvantages are incorrect tray location, lengthy procedure and protracted endurance for the patient. The advantage of the one-stage impression is expediency and guaranteed correct seating, but timing is critical. The wash must be placed simultaneously on to the abutment while the assistant mixes and loads the putty or heavy-bodied material. In addition, once mixed, the tray must be inserted immediately to prevent the material reaching the elastic stage, which can flex the tray (if plastic) and produce distortions.[4]

Passive vs. non-passive

Most elastomeric materials recoil after the tray is removed from the mouth. A non-passive impression made by continuously applying pressure to the tray while the material is setting, causes pronounced recoil, with the detrimental manifestation that the crown fits the plaster die, but not the intra-oral abutment. To circumvent the latter, once the tray is correctly seated, pressure is relieved, allowing the material to set passively. Since the material polymerises without external pressure with a passive impression, post-removal recoil is significantly reduced.[5]

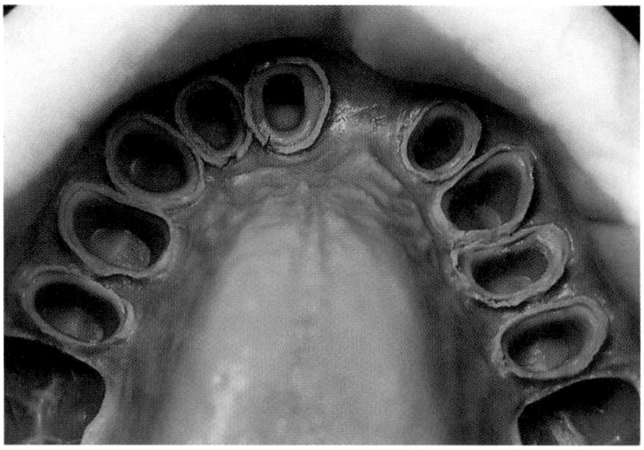

Warm vs. cold environment

When attempting impressions for multiple units, a prolonged working time is clearly desirable. Chilling an impression material facilitates this, but increases the viscosity with possible alteration or retardation of the material setting reaction. Recently, a new impression material has been introduced, Flexitime (Heraeus Kulzer, Hanau, Germany), which facilitates a variety of clinical situations. Because the setting reaction is initiated by the warm oral ambient temperature, polymerisation only starts when the material is placed in the mouth. The working time ranges from 30 seconds to $2\frac{1}{2}$ minutes, but setting is always $2\frac{1}{2}$ minutes after tray insertion, allowing impressions of single as well as multiple preparations (Fig. 8.7).

Manual vs. automated mixing

Using mechanical or automatic mixing equipment ensures a homogenous, void-free mix, greatly enhancing the quality of the final impression. A variety of materials, including polyethers and addition silicones, are available in cartridges for these machines. The only drawback is the initial capital outlay for equipment purchase.

Figure 8.7 Flexitime (Heraeus Kulzer) full maxillary arch impression.

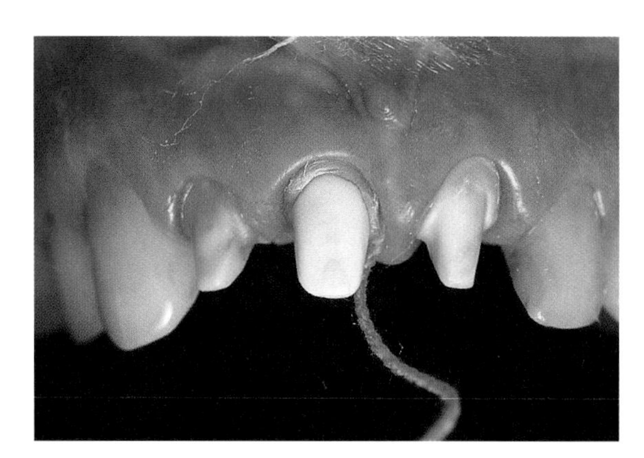

Figure 8.8 Retraction cord being placed around prepared teeth.

Physical vs. chemical gingival retraction

Physical retraction of the gingival crevice involves using retraction cord(s) (Fig. 8.8). This is an effective and predictable method for achieving transient opening of the sulcus, allowing an impression material to record the preparations' margins (Fig. 8.9). In addition, gingival retraction is less traumatic than electrosurgery or rotary gingival curettage, with diminished chances of ensuing gingival recession.[6,7] However, excessive pressure during cord placement may inadvertently damage the delicate epithelial lining of the crevice or violate the biologic width.

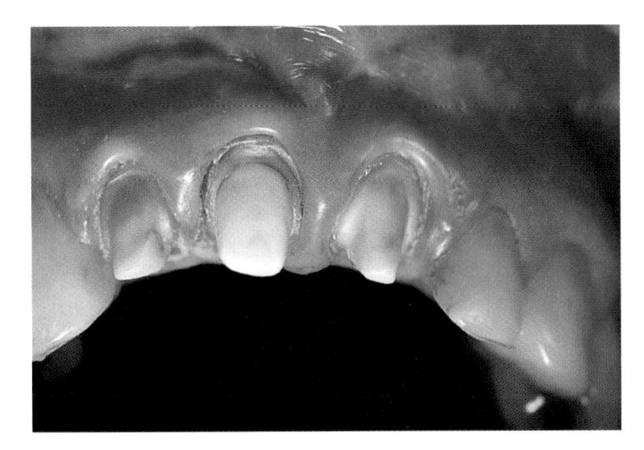

Figure 8.9 Retraction cord in situ to deflect gingival crevice and act as a physical barrier protecting the biologic width.

Another concern with retraction cords is using haemostatic agents. Recent research concludes that using the commonest haemostatic agents, such as racemic epinephrine, aluminum sulphate, aluminum chloride, aluminum potassium sulphate or ferric sulphate, has no effect on setting reactions of polyvinyl siloxanes (addition silicones).[8] Additionally, aluminum chloride is effective for achieving chemical and mechanical tissue displacement,[9] whereas epinephrine causes local necrosis and possible unwanted systemic side effects.[10]

A recently introduced chemical retraction agent (Expasyl, Kerr) combines aluminium chloride and kaolin. The aluminum chloride acts as the astringent, while the hygroscopic kaolin expands once in contact with crevicular fluid for achieving the desired gingival deflection. Whilst circumferential enlargement of the sulcus is achieved, subsequent removal of the material by rinsing can be problematic. Lastly, chemical retraction alone does not offer a physical barrier, as with retraction cords, for safeguarding the biologic width.

Impression materials

The dental market is awash with impression materials and selection depends on the intended use of the impression. Irreversible hydrocolloids may be acceptable for diagnostic or opposing arch impressions, but are inappropriate for precision-fabricated restorations. The properties of five commonly used impression materials for prosthodontics are summarised below and in Table 8.1.

Definitions

- Tear resistance – ability of an impression material to resist tearing in small cross sections, especially intra-sulcular areas
- Elastic recovery – the degree of recoil of a material without permanent elastic deformations, e.g. from a tooth preparation undercut
- Dimensional stability – ability to withstand stress without permanent deformation, e.g. a heavy-bodied or putty formulation

Reversible hydrocolloids

A decade ago, reversible hydrocolloids were the vogue. These materials are hydrophilic, allowing impression making in a relatively moist environment, and extremely accurate with good tear resistance. However, due to poor long-term stability, immediate pours are mandatory. In addition, a custom tray and heating/cooling apparatus are required, prolonging clinical time with additional procedures. Another factor is that multiple pours may not be feasible, and these are necessary for most contemporary all-ceramic restorations.

Polysulphides

Polysulphides were the first elastomeric impression materials, with excellent tear resistance, ideal for capturing subgingival crown margins. However, inferior elastic recovery necessitated immediate pours, while poor dimensional stability mandated using custom trays, both affecting the accuracy of the impression.

Table 8.1 Properties of popular impression materials.

Property	Reversible hydrocolloids	Polysulphides	Condensation silicones	Polyethers	Addition silicones
Tray	Custom	Custom	Custom/stock	Custom/stock	Custom/stock
Handling	Specific equipment necessary Multiple pours?	Soft	Soft	Rigid, unpleasant taste Multiple pours?	Soft, multiple pours possible, avoid latex gloves,[11] and acrylic monomers
Hydrophilic	Yes	No	No	Yes	No
Tear resistance	Good	Good	Poor	Good	Average
Elastic recovery	Average	Average	Good	Good	Good
Long-term stability	Poor	Poor	Poor	Good	Good
Disinfection	Non-water soluble	Water soluble (e.g. NaOCl)	Water soluble (e.g. NaOCl)	Non-water soluble	Water soluble (e.g. NaOCl)
Immediate pour	Yes	Yes	No	No	No
Accuracy	Good	Average	Average	Good	Good

Condensation silicones

These materials have enhanced elastic recovery compared to polysulphides, but suffer from poor tear resistance (Fig. 8.10). Hence, recording subgingival margins is trying and often results in torn material left in the gingival crevice, yielding inaccurate margins.

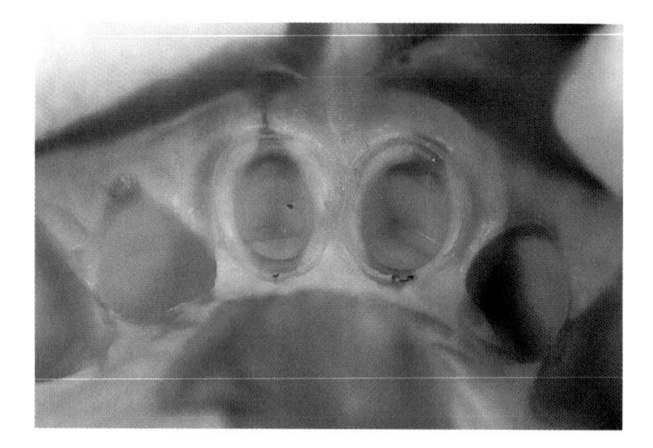

Figure 8.10 Condensation silicone impression (Optosil, Xantopren, Heraeus Kulzer).

Polyethers

Polyethers have superior tear resistance compared to condensation silicones, with excellent dimensional stability and accuracy. Another benefit is the hydrophilic property, allowing impressions to be made in relatively moist conditions. Initially, polyethers were unavailable in a heavy body, but newer formulations have putty components, obviating the need for using a custom tray. Another disadvantage was rigidity, making removal from undercuts extremely difficult, e.g. locking into gingival embrasures around periodontally compromised teeth. This limitation is also significant if multiple pours are necessary, since material rigidity causes breakage of plaster casts upon removal of the impression. The latest generations are 'soft polyethers' for increased patient comfort, and ease of retrievability from the mouth (Fig. 8.11). Newer versions are also insipid, eliminating the undesirable taste of older polyethers.

Polyvinyl siloxanes (addition silicones)

The most ubiquitous impression materials currently used for prosthodontics are the addition silicones. The large number of viscosities (Figs. 8.12 & 8.13) makes these materials extremely versatile for many clinical situations (Figs. 8.14–8.19). The beneficial properties are excellent elastic recovery, dimensional stability, the materials are tasteless and relatively soft (allowing removal from undercuts), stock or custom trays can be used and there is good detail

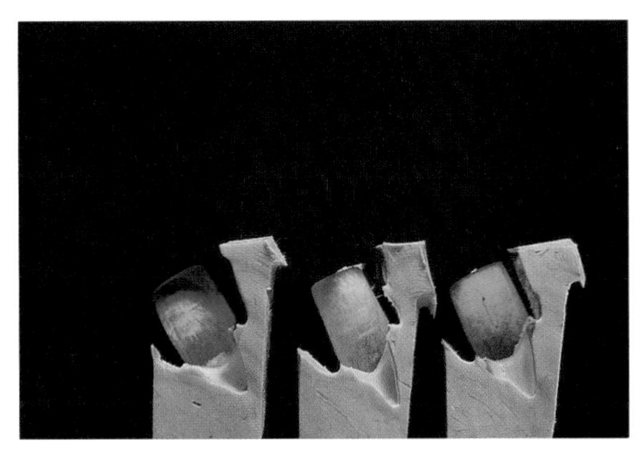

Figure 8.13 Sectioned impression and dies using three addition silicone viscosities for patient in Figure 8.12.

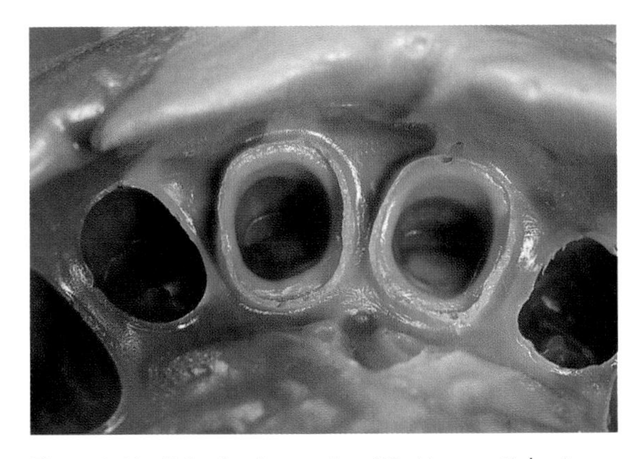

Figure 8.11 Polyether impression (P2, Heraeus Kulzer).

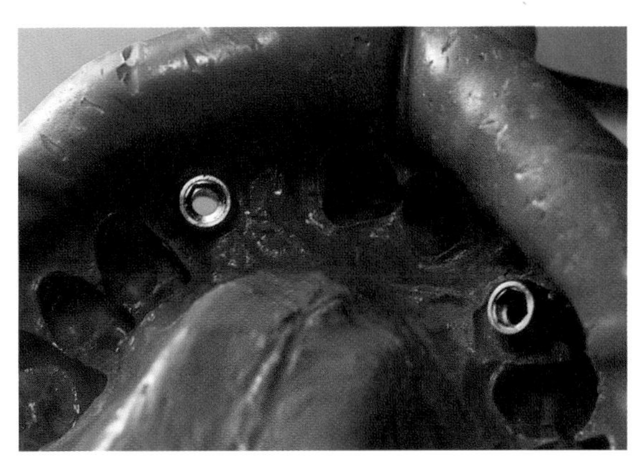

Figure 8.14 Use of addition silicones: implant-supported restorations.

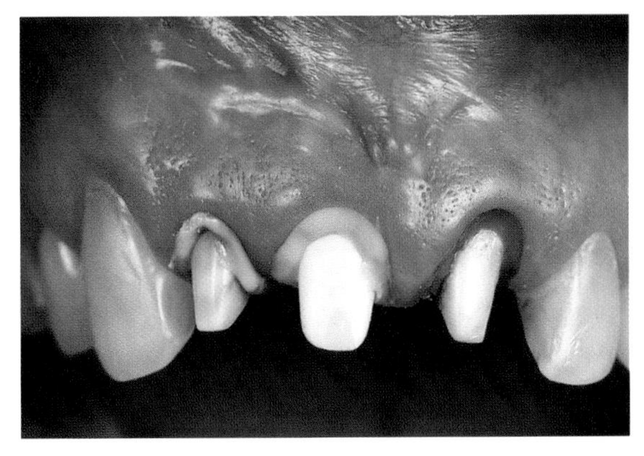

Figure 8.12 Addition silicones are available in a variety of viscosities: monophase, medium and light-bodied consistencies.

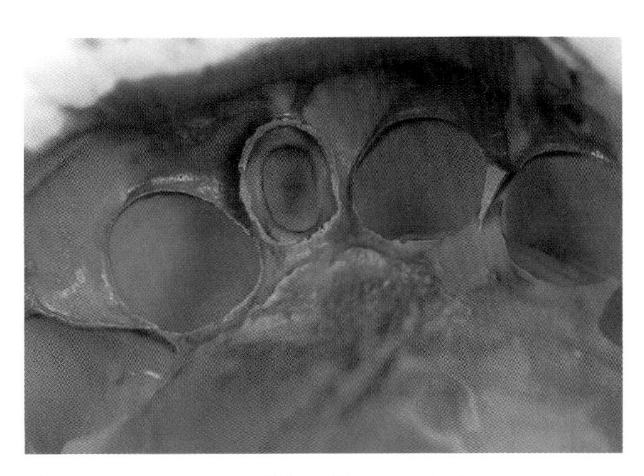

Figure 8.15 Use of addition silicones: single units.

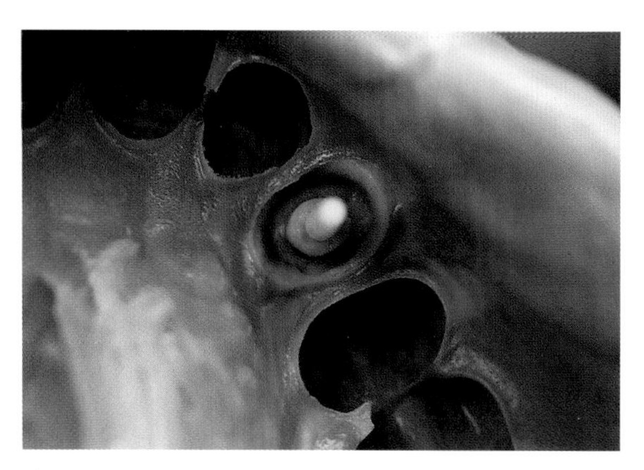

Figure 8.16 Use of addition silicones: indirect post/cores.

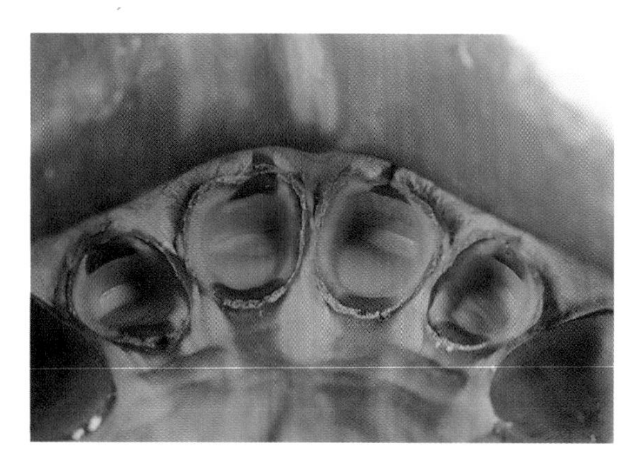

Figure 8.17 Use of addition silicones: multiple units.

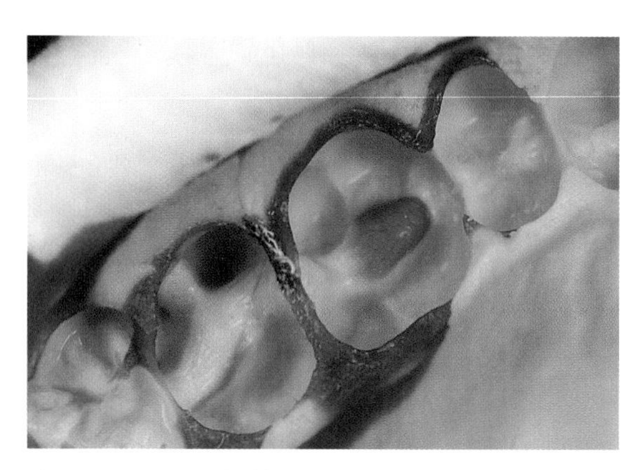

Figure 8.18 Use of addition silicones: porcelain inlays.

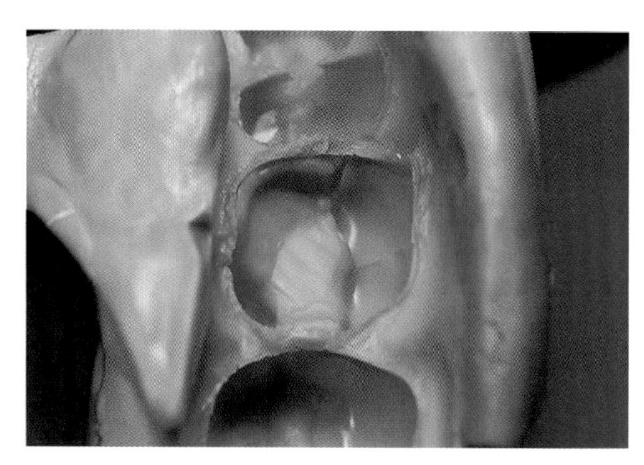

Figure 8.19 Use of addition silicones: porcelain onlays.

reproduction (accuracy). The tear resistance of addition silicones is less than that of polysulphides. However, a balance is necessary. The high tear resistance of polysulphides, but poor elastic recovery, means that although the material will not tear, it will permanently deform. Conversely, the addition silicones have good elastic recovery and lower tear resistance, meaning that the material will tear before permanent deformation. The latter is crucial for accurately reproducing prepared abutments. These properties are a major reason for their popularity for contemporary dental procedures.[12] The main disadvantage is that polyvinyl siloxanes are intrinsically hydrophobic, but the recently introduced Provil novo (Heraeus Kulzer, Hanau, Germany) claims to be 'hydroactiv', by initially 'wetting' the abutment tooth, thereby overcoming the stringent arid environment necessary for addition silicones.

Primary determinant

The above discussion has focused on the secondary determinants influencing an accurate impression. However, even if all these factors are optimally prevalent, absence of the primary determinant makes an accurate impression elusive. The single factor, which is quintessential for a precise impression, is attaining and

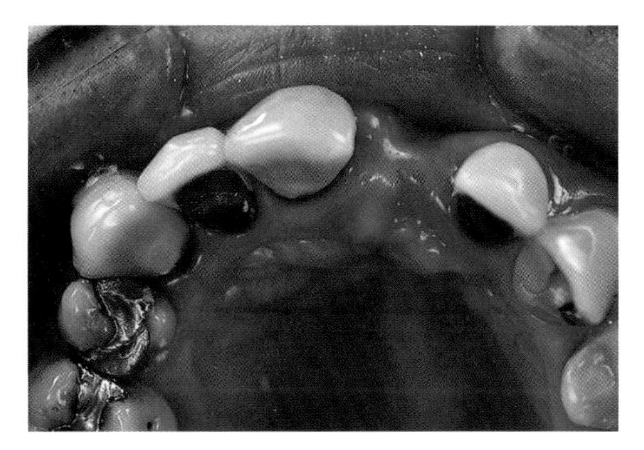

Figure 8.20 Achieving periodontal health: pre-operative defective crowns.

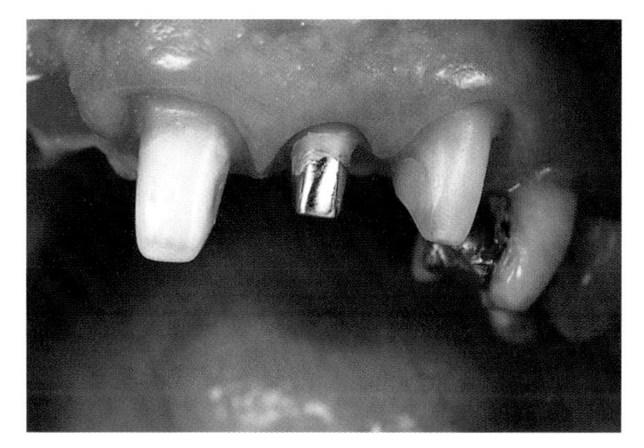

Figure 8.22 Achieving periodontal health: post/core build-up. Following tooth preparation and temporarisation, the gingiva is stable and healthy, ready for impression making.

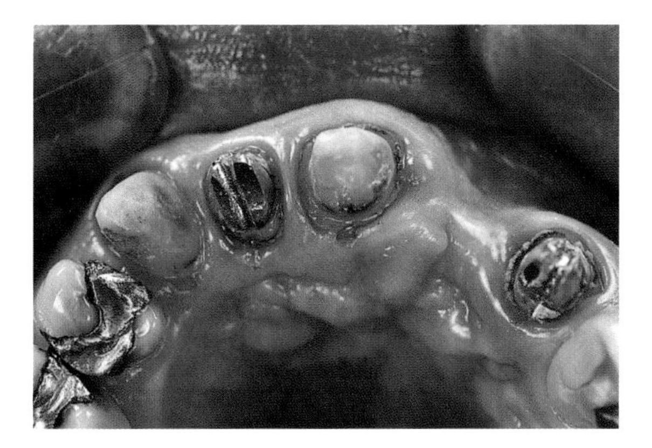

Figure 8.21 Achieving periodontal health: crown removal.

maintaining periodontal health; this is termed the primary determinant (Figs. 8.20–8.22). The period for gingival healing varies enormously from 3–21 days, and is influenced by patient and operator factors.[13]

Patient factors (risk assessment)

- Genetic predisposition
- Age
- Gender, e.g. pregnancy, osteoporosis
- Race
- Systemic illness, e.g. diabetes, compromised immune system, psychological stress[14]
- Dental biotype and bioform
- Type of oral pathogens
- Local trauma, or previous pathology with compromised vascularity, e.g. periapical lesions
- Socio-economic status
- Oral hygiene
- Local irritants, e.g. smoking, tobacco or betel nut chewing

All the above factors are beyond the clinician's control, and first nine are beyond the patient's control.[15] Although unchangeable, these risk factors should be borne in mind since these affect the rate of healing and may necessitate revising the proposed treatment plan (see discussion on risk assessment in Chapter 1). For example, an elderly patient, with systemic ailments, will have a protracted healing time. Also, a thin scalloped biotype will negate extensive soft tissue manipulation for fear of gingival recession, especially in aesthetically sensitive areas. Finally, low socio-economic status patients may not regard dental care a priority, and proposing sophisticated treatment modalities may be futile because of a high risk of failure (poor compliance and maintenance).

The last two items, oral hygiene and local irritants, are the only two factors that a patient can change, and which the clinician can influence by oral health education, emphasising the importance of maintaining a natural dentition.

Operator factors

- Prevention and prophylaxis, e.g. scaling and polishing
- Biologic width integrity
- Correct emergence profile
- Atraumatic clinical protocols, e.g. non-haemorrhagic procedures, calculated and precise tooth preparation, accurate impressions and cementing techniques
- Therapeutic temporary restorations

The operator factors are entirely controllable by clinical decisions and protocols, influencing whether or not periodontal health is achieved and maintained.

Prophylaxis

Scaling, polishing or root planing, with or without pharmaceutical adjuncts, are the first prerequisites for achieving periodontal health. Often, these vital procedures are either omitted or ignored, due to the overwhelming desire for commencing treatment. A little time spent at the start is not only beneficial for long-term oral health, but expedites all ensuing clinical stages. An adequate time following thorough prophylaxis is necessary to assess home oral hygiene measures and verify gingival health (Figs. 8.23–8.26). This also confirms the patient's responsibilities and commitment to the proposed treatment. If, however, compliance during this phase is poor, the treatment plan may require

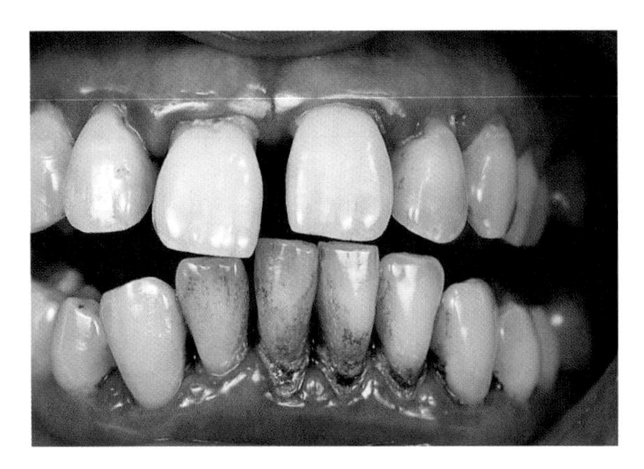

Figure 8.23 Pre-operative calculus and plaque deposits.

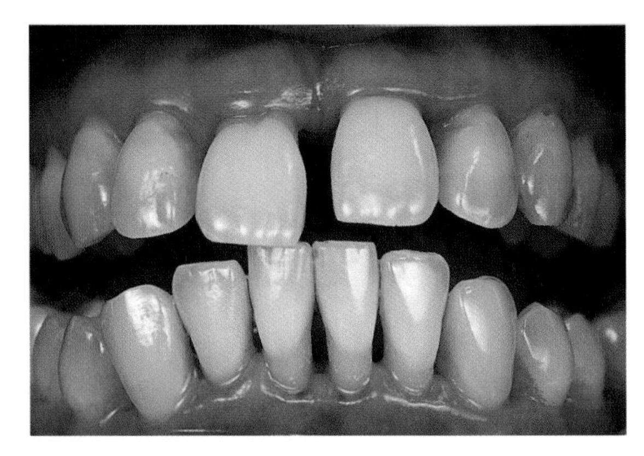

Figure 8.24 Post-operative after scaling and oral hygiene instruction of patient in Figure 8.23.

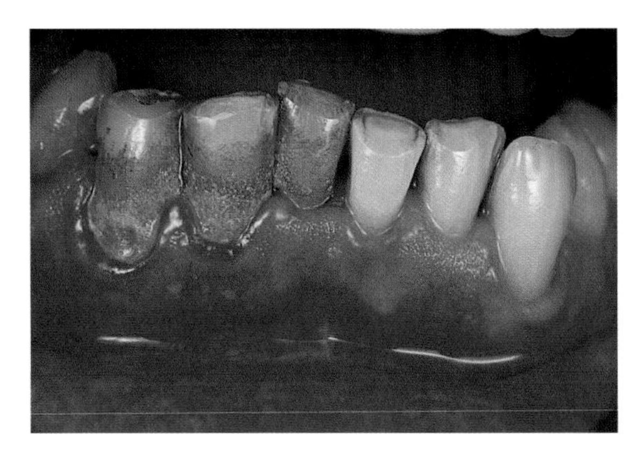

Figure 8.25 The left anterior mandibular teeth have been scaled, showing gingival health (pink colour, stippling, knife-edge FGMs). Compare with the right side, which has deposits and inflammation.

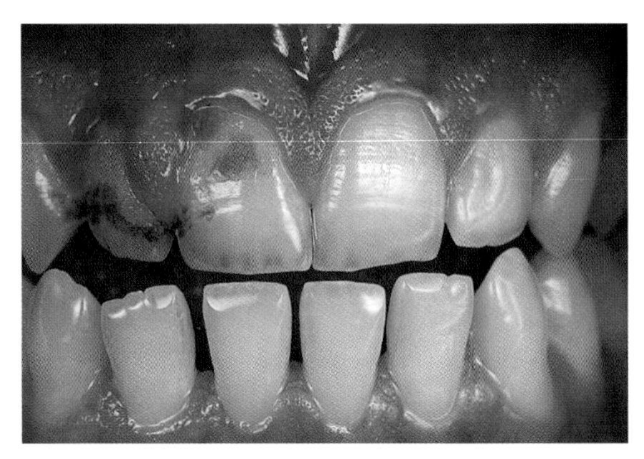

Figure 8.26 The anterior mandibular and left maxillary teeth have been scaled. Compare with the right maxillary teeth, which have calculus and periodontal inflammation.

modification to less sophisticated options, in order to avoid disappointments at later phases of treatment.

Biologic width integrity

The biologic width is discussed in Chapter 2, and is nature's way of protecting the two essential elements which ensure the survival of a tooth: the alveolar bone and the periodontal ligament. If these are compromised, the survival of the tooth is jeopardised. A shield is obviously only effective when intact. If damaged or destroyed, its function is reduced or nullified. Hence, any insult to this shield, bacterial or iatrogenic, diminishes its ability to fulfil the intended function. Clinical procedures potentially hazardous to the biologic width are retraction cord placement, tooth preparation, impressions, location of crown margins and cementation. Therefore, any restorative procedure either should be supragingival, or confined to dimensions of the gingival sulcus for respecting biologic width dimensions.

If location of the crown margins is subgingival, it is necessary to verify the crevice depth, so that impression procedures do not violate the epithelial attachment. Chapter 2 discussed the rationale for either using the alveolar bone crest (ABC), or a healthy free gingival margin (FGM) as a reference point. If the ABC is used as a landmark, the sulcus depth must be verified. Measuring pocket depths with a periodontal probe is inaccurate, because it is often difficult to assess the position of the probe tip, which may have penetrated beyond the crevice base into the epithelial or connective tissue attachments. The probe depth also depends on the force applied, tooth and probe angulations and prevalent inflammation. The ideal method to determine sulcus depth is to sound bone around an anaesthetised tooth and measure the entire dentogingival complex. Assuming ideal tooth anatomical variables, a mid-facial reading of 3 mm indicates a sulcus depth of 1 mm (entire dentogingival complex = 3 mm, minus 2 mm for biologic width = 1 mm sulcus depth). An interproximal measurement of 5 mm, indicates a 3 mm sulcus depth (entire dentogingival complex = 5 mm, minus 2 mm for biologic width = 3 mm sulcus depth).

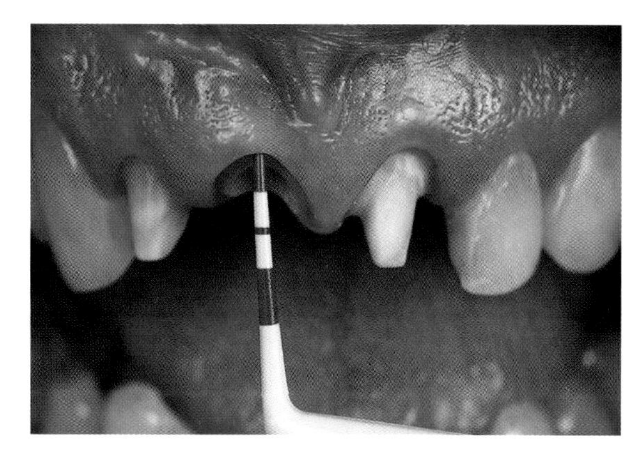

Figure 8.27 Periodontal probe measuring sulcus depth, using a healthy FGM as a reference point.

Alternatively, if the FGM is used, the crown margins should be placed 0.5 mm within the sulcus from the most apical zenith of the FGM, coronal to the epithelial attachment (Fig. 8.27). It is evident that whichever landmark is used, ABC or FGM, the margins are located coronal to the epithelial attachment. Similarly, the impression procedures are also limited to the dimensions of the sulcus.

Another factor to consider is the periodontal biotype, e.g. a thin, scalloped biotype will predispose to gingival recession, while a thick, flat biotype predisposes to periodontal pocket formation or persistent inflammation.[16] For anterior restorations, delicate tissue manipulation is necessary with thin scalloped biotypes for avoiding gingival recession, which could compromise aesthetics.

Emergence profile

The emergence profile of a crown is the junction of its cervical aspect, which meets the prepared tooth margin (Fig. 8.28).[17] An ideal emergence profile is attained when the crown and tooth margins meet at a tangent. Or, put another way, the crown margin lies at 180° to the root surface, apical to prepared tooth margins, ensuring that the crown is neither over- nor under-contoured. If the TTR was correctly fabricated, gingival health should be apparent. If the FGM is blanched or flaccid and unsupported, the gingiva

Figure 8.28 Emergence profile: sagittal view of a crown silhouette showing that its margins are on a tangent with the root apical to the finish line.

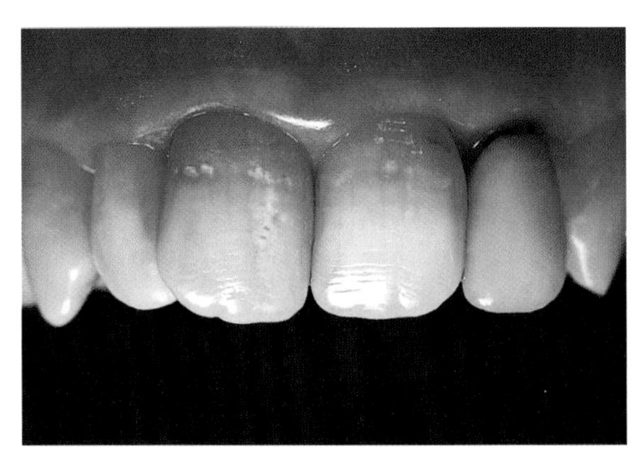

Figure 8.30 Atraumatic clinical protocol: pre-operative defective crown on left maxillary lateral.

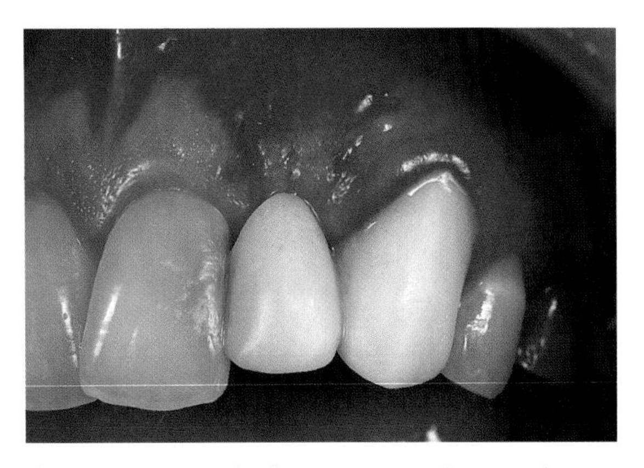

Figure 8.29 Gingival inflammation around incorrectly contoured temporary crown on left maxillary canine.

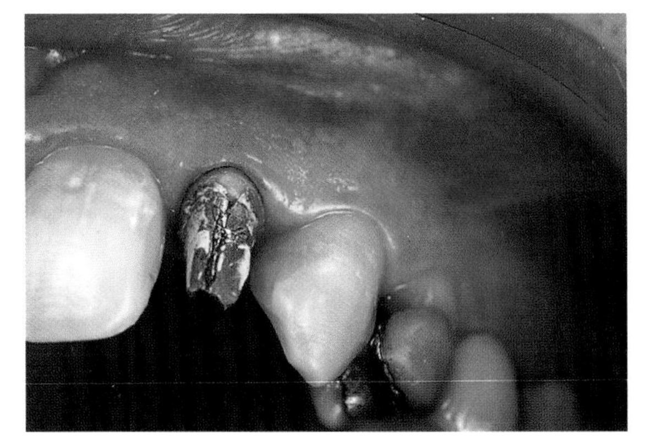

Figure 8.31 Atraumatic clinical protocol: retraction cord in sulcus and crown removal.

will be inflamed, and this requires resolution before biological impressions are attempted (Fig. 8.29).

Atraumatic clinical protocols

Following prophylaxis and achievement of periodontal health and stability, all clinical procedures should be performed atraumatically, minimising soft and hard tissue damage. These include crown removal, tooth preparation, retraction cord placement, impression making and cementation.[18] Ideally, whenever possible, a non-haemorrhagic approach is adopted, with the rationale that minimising trauma during treatment not only accelerates the healing process, but also helps maintain existing health (Figs. 8.30–8.34).

Therapeutic temporary restorations

A detailed explanation for fabricating temporaries is outlined in Chapter 7. To summarise, a temporary restoration should respect the biologic width, have a correct emergence profile and act as a template for the definitive restoration (Fig. 8.35). The fruits of these labours are realised when attempting impressions. Meticulous attention to detail during fabricating, adjusting and maintaining a temporary prosthesis results in optimal soft tissue health, a prerequisite for both dental and gingival impressions.

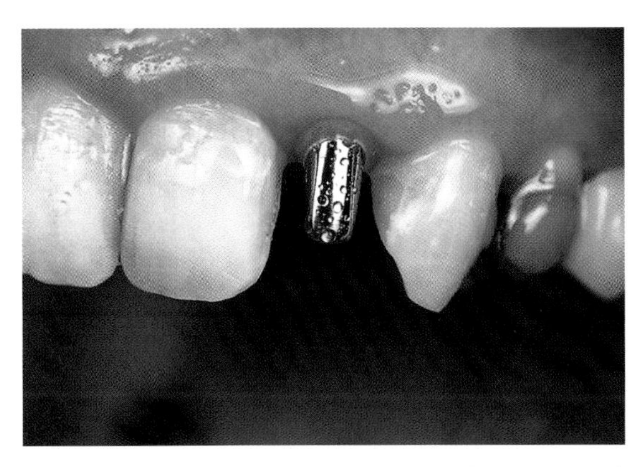

Figure 8.32 Atraumatic clinical protocol: refined cast metal core using a haemorrhage-free protocol.

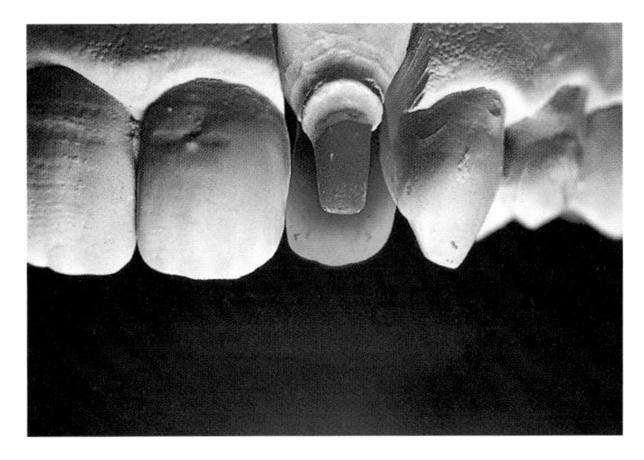

Figure 8.33 Atraumatic clinical protocol: definitive crown-to-tooth preparation relationship.

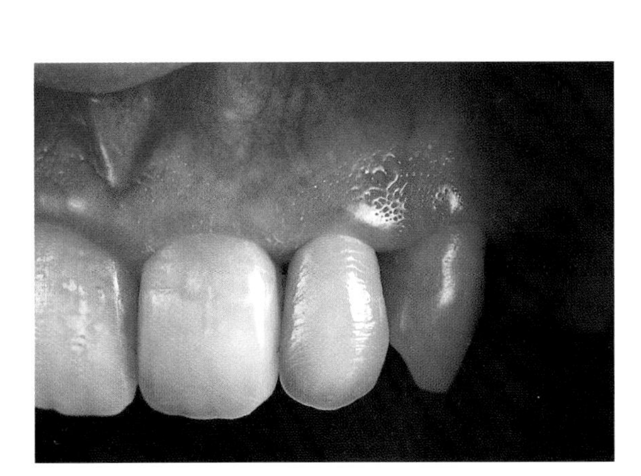

Figure 8.34 Atraumatic clinical protocol: cemented definitive crown.

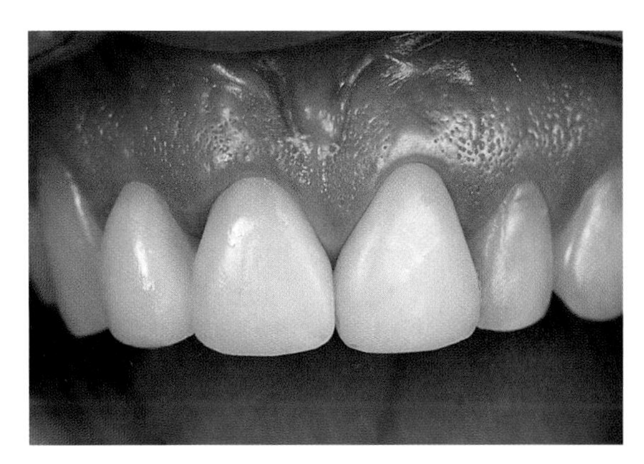

Figure 8.35 Chairside temporary acrylic crowns on teeth #12, 11 and 21, which will be adjusted and used as templates for the final restorations.

CLINICAL PRACTICE

Once the primary determinant, gingival health, is attained and maintained, biological impressions are contemplated. Two types are required, the dental and gingival biological impressions.

Dental biological impressions

The dental biological impression is for recording the prepared tooth margins. To achieve this, gingival retraction using the double cord technique is necessary for exposing the preparation margins, maintaining an arid environment and accommodating an adequate bulk of impression material.[19] In order to avoid distortion of the impression material a minimum sulcus opening of at least 0.2 mm is required,[20] and typically, a gingival deflection of 0.3–0.4 mm is routine.[21] Finally, it is necessary to record the apical part of the root beyond the preparation margins, allowing the ceramist to construct a correct crown emergence profile. The double cord technique is shown in Figure 8.36. The first thin cord (Ultradent # 000) is delicately introduced into the sulcus to vertically retract the gingiva apically, and maintain a dry field by absorbing the crevicular fluid. This cord should disappear into

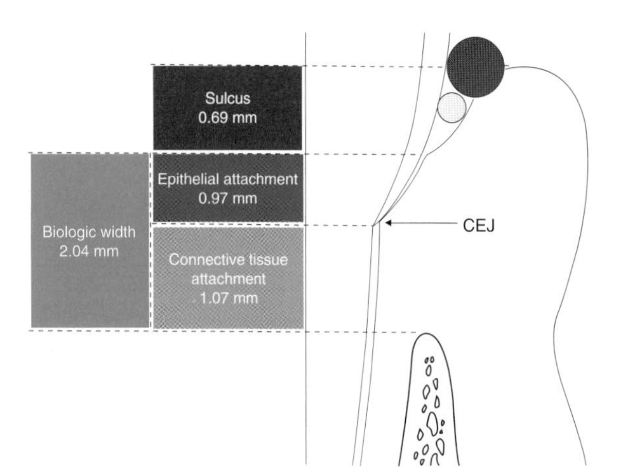

Figure 8.36 Double retraction cord technique.

the sulcus and be invisible from the facial aspect. The second thicker cord (Ultradent # 1), pre-impregnated with an astringent, e.g. buffered aluminium chloride, is introduced to half its width to transiently horizontally (laterally) open the gingival crevice. Instead of using a pre-impregnated cord, a dry cord can be placed into the sulcus, and then dabbed with astringent, which swells the cord and dilates the crevice. After 5 minutes, the second cord is removed, while the first stays in situ. An impression is now possible to record the preparation margins, and an apical part of the tooth beyond the finish line (Figs. 8.37 & 8.38).

To ensure predictable and consistently accurate impressions, the following sequence is necessary:

(1) Establish presence of primary determinant, i.e. gingival health
(2) Choose appropriate secondary determinates:
  - Stock tray for up to three units, custom tray for more than three units
  - Full intra-arch impressions
  - Avoid excessively large holes in trays, minimising intra-oral excess material spillage (or use closed-tray technique)
  - One-stage technique
  - Passive setting of impression material
  - Avoid chilling impression material
  - Use automixing units
  - Use either retraction cord as a physical barrier in sulcus or chemical retraction
  - Use either polyether or addition silicone materials for convenience, expediency and accuracy
(3) After tooth preparation (Fig. 8.39), seal exposed dentine tubules, mitigating post-operative sensitivity[22] using either a sixth or seventh generation self-etching DBA[23] or a fifth generation DBA by etching, priming and sealing. To avoid interaction of the oxygen inhibition layer with acrylic monomer and impression materials, light-cure the bonding agent through a glycerine gel cover[24]
(4) Ascertain sulcus depth for selection of the appropriate diameters of the retraction cords. For the double retraction cord technique, both cords are placed within the dimensions of the prevailing sulcus depth. The first cord is thinner than the second cord
(5) Assuming normal anatomical relationships, the first cord is usually # Ultradent 000. Applying gentle pressure with a thin flat plastic instrument, introduce the dry cord into the friable sulcus without causing haemorrhage (Fig. 8.40) (Hint 8.1)
(6) Next, a second thicker cord, usually Ultradent # 1 pre-impregnated with an astringent, e.g. buffered aluminium chloride, is placed to half its width (Hint 8.2). This second cord should be visible from the facial aspect (Fig. 8.41) (Hint 8.3)
(7) After 5 minutes, ease second cord from the sulcus, leaving the first thinner cord in situ (Figs. 8.42 & 8.43) (Hint 8.4)
(8) Copiously apply tray adhesive to the appropriate size tray (Hint 8.5)[25]
(9) While injecting the low viscosity wash on to the prepared abutment(s) (Fig. 8.44), ask assistant simultaneously to load the heavy-body material into impression tray (Hint 8.6)
(10) After correct seating and location of the tray, relieve pressure allowing passive polymerisation of the impression materials (Hint 8.7)
(11) Once set, rapidly remove tray avoiding viscoelastic distortions of impression materi-

als. Rapid removal reduces the time the material is under stress and therefore reduces permanent distortions[26]

(12) Check impression for absence of voids and defects, and faithful reproduction of the part of the root surface apical to the preparation margins (Hint 8.8)

(13) Disinfect with appropriate antiseptic solution, e.g. glutaraldehyde or sodium hypochloride (Hint 8.9)[27]

(14) Pour impression using dental plaster/stone (addition silicones are compatible with most dental plasters for model and die fabrication) (Fig. 8.45)

(15) Addition silicones allow multiple pours for up to 1 week, and both addition silicones and polyethers can be stored in temperature ranges of 4–40°C without affecting dimensional stability[28]

(16) Take facebow and bite registrations (Figs. 8.46 & 8.47).

Gingival biological impressions

The gingival impression is for assessing the relationship between soft tissues and the artificial prostheses. This impression is essential for anterior teeth where 'pink' or soft tissue aesthetics are of paramount concern, but less relevant for

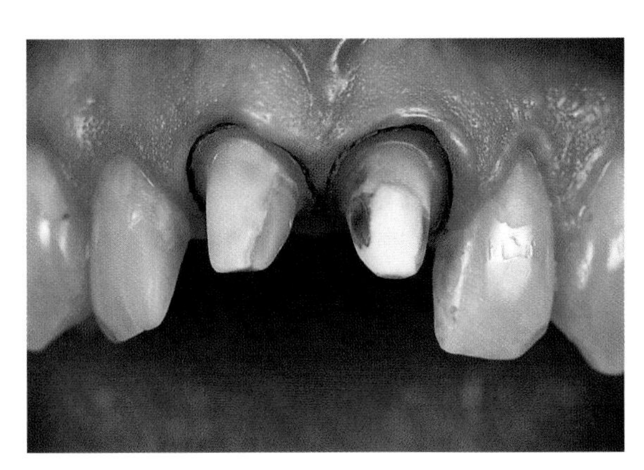

Figure 8.37 Retraction cord in situ to deflect gingival margins for recording the root surface apical to the finish line.

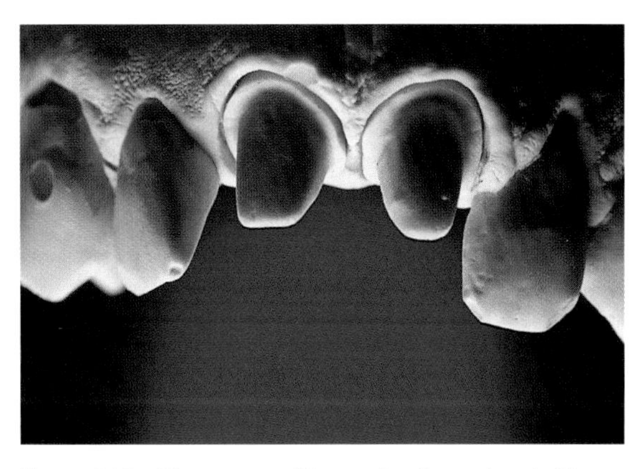

Figure 8.38 Plaster cast of impression for patient in Figure 8.37 showing that the area apical to the crown margins is accurately reproduced, which will be used by the ceramist to obtain a correct emergence profile.

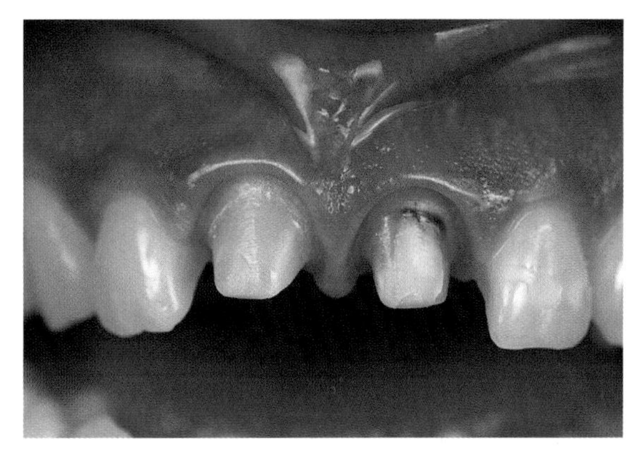

Figure 8.39 Double retraction cord technique for dental biological impressions: completed tooth preparations on maxillary central incisors with a healthy periodontium.

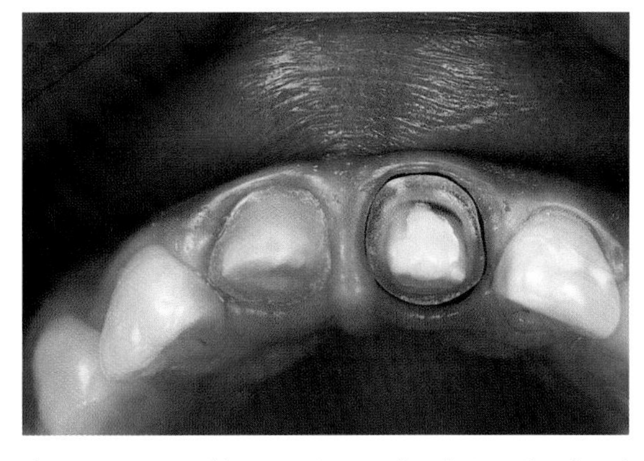

Figure 8.40 Double retraction cord technique for dental biological impressions: the sulcus around the left central will be deflected, while that on the right central will remain undeflected for comparison. First thin, dry cord placed into the gingival crevice.

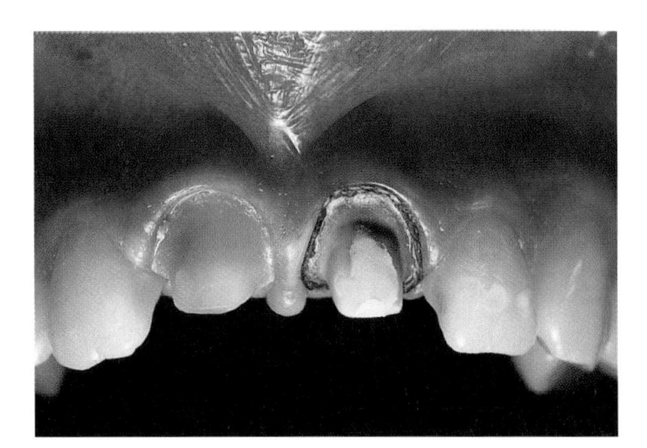

Figure 8.41 Double retraction cord technique for dental biological impressions: second thicker cord placed to half its width.

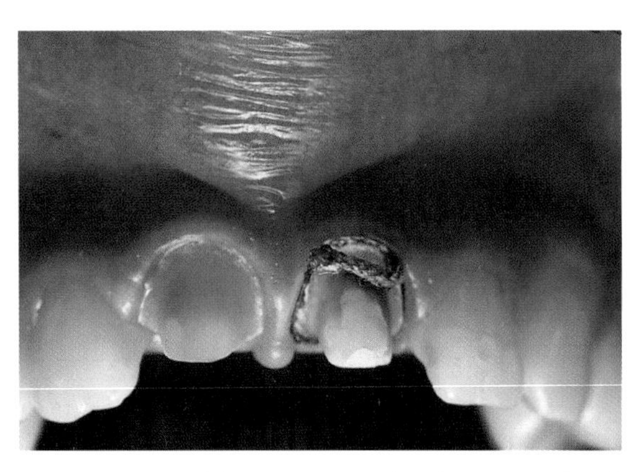

Figure 8.42 Double retraction cord technique for dental biological impressions: second cord removed after 5 minutes, leaving the first thinner cord in the sulcus.

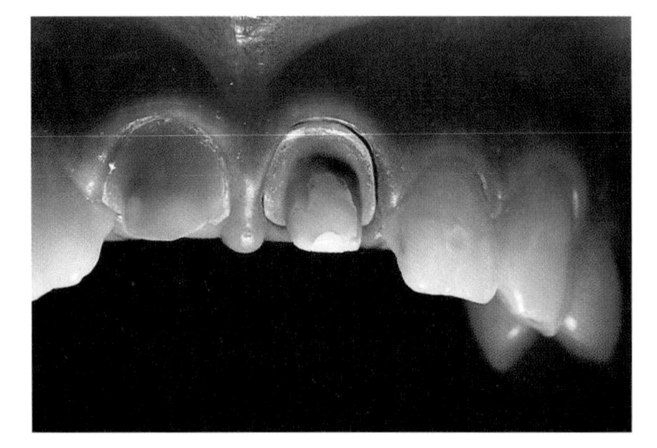

Figure 8.43 Double retraction cord technique for dental biological impressions: retracted sulcus on left central incisor, compare with un-deflected sulcus around right central.

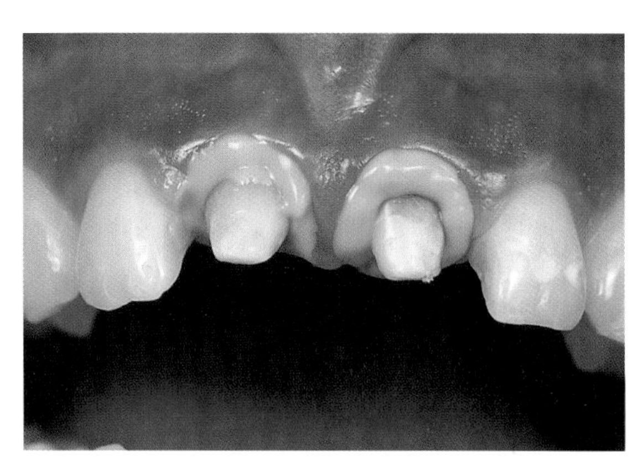

Figure 8.44 Double retraction cord technique for dental biological impressions: light-bodied impression material placed around preparations immediately following gingival retraction.

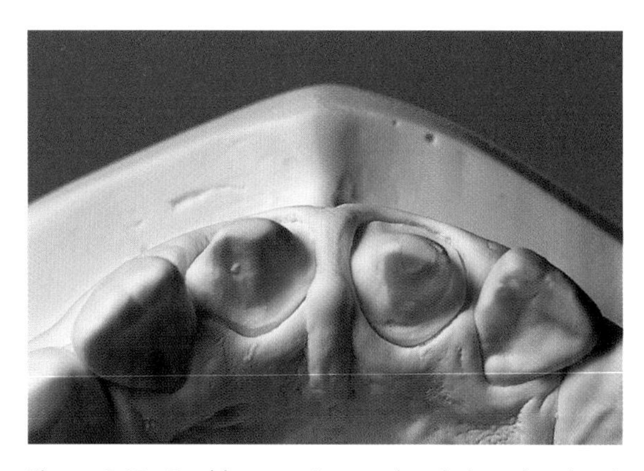

Figure 8.45 Double retraction cord technique for dental biological impressions: plaster cast showing accurate recording of the root surface apical to the finish line.

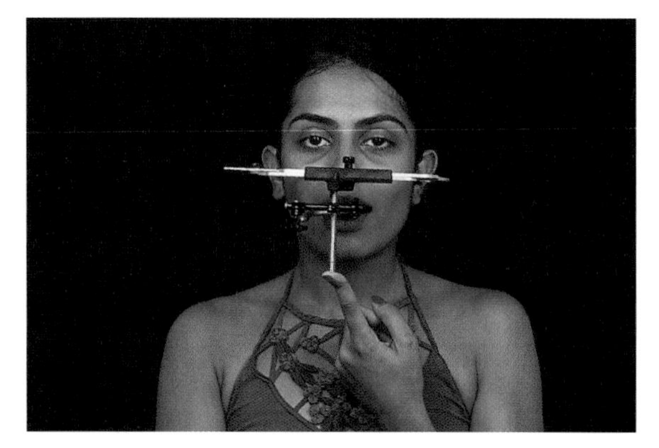

Figure 8.46 Double retraction cord technique for dental biological impressions: facebow registration for semi-adjustable articulator.

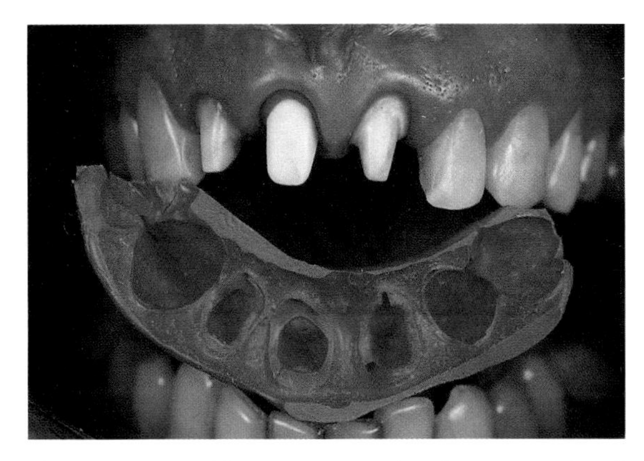

Figure 8.47 Double retraction cord technique for dental biological impressions: silicone bite registration.

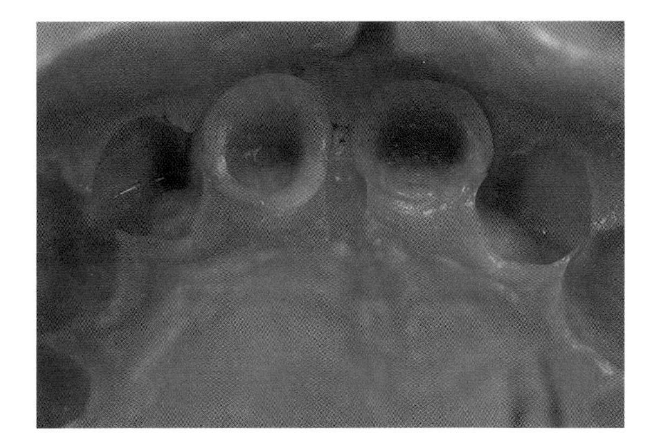

Figure 8.48 Gingival biological impressions: crowns picked up in a soft silicone impression material.

posterior extra-coronal and all intra-coronal restorations.

The gingival biological impression is made either at the bisque try-in stage of the definitive restoration, or with the TTRs (Fig. 8.48). The purpose is recording undeflected, healthy gingival architecture in a natural resting state. This allows correct interproximal contact points (Fig. 8.49), by contouring the crowns in relation to the bone crest, ideally 5 mm or less for complete papilla,[29] and ensuring ideal transmucosal support of the FGM by the cervical part of the crown, preventing a horizontally under- or over-contoured crown.

Clinically, steps for a gingival impression are similar to the dental impressions. The essential difference with gingival impressions is that retractions cords are omitted.

(1) Establish presence of primary determinant, i.e. gingival health
(2) Choose appropriate secondary determinates as for dental impressions
(3) A monophase consistency of either polyether or addition silicone is the ideal material for gingival biological impressions
(4) Ensure tooth abutment is clean and free of temporary cement
(5) Place crowns (bisque stage definitives or TTR) on to prepared abutments
(6) Copiously apply tray adhesive to appropriate size tray
(7) Mix monophase impression material and load into tray
(8) After correct seating and location of the tray, relieve pressure, allowing passive polymerisation of the impression materials
(9) Once set, rapidly remove tray avoiding viscoelastic distortions of impression materials. Rapid removal reduces the time the material is under stress and therefore reduces permanent distortions
(10) Check impression for absence of voids and defects
(11) The crowns should be picked up in the impression, if not, remove from the abutment(s) and carefully seat into impression
(12) Disinfect with appropriate antiseptic solution, e.g. glutaraldehyde or sodium hypochloride
(13) Pour impression using dental plaster/stone (addition silicones are compatible with most dental plasters for model and die fabrication or create soft tissue emulating the gingivae (Figs. 8.50 & 8.51)
(14) Addition silicones allow multiple pours for up to 1 week, and both addition silicone and polyethers can be stored at temperatures of 4–40°C without affecting dimensional stability.

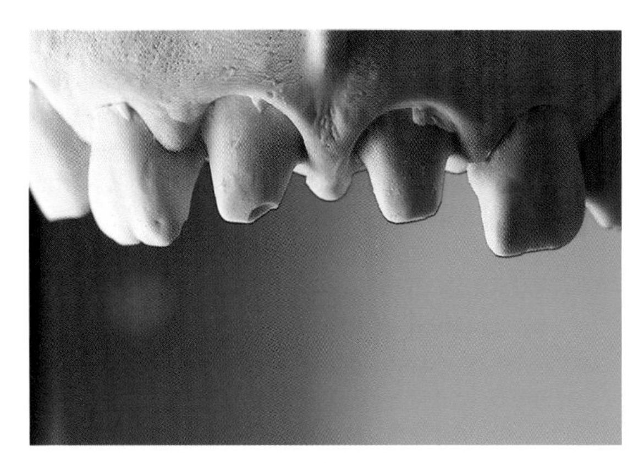

Figure 8.49 Gingival biological impressions: plaster cast showing that the gingival impression records the soft tissues in a healthy, non-deflected state.

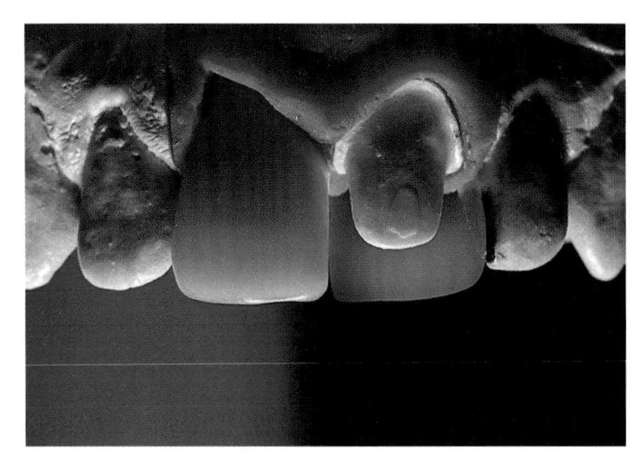

Figure 8.50 Gingival biological impressions: silicone soft tissue model to contour transmucosal part of the crown.

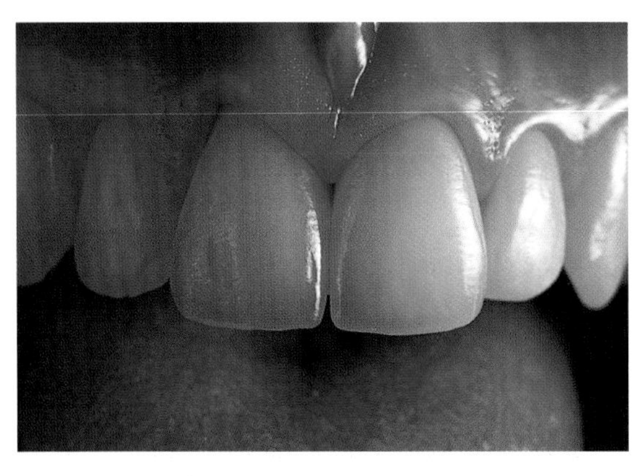

Figure 8.51 Gingival biological impressions: correctly contoured crowns for patient in Figure 8.50.

Hints and Tips

- Hint 8.1 – The first thinner cord should entirely disappear into the sulcus, and be invisible from the facial aspect
- Hint 8.2 – The second, thicker cord should be impregnated with the haemostatic agent 10–15 minutes before use
- Hint 8.3 – Instead of pre-soaking the second cord in a haemostatic agent, it can be placed and soaked later with haemostatic agent using cotton wool pellets. This protocol swells the cord, facilitating mechanical dilatation of the sulcus
- Hint 8.4 – Moistening the second cord with water before removal prevents unwanted haemorrhage
- Hint 8.5 – Air-drying the tray adhesive ensures tenacity, and prevents pooling which causes the adhesive to act as a lubricant rather than an adhesive
- Hint 8.6 – When mixing addition silicone putty manually, use vinyl instead of latex gloves, which retard setting reaction
- Hint 8.7 – Using a timer or stopwatch ensures precise intra-oral setting reaction, usually 3 minutes (depending on proprietary product)
- Hint 8.8 – If the first, thinner cord is picked up in the impression, loose parts can be cut with scissors. However, attempting to pull tenacious cord embedded in the impression material causes tears, leading to inaccuracies of the crown margins or the area apical to the margins; these areas are essential for creating a correct emergence profile
- Hint 8.9 – Disinfecting for 30–60 minutes results in no distortion, but long-term, overnight soaking (>18 hours) causes irreversible distortion of the impression material

References

[1] Shavell, H.M. (1988) Mastering the art of tissue management during provisionalization and biological final impressions. *Int J Periodont Rest Dent*, **8(3)**, 24–43

[2] Touati, B. and Etienne, J.-M. (1998) Improved shape and emergence profile in an extensive ceramic rehabilitation. *Pract Periodont Aesthet Dent*, **10(1)**, 129–135

[3] Ceyhan, A.J., Johnson, G.H. and Lepe, X. (2003) The effect of tray selection, viscosity of impression materials, and sequence of pour on the accuracy of dies made from dual-arch impressions. *J Prosthet Dent*, **90(2)**, 143–149

[4] McCabe, J.F. and Carrick, T.E. (1989) Rheological properties of elastomers during setting. *J Dent Res*, **68**, 1218–1222

[5] Sadan, A. (2001) The one-step versus the two-step impression technique. *Pract Proced Aesthet Dent*, **13(4)**, 282

[6] Ruel, J., Schuessler, P.J., Malament, K. and Mori, D. (1980) Effects of retraction procedures on the periodontium in humans. *J Prosthet Dent*, **44**, 508–515

[7] Azzi, R., Tsao, T.F., Carranza, F.A. and Kennedy, E.B. (1983) Comparative study of gingival retraction methods. *J Prosthet Dent*, **50**, 561–565

[8] de Camargo, L.M., Chee, W.W.L. and Donovan, T.E. (1993) Inhibition of polymerisation of polyvinyl siloxanes by medicaments used on gingival retraction cords. *J Prosthet Dent*, **70**, 114–117

[9] Weir, D.J. and Williams, B.H. (1984) Clinical effectiveness of mechanical-chemical tissue displacement methods. *J Prosthet Dent*, **51**, 326–329

[10] Pelzner, R.B., Kempler, D., Stark, M.M., Lum, L.B., Nicholson, R.J. and Soelberg, K.B. (1978) Human blood pressure and pulse rate response to racemic epinephrine retraction cord. *J Prosthet Dent*, **39**, 287–292

[11] Kahn, R.L. and Donovan, T.E. (1989) A pilot study of polymerisation inhibition of poly(vinyl siloxane) materials by latex gloves. *Int J Prosthodont*, **2**, 128–130

[12] Tjan, A.H.L., Whan, S.B., Tijan, A.H. and Sarkissian, R. (1996) Clinically orientated evaluation of the accuracy of commonly used impression materials. *J Prosthet Dent*, **56**, 4–8

[13] de Gennaro, G.G., Landesman, H.M. and Calhoun, J.E. (1982) Comparison of gingival inflammation related to retraction cords. *J Prosthet Dent*, **47**, 384–386

[14] Torabi-Gaarden, R., Breivik, T., Hansen, F., Malt, U.F. and Gjermo, P.E. (2004) Negative life events, anxiety, depression and coping ability (stress) as related to chronic periodontitis. *Perio*, **1(1)**, 35–42

[15] Wilson, T.G. and Kornman, K.S. (1996) *Fundamentals of Periodontics*. Quintessence Publishing Co. Inc., Carol Stream, IL

[16] Olsson, M. and Lindhe, J. (1991) Periodontal characteristics in individuals with varying form of the upper central incisors. *J Clin Periodontol*, **18(1)**, 78–82

[17] Martignoni, M. and Schonenberger, A. (1990) *Precision Fixed Prosthodontics: Clinical and Laboratory Aspects*. Quintessence Publishing Co. Inc., Chicago

[18] Ahmad, I. (2001) Replacing defective porcelain fused to metal crowns with galvano-ceramic restorations as an alternative to all-ceramic crowns: a clinical case study. *Independent Dentistry*, November, 2001

[19] Perakis, N., Belser, U.C. and Magne, P. (2004) Final impressions: a review of material properties and description of a current technique. *Int J Periodontics Restorative Dent*, **24**, 109–117

[20] Laufer, B.Z., Baharav, H., Ganor, Y. and Cardash, H.S. (1996) The effect of marginal thickness on the distortion of different impression materials. *J Prosthet Dent*, **76**, 466–471

[21] Ramadan, F.A. (1968) *The Linear Effectiveness of Dental Tissue Displacement Materials*. Thesis, St Louis University Dental School

[22] Paul, S.J. and Scharer, P. (1997) The dual bonding technique: a modified method to improve adhesive luting procedure. *Int J Periodontics Restorative Dent*, **17**, 536–545

[23] Ahmad, I. (2003) Evaluating dentine bonding agents: an update. *Pract Proced Aesthet Dent*, **15(7)**, 531–538

[24] Magne, P. and Belser, U. (2002) Immediate dentin bonding. In: *Bonded Porcelain Restorations in the Anterior Dentition – A Biomimetric Approach*. pp. 270–273. Quintessence, Berlin

[25] Bindra, B. and Heath, J.R.I. (1997) Adhesion of elastomeric impression materials to tray. *J Oral Rehabil*, **24**, 63–69

[26] Hondrum, S.O. (1994) Tera energy properties of three impression materials. *Int J Prosthodont*, **7**, 517–521

[27] Rios, M., Morgano, S.M., Stein, R.S. and Rose, L. (1996) Effects of chemical disinfectant solutions on the stability and accuracy of the dental impression complex. *J Prosthet Dent*, **76**, 356–362

[28] Corso, M., Abanomy, A., Di Canzio, J., Zurakowski, D. and Morango, S.M. (1998) The effect of temperature changes on the dimensional stability of polyvinyl siloxane and polyether impression materials. *J Prosthet Dent*, **79**, 626–631

[29] Tarnow, D., Magner, A. and Fletcher, P. (1992) The effect of the distance from the contact point to the crest of bone in the presence or absence of the interproximal dental papilla. *J Periodontol*, **63**(**1**), 995–996

9 Try-in procedures

The try-in stage is the most interactive stage in the provision of artificial restorations, involving the clinician, ceramist, dental nurse, hygienist, the patient and patient's family and friends. Whilst biological and technical aspects are the concerns of the clinician and ceramist, respectively, aesthetics and visual assessment by the entire dental team, the patient and their entourage is invaluable for avoiding later disappointments and misgivings.

At the try-in procedure, the clinician has a last chance to rectify a restoration prior to cementation. Most aspects of the prosthesis should have been finalised with the therapeutic restorations, including occlusion, phonetics and aesthetics (form, size and position). While the latter can be re-assessed, some items can only be evaluated at the try-in stage. These include correct die trimming, sufficient space for a cement vent by using die spacers, intaglio surface purity, unimpeded seating, margin integrity, proximal contacts, emergence profile, cervical trans-gingival contour (horizontal and vertical under- or over-contouring), texture, lustre and colour with different lighting conditions (Fig. 9.1).

Basically, two types of refinements may be necessary: material additions and removals. As a generalisation, additions usually require a remake, whilst removals, if minimal, can be carried out chairside. If removals are required, these should be kept to an absolute minimum. As previously mentioned, any adjustment to ceramics initiates flaws, which propagate to eventual fracture. This is particularly relevant for thin cross-sectional or uni-layer ceramics, unsupported by high-strength ceramic cores. If adjustments are limited, these can be subsequently 'sealed' by either polishing and/or re-glazing in the dental laboratory. Adjustments are carried out using a 12-fluted tungsten carbide finishing bur with copious irrigation, or aluminium oxide abrasive discs followed by silicone tips and rubber cups loaded with diamond polishing paste. However, if extensive adjustments are envisaged, a remake is a better option, saving clinical time and ensuring long-term viability of the restoration. The try-in stage consists of the extra – and intra-oral evaluation.

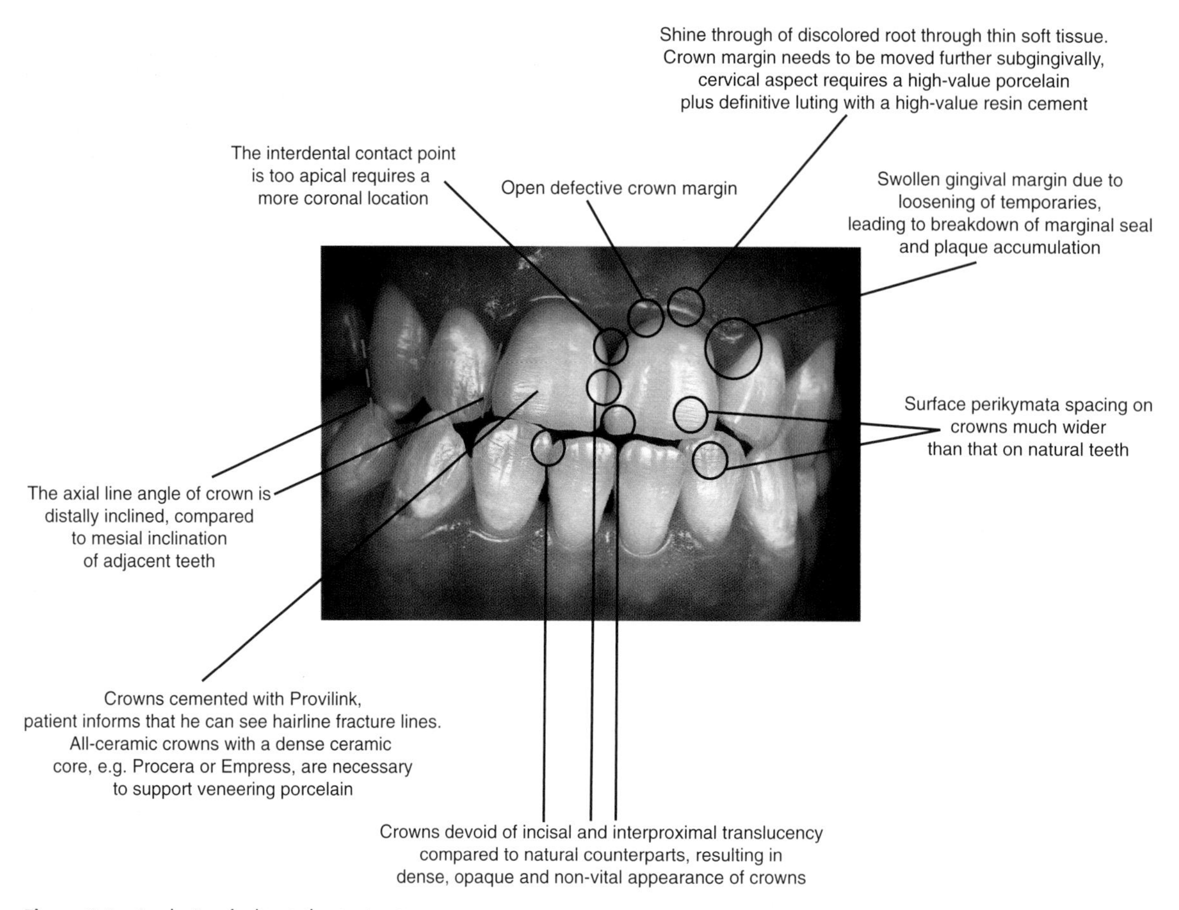

Figure 9.1 Analysing faults at the try-in stage.

CLINICAL PRACTICE

Extra-oral evaluation

Most all-ceramic systems require at least two pours of the dental biological impression. The first plaster cast is left untrimmed, and, if necessary, mounted on to an articulator using a facebow and bite registrations. The second cast is trimmed and the die sectioned for fabricating the definitive restoration (Figs. 9.2 & 9.3). An advantage of using addition silicone impression materials is that multiple pours are possible, and these may be difficult with reversible hydrocolloids and some polyethers. Although the master cast can be duplicated by making impressions in the dental laboratory, this practice should be resisted. The greater the number of laboratory stages, the greater the possibility of introducing error. Ideally, all pours should be made from the original intra-oral impression, keeping laboratory stages to an absolute minimum.

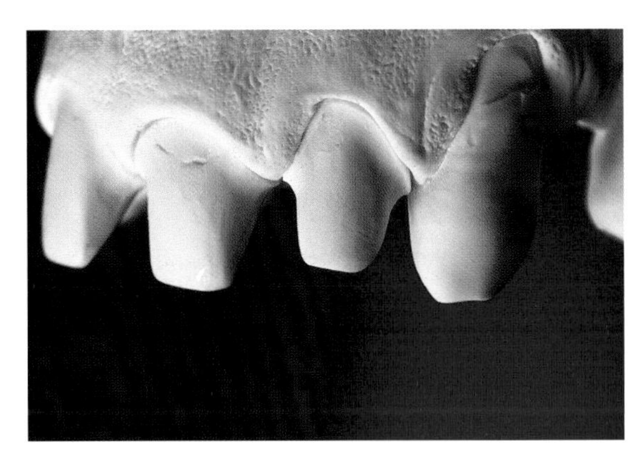

Figure 9.2 Untrimmed cast from the dental biological impression.

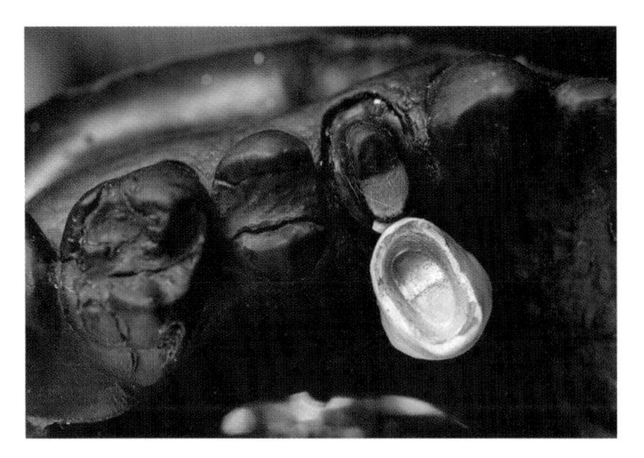

Figure 9.4 Inspection of the intaglio surface for defects.

Figure 9.3 Correctly trimmed die from the dental biological impression for fabricating an all-ceramic crown.

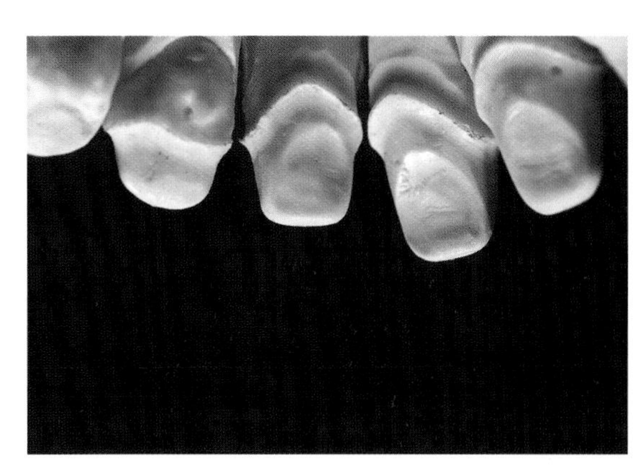

Figure 9.5 The finish line is marked using a fine pencil.

Inspection of restoration on trimmed die

(1) Inspect intaglio surface for air blows or blebs that impede correct seating on the die (Fig. 9.4). For all-ceramic units, passive seating is essential to prevent initiation of crack formation. If a milled coping is used as a substructure, it should have an ideal cement spacing of less than 100 µm. A tight fit is detrimental, causing stress within the ceramic, while larger discrepancies create a wider cement thickness layer, which may yield under functional loads. In both scenarios, a remake is advisable

(2) Correct die trimming is essential to delineate the crown margins especially if CAD/CAM technology with a scanner is utilised. The finish line should be marked with a fine pencil (Fig. 9.5). In order to define the circumferential finish line, an apical hollow beyond the finish line is created by trimming the plaster cast 0.5 mm horizontally and 1–2 mm vertically (Fig. 9.6). The margin integrity is severely compromised unless this stage is meticulously performed. Having confirmed that the die is correctly trimmed, the crown is inspected under magnification, ensuring validity of the cervical margins. Since the die is trimmed by removing the plaster apical to the finish line, the emergence profile can only be assessed on the untrimmed cast

(3) Ensure die spacer is sufficient to accommodate cement lute (Fig. 9.7)

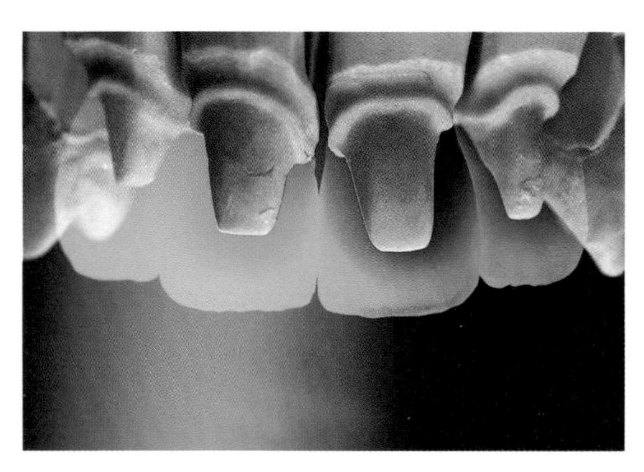

Figure 9.6 Creating an apical hollow beyond the crown margins delineates the finish line.

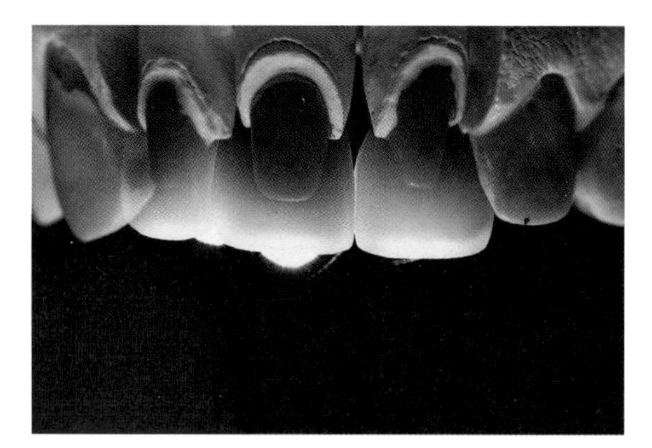

Figure 9.8 Correct emergence profile of three all-ceramic crowns.

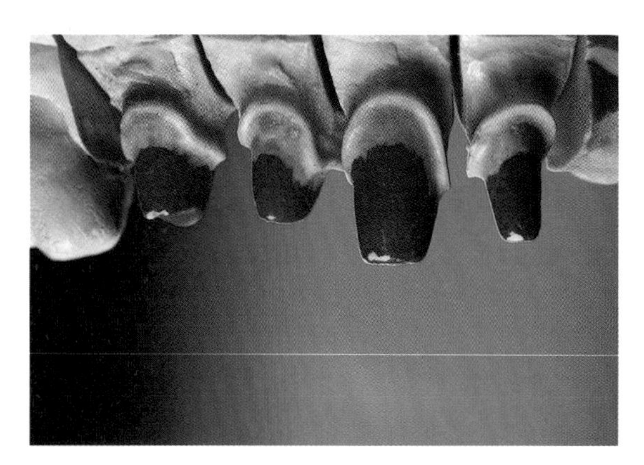

Figure 9.7 Die spacer for adequate cement space.

Inspection of restoration on untrimmed die

The remainder of the assessment is performed by placing the restoration on to the untrimmed die:

(1) Verify that emergence profile is on a tangent to an area apical to the finish line in both the horizontal and vertical planes (Fig. 9.8). Also, on a soft tissue model, ensure that the transgingival contour is sufficient to support the FGM. Minor over-contouring can be trimmed with appropriate rotary instruments, but deficiencies will require additions or remake in the dental laboratory
(2) Ensure occlusion is correct in CR, CO and lateral and protrusive excursions (anterior guidance), particularly if mounted on to an articulator, using thin, coloured articulation papers (40 μm – Bausch, Koeln, Germany) and shim stock (8 μm – Hanel, Langenau, Germany). Where difficulties are envisaged, a bisque try-in may be prudent to make adjustments intra-orally, before returning the restoration to the laboratory for polishing and glazing
(3) Aesthetics are better assessed intra-orally, but a cursory check of the following is helpful: colour, characterisations, morphology, size (Figs. 9.9–9.11)
(4) Contacts. For posterior teeth, contacts should be coronal to the interproximal col, preventing gingival entrapment and allowing ease of oral hygiene procedures. They should be tight and wide to prevent food impaction, without placing undue pressure on adjacent dentition. For anterior teeth, the contacts influence aesthetics with regard to the degree of papilla fill, and are best assessed intra-orally.

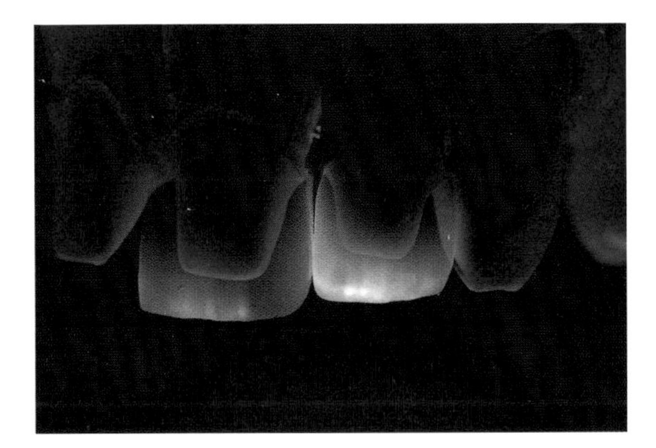

Figure 9.9 Incisal translucency and characterisations of two all-ceramic units.

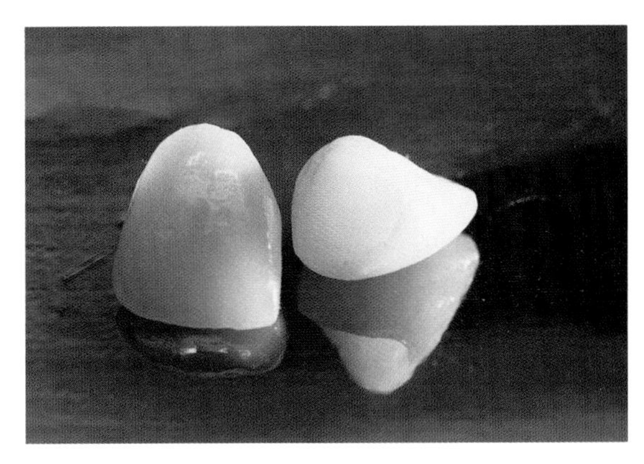

Figure 9.10 Assessing surface texture and lustre.

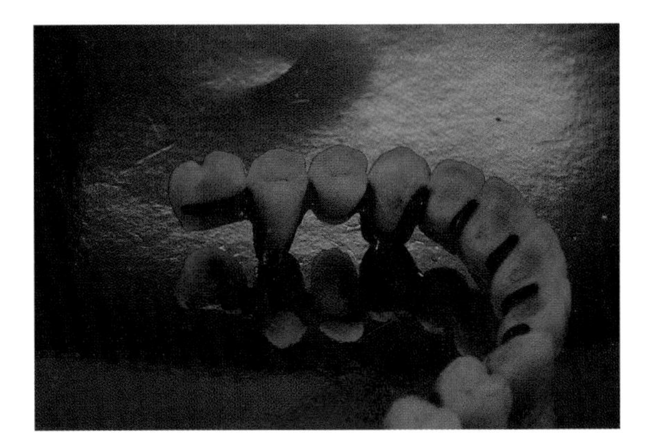

Figure 9.11 Ultraviolet illumination checks fluorescence of the veneering porcelain.

Intra-oral evaluation

(1) Remove therapeutic temporary restoration, provisional cement and clean abutment with a mixture of pumice and chlorhexidine paste
(2) Place definitive restoration on to abutment
(3) Confirm marginal integrity using a silicone paste, such as Fit Checker (GC)
(4) Check emergence profile and the transgingival contour, ensuring that the FGM is adequately supported by the cervical part of the restoration. Over-contoured restorations blanch the gingivae, while under-contouring results in unsupported and flaccid FGMs. If gross alterations are necessary, place crown(s) on to abutment(s) and make a gingival biological impression, allowing the ceramist to visualise the healthy, stable FGM, and adjust contour accordingly (Fig. 9.12) (Hint 9.1)
(5) Check occlusion with articulation paper, in a similar manner to extra-oral assessment. The best method of checking occlusion is in the mouth, no articulator can substitute intra-oral verification. CR, CO and excursions are checked, with particular attention to avoid introducing new defective contacts (see Chapter 2) (Hint 9.2)
(6) Finalise aesthetics, including colour (Hint 9.3), morphology, size, surface texture, comparing to adjacent and antagonist teeth (Fig. 9.13). Finally, check alignment of the restoration(s) in relation to lips and facial landmarks, e.g. interpupillary line
(7) Phonetics – check 'm', 'f', 'v', 'th' and 's' sounds (see Chapter 2)
(8) Contacts. For posterior teeth, contacts should be coronal to the interproximal col, preventing gingival entrapment and allowing ease of oral hygiene procedures. They should be tight and wide to prevent food impaction, without placing undue pressure on adjacent dentition. For anterior teeth, the contacts influence aesthetics with regard to the degrees of papilla fill. Ensure that the contact point is 5 mm or less from the bone crest,

mark position on the restoration and make adjustments accordingly

(9) If alterations are necessary return restoration to dental laboratory; otherwise, proceed to cementation of the restoration (see Chapter 10).

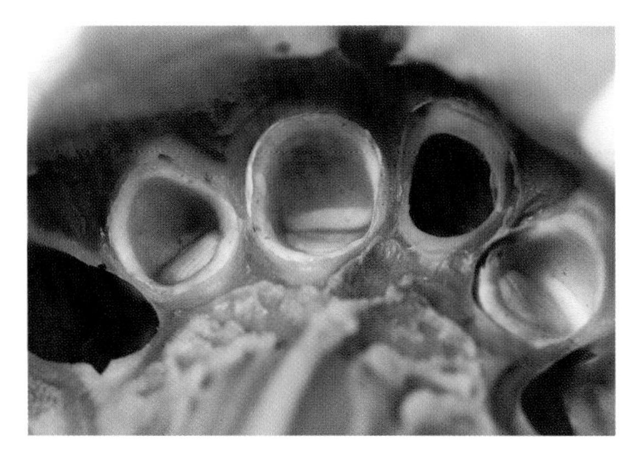

Figure 9.12 Gingival biological impression with definitive crowns to verify correct cervical contours and interproximal contact points.

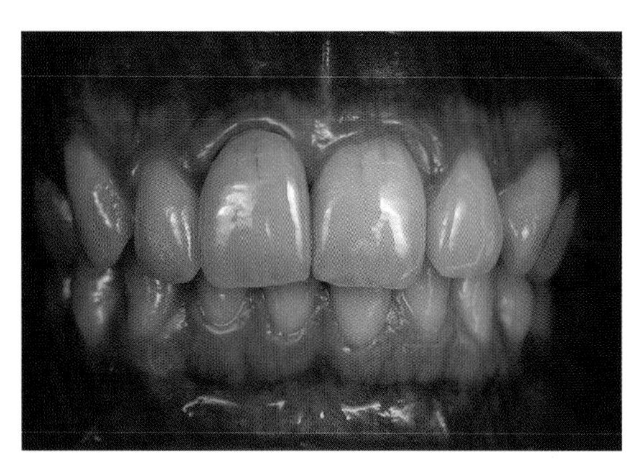

Figure 9.13 Incorrect colour: the crown on the right central incisor is too grey and has a lower value compared with the natural contralateral incisor.

Hints and Tips

- Hint 9.1 – A gingival biological impression is best achieved using a monophase or soft addition silicone impression material
- Hint 9.2 – Using different coloured articulation papers expedites occlusal assessment, e.g. red for CO, black for CR and blue for lateral and protrusive excursions. Shim stock is invaluable for ensuring tight contralateral contacts for posterior restorations, while for anteriors a light contact is desirable
- Hint 9.3 – To 'optically connect' the restoration with the underlying tooth for colour assessment, fill the crown with chlorhexidine paste prior to seating

10 Cementation and dentine bonding agents

Theoretically, the purpose of a luting or cementing agent is uniting a dental restoration with the underlying tooth, hermetically sealing it from the oral cavity. In reality, this ideal is often unfulfilled because of a variety of factors, including preparation design, the material from which the restoration is fabricated, choice of cement and clinical technique. Contemporary restorations, particularly all-ceramic prostheses, dictate a change in mind-set regarding cementation protocols. Many older cements and techniques are considered redundant, and newer ceramic restorations require technique-sensitive procedures for obtaining a lasting and durable bond to the abutment (implant or natural tooth).

SCIENTIFIC RATIONALE

The number of cements currently available is daunting, leading to confusion regarding choice for a specific restoration and clinical scenario. In order to make selection easier, this chapter discusses types of cements, their evolution and properties, followed by guidelines for choosing appropriate agents depending on the restoration. Finally, theory is applied to clinical protocols for cementing dental prostheses.

Types and properties of luting agents

The literature is unanimously emphatic that the type of bond (chemical or micromechanical), its durability and quality between the restoration and abutment is dependent on choice of luting agent and the technique employed for cementation.[1] The starting point is discussing the various classes of cements currently available. Below is a list of cements, in chronological order of development over the past decades, together with a brief summary of their advantages and disadvantages.

Zinc oxide eugenol (ZOE)

Advantages of ZOE include retrievability (primarily used for temporary restorations) and it is palliative to freshly cut and exposed vital dentine. There are many formulations, including transparent ones for improved aesthetics, and non-eugenol varieties if using DBAs, which prevent dentine contamination and formation of the hybrid layer.

Disadvantages of ZOE include high solubility, lack of adhesion (absence of chemical bond to tooth substrate and fitting surface of prosthesis) and poor marginal integrity with increased leakage. It is unsuitable for provisional cementation of all-ceramic prostheses, due to the lack of chemical adhesion to the underlying tooth substrate. Proprietary products include TempBond (Kerr, Orange, CA, USA).

Zinc phosphate (ZP)

Advantages of ZP include a proven track record with long-term clinical use, ease of use, it is expedient and technique forgiving. Disadvantages include high solubility, lack of adhesion (absence of chemical bond to tooth substrate and restoration interface), poor marginal integrity and increased leakage. There are numerous proprietary products.

Polycarboxylate (PC)

Advantages of PC include reduced pulpal irritation and greater plastic deformation compared to ZP and chemical adhesion to tooth substrate via free carboxylic acid groups with calcium.[2] Disadvantages include a short working time and the tooth requires conditioning prior to cementation. There are numerous proprietary products.

Glass ionomer (GI)

Advantages of GI include fluoride release (cariostatic), similar coefficient of thermal expansion to natural tooth structure and chemical adhesion to dentine and enamel. Disadvantages include poor mechanical properties, e.g. low tensile strength and fracture resistance, and susceptibility to moisture during initial setting (therefore an arid environment is a prerequisite). A proprietary product is Ketac-Cem (3M ESPE, Seefeld, Germany).

Resin-modified glass ionomer (RGI)

Advantages of RGI include improved tensile and compressive strength compared to ZP and GI and resistance to water contamination during initial setting reaction compared to GI. Disadvantages include that RGI is hydrophilic. Water adsorption and hygroscopic expansion lead to crack formation, cement deterioration and intermediate leakage (between ZP and DR). A proprietary product is Fuji Plus (GC, Tokyo, Japan).

Dual-polymerisation resins (DR)

Advantages of DR are enhanced mechanical and aesthetic properties and chemical adhesion to the tooth with DBA and ceramics with appropriate pre-treatment of intaglio surface (depending on type of ceramic, e.g. silica, alumina or zirconia). Disadvantages are the protracted clinical protocols and therefore increased cost, and the technique-sensitive procedures required. A proprietary product is Variolink II (Ivoclar-Vivadent, Schaan, Liechtenstein).

Self-adhesive, dual-polymerisation resins (SADR)

Advantages of SADR include ease of handling, no pre-treatment of tooth or fitting surface, high compressive strengths and diametral tensile strength,[3] good aesthetic properties, chemical adhesion to tooth (with DBA) and intaglio surface by multifunctional monomer, 10-methacryloyloxydecyl dihydrogen phosphate (MDP) and high shear bond strength (SBS) with all restorative materials. A disadvantage is reduced fracture strength after artificial ageing.[4] Proprietary products include Rely X Unicem (3M ESPE, Seefeld, Germany), Panavia F and Panavia F2.0 (Kuraray, Osaka, Japan).

Self adhesive, auto-polymerisation resins (SAAR)

Advantages of SAARs are that they are ideal for metal–ceramic and highly opaque all-ceramic restorations (light-curing not necessary), and have favourable mechanical and aesthetic properties. They can be used for adhesion to:

- Tooth with DBA
- Metal substructure of metal–ceramic crowns intaglio surface by chemically bonding to metal oxides[5] with the multifunctional monomer, MDP
- Alumina (Procera) pre-treated with air abrasion and silane or ceramic primer
- Zirconia[6] with air abrasion and ceramic primer

A disadvantage is that some of the newer generations of DBAs (sixth and seventh), which contain acidic components to etch, prime and seal dentine tubules simultaneously, form a residual 'acidic inhibition' layer retarding the setting reaction of auto-curing luting agents. Whilst light-cured polymerisation is immediate, with auto-curing the process is slower, allowing the acidic layer to interfere with complete setting at the cement–tooth interface, creating a fragility zone.[7] This non-homogenous zone has poor mechanical and physical properties. There is no long-term clinical data about this. A proprietary product is Panavia 21 (Kuraray, Osaka, Japan).

Ceramic primers (CP)

- Porcelain Liner-M in combination with Super-Bond C&B (Sun Medical, Shiga, Japan)
- Porcelain Bond Activator in conjunction with Clearfil SE Bond or Clearfil Protect Bond in combination with Panavia F, Panavia F 2.0, or Panavia 21 (Kuraray, Tokyo, Japan)
- Rely X Ceramic Primer in combination with Rely X Unicem (3M ESPE, Seefeld, Germany)

Efficacy of cementing agents

It is important to realise that most studies assessing properties of cementing agents, e.g. durability, are in vitro based, simulating mechanical wear and ageing by cyclic loading and thermocycling, respectively. Whilst these thermomechanical fatigue models are invaluable for comparing different products, they are not a true assessment of clinical durability, failing to account for negative factors, such as multidirectional non-axial occlusion forces, thermal stresses and saliva immersion. This is especially significant with intra-oral stresses, since most cement failures are attributed to tensile rather than compressive forces. In vivo studies are the gold standard, but are difficult to standardise, and are costly and time consuming. The key elements for assessing suitability of various agents are adhesion, mechanical properties, marginal integrity (leakage) and retention.

Adhesion

Adhesion is categorised into true chemical bonding and micromechanical interlocking, involving two interfaces (Fig. 10.1):

- Cement–tooth (enamel and/or dentine) interface
- Cement–restoration (metal and/or ceramic) interface

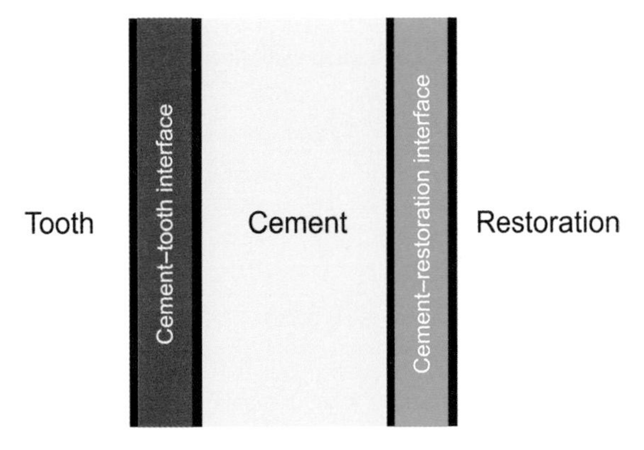

Figure 10.1 The cement–tooth and cement–restoration interfaces.

In addition, the integrity of the intermediate cement layer between these two interfaces is essential for a successful union between tooth and the restoration. Successful adhesion, at either the cement–tooth or the cement–restoration interface, relies on formation of chemical bonds as well as micromechanical interlocking. Whichever is achieved depends on the restorative material from which the prosthesis is fabricated, and the cement utilised. Ideally, a chemical bond is desirable at both interfaces as opposed to micromechanical interlocking, but often the latter compromise is apparent due to the restorative material and less than ideal clinical protocols. Table 10.1 summarises types of adhesion with different cements at both the cement–tooth and cement–restoration interfaces.

Modes of de-cementation are defined as adhesive or cohesive failures. Adhesive failures occur between the cement–tooth or cement–restoration interfaces, while cohesive failures are encountered within the intermediate cement layer or the underlying tooth substrate (Fig. 10.2). The majority of failures are adhesive, usually between the cement–tooth interfaces. This is the weakest link of the crown/tooth complex, due to the weak dentine bond at the cement–dentine interface (especially the fragile hybrid layer).[8] Conversely, the bond strength at the cement–crown interface (e.g. with ceramic etching/silane or ceramic priming) exceeds that of the dentine bond with natural tooth.[9]

The bond strength (expressed as shear bond strength – SBS) is dependent on not only the type of cement but also on tooth preparation design, including retention and resistance form, margin geometry (finish line) and degree of taper (convergence angle). In addition, the SBS varies initially and following ageing. The non-resin cements, such as ZOE, ZP, GI and RGI, exhibit deterioration of SBS after exposure to water and thermal cycling, while the resin cements, such as DR, SADR, may exhibit an increase in SBS due to postpolymerisation, which enhances mechanical resilience. However, protracted ageing of the resins has revealed complete adhesive failure modes at the cement–ceramic interface following thermal cycling.

Another point worth noting is that with RGIs failure can occur at both cement–dentine and cement–crown interfaces, while resin cements with an adhesive cementation technique only have deterioration at the cement–dentine interface. Finally, cements containing an adhesive phosphate monomer (MDP), used in conjunction with air abrasion for alumina and zirconia ceramics, exhibit increased initial and long-term bond strengths.

Occlusal stresses

The mean human masticatory force is 40 N, but in the posterior regions, the forces can vary from 200–540 N, depending on facial anatomy and age.[10] All-ceramic restorations inherently suffer from brittleness and are susceptible to tensile and torsional stresses.[11] In order for a restoration to

Table 10.1 Types of adhesion with different cements.

Interface	Micro-mechanical interlocking	Chemical bonding
Cement–tooth	ZOE, ZP, DR[i]	PC, GI, RGI, DR[iii], SADR[iii], SAAR[iii]
Cement–restoration	ZOE, ZP, PC, GI, RGI, DR[ii]	DR[iv], SADR[iv], SAAR[iv]

[i] without DBA.
[ii] without pre-treatment of intaglio surface.
[iii] with DBA. The bond between dentine and resin cements is via dentine adhesion using a DBA. This is not a true chemical bond, but micromechanical in nature, involving formation of the hybrid and adhesive layers, which 'connect' to resin cements.
[iv] with appropriate pre-treatment of intaglio surface depending on restorative material.

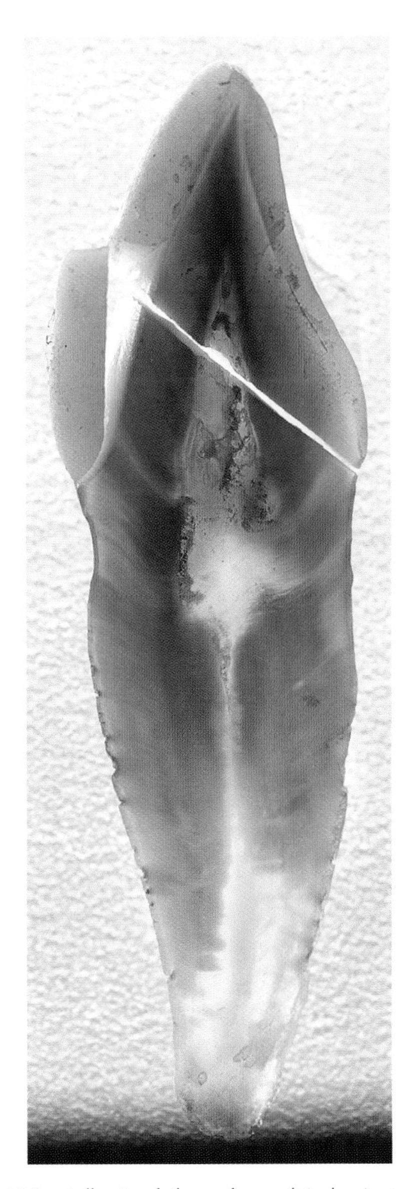

Figure 10.2 Adhesive failure of porcelain laminate veneer.

survive, it is desirable that it matches or exceeds these forces. Many currently available all-ceramic systems can withstand the maximum masticatory forces encountered on posterior teeth, with fracture resistance comparable to natural teeth.[12] The fracture strength of a ceramic depends on inherent flexural strength and MOE, and the skill of the ceramist during fabrication and manipulation of the material. For example, autoglazing may be inadequate for sealing microsurface irregularities, whereas over-glazing may close surface defects exposed to the oral environment and minimise potentially catastrophic fractures.

Marginal integrity and leakage

Marginal discrepancies and leakage at the cement–tooth or cement–restoration interfaces are susceptible to periodontal disease, secondary caries, staining (poor aesthetics), post-operative sensitivity, crown dislodgement and ultimate failure of the restoration. Therefore, the sealing ability of a luting agent is crucial for longevity and durability. The first aspect to consider is correct seating on to the abutment tooth. Crown elevation due to improper location or seating introduces vast discrepancies, and compromises aesthetics due to staining of the cement line. Nevertheless, as one study points out, the thickness of the cement line is not directly related to the extent of microleakage.[13]

Secondly, light polymerisation increases SBS of dual-polymerisation cements, allowing complete setting with superior physical and mechanical properties, especially for subgingival margins. However, photoactivation causes rapid curing creating higher stresses at the bonded interfaces, increasing the risk of microleakage compared to auto-cured cements, which have time for viscous flow.[14]

The next factor is margin opening due to ageing. In vitro studies simulate ageing using thermal and mechanical stresses by thermocycling and cyclic loading, respectively. The result of ageing manifests as marginal integrity deterioration, and is influenced by the type of luting agent. This is particularly evident with metal–ceramic crowns, where ageing increases leakage.[15] However, a recent study reveals that all-ceramic crowns cemented with resin cements have little differences in marginal discrepancy after simultaneous thermocycling and cyclic loading. This is explained by the fact that the vertical, in vitro cyclic loading causes compressive stresses, closing margins. However, during mastication, both vertical and horizontal (tensile) stresses are encountered, which are not reproduced in the in vitro set-up. The same study also emphasises intermediate and severe leakage with RGI and ZP cements, respectively.[16]

Retention

Retention is the ability of a restoration to resist displacement in the opposing direction to insertion. It is primarily dependent on the geometry of the preparation, including the height, width, surface area and degree of taper. The item that has attracted most attention is the degree of taper.[17] It is important to clarify terminology regarding the angulations and configurations of a tooth preparation. Taper refers to the angle of a single wall, usually mesial or distal, while the convergence angle refers to the combination of the tapers for a given preparation. For example, the ideally quoted convergence angle of 12° is derived by the addition of the two axial walls (6° mesial and 6° distal tapers). Decreasing the taper increases retention and surface area, but excessively parallel (small tapers) preparations cause incorrect seating.

Another factor determining the degree of retention is the choice of cement. Conventional ZP cements are luting agents, which rely on interlocking irregularities of the intaglio and tooth surfaces for retention, while GI and resin cements create chemical bonds with artificial prostheses. With ideal tapers of 6–12°, the choice of cement becomes irrelevant to retention of the crown. Hence, retention is not compromised when the taper increases from 6° to 12°. But because conventional cements do not offer adhesion, cement dissolution may predispose to microleakage over time. In clinical practice, the average taper of a tooth preparation ranges from 14–20°, making the choice of cement a crucial factor for retention.[18] For example, taper increases from 6° to 24° decrease retention of all cements; ZP by 42%, GI by 38% and resin cements by 20%. In addition, GI and ZP cements offer similar retention (3.6 MPa), half the values compared to resin cements (6.5 MPa), irrespective of taper angle. Furthermore, for a 24° taper, resin cements offer retention comparable to luting with ZP with a 6° taper.

The clinical significances are as follows:

- Resin cements offer superior retention
- ZP and GI cements offer similar retention values with tapers of 6–12°, and the choice of cement is irrelevant (with the disadvantages of absence of adhesion, weaker mechanical properties, microleakage, marginal staining, and post-operative sensitivity)
- When the taper increases to 24°, resin cements offer better retention than both ZP and GI luting agents.[19] Using resin luting agents for less than ideal tooth preparations offers superior marginal adaptation,[20] and higher fracture resistance,[21] especially if the restoration is susceptible to high occlusal loads[22]

Table 10.2 suggests the ideal choice of cement for different types of restorations.

Table 10.2 Choice of cements for different restorations.

Material	Ideal cement choice
Acrylic or composite (temporary crown)	ZOE, ZP
High-gold alloy	SAAR
Semi- or non-precious alloy	SAAR
Silica ceramics[i]	DR, SADR, SAAR
Alumina ceramics[ii]	SAAR
Zirconia ceramics[iii]	SAAR
Implant-supported prostheses	ZOE[iv]

[i] Silica ceramics – e.g. feldspathic, leucite reinforced glass ceramic (Empress 1 – Ivoclar-Vivadent, Liechtenstein), lithium disilicate glass ceramic (Empress 2 – Ivoclar-Vivadent, Liechtenstein).

[ii] Alumina ceramics – e.g. densely sintered pure aluminum oxide ceramic (Procera, Nobel Biocare, Sweden), glass infiltrated alumina (In-Ceram, Vita, Germany).

[iii] Zirconia ceramics – e.g. Cercon (Dentsply, Germany), Lava (3M-ESPE, Germany), Procera Zircon (Nobel Biocare, Sweden).

[iv] Alternatively, use acrylic/urethane polymer proprietary implant cement (ImProv, Nobel Biocare, Sweden).

Pre-treatment of abutment

Two surfaces require pre-treatment, firstly the cut dentine and enamel following tooth preparation, and secondly the intaglio or fitting surface of the restoration. Traditionally, before the advent of DBAs, the prepared tooth surface was left untreated, an impression made, temporary fabricated and the definitive restoration luted with a conventional cement. The introduction of DBAs, and their development over the last half-century, have revolutionised cementation protocols. Today, DBAs are pivotal, not only for direct composite and amalgam restorations, but for nearly all indirectly fabricated laboratory prostheses.

Two modes for pre-treatment of the prepared tooth abutment using DBAs are possible, either at cementation of the definitive prosthesis, or immediately after tooth preparation.[23] Numerous studies have concluded that application of a DBA after preparation produces a wider hybrid layer with longer and abundant resin tags. These tags have a lower MOE than the overlying resin cement with inherent elastic buffering capacity, absorbing shocks and stresses placed on the artificial restoration.[24] Furthermore, the mircotensile bond strength is greater, with reduced microleakage and post-operative sensitivity.

Dentine bonding agents

Introduction and development of DBAs have revolutionised many clinical procedures, including cementation. Their use is commonplace in contemporary dental practices for numerous applications and therapies. In addition, luting all-ceramic restorations using DBA and resin cements improves longevity.[25]

Buonocore conceived bonding to enamel over half a century ago with the introduction of acid etching.[26] Although composite fillings of the period were relatively inferior compared to contemporary analogues, the technique for interlocking a resin to enamel prisms is still applicable today, as it was in 1955. Adhesion to dentine, on the other hand, has proved far more elusive. The reason is that bonding to an inorganic substance, such as enamel, is far easier than the organic and inorganic complex prevalent in dentine. While the theoretical mechanism of dentine bonding is understood, the practical achievement is still unattainable. The following discussion highlights current thinking and evolution of DBAs.

Dentine bonding mechanism

Traversing from enamel to the dental pulp, there is an increase in both the organic phase and water content (Figs. 10.3 & 10.4). The inorganic enamel is hydrophobic, while the dentine and pulp are hydrophilic. A viable bond is only possible in a hydrophobic environment, hence the ease of bonding to enamel. For dentine, the envi-

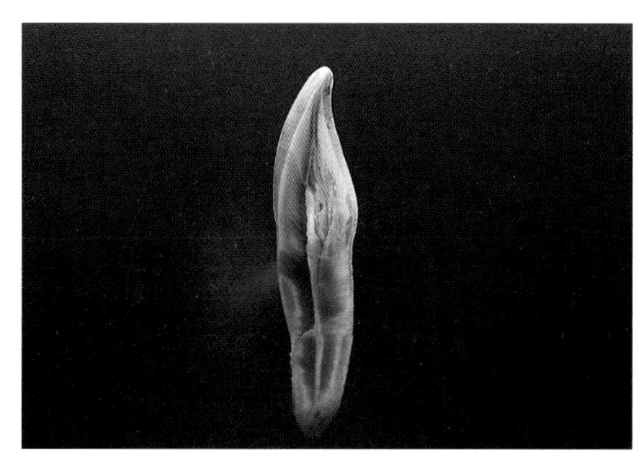

Figure 10.3 Sectioned natural tooth (transmitted light) showing enamel and dentine strata.

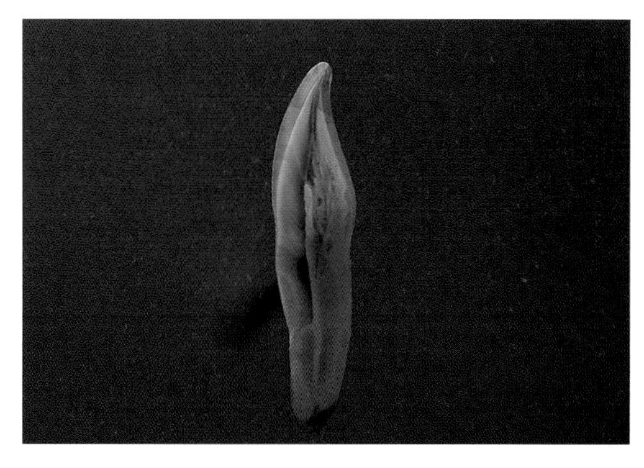

Figure 10.4 Sectioned natural tooth (ultraviolet light) showing enamel and dentine strata.

ronment must be transiently converted into a hydrophobic state conducive for successful bonding, which is the basic aim of all DBAs.

Technological and material advances have improved the efficiency of dentine bonding, for example, the total etch technique and use of hydrophilic primers in bonding agents.[27,28] Dentine bonding, or adhesion, is micro-mechanical in nature, succinctly described as follows. The first step is removing the smear layer (Fig. 10.5) by conditioning to demineralise the inorganic phase and expose the dentine tubules (Fig. 10.6) and collagen fibres (Fig. 10.7), constituents of the organic phase of dentine. Next, the surface is primed by monomers (to create a hydrophobic environment), which facilitates the last stage of resin impregnation and penetration to encapsulate and stabilise the collagen network.[29] The resultant entity is a resin-reinforced dentine, which has differing nomenclature, depending how the latter is envisaged: hybrid layer (union of resin and collagen fibres)[30], interdiffusion zone (permeation of dentine by resin)[31] or RIDL (resin-infiltrated dentine layer).[32] The terminology is irrelevant, but the significance is that a micromechanical connection is made between dentine and the resin that functions as a viable bond (Fig. 10.8).

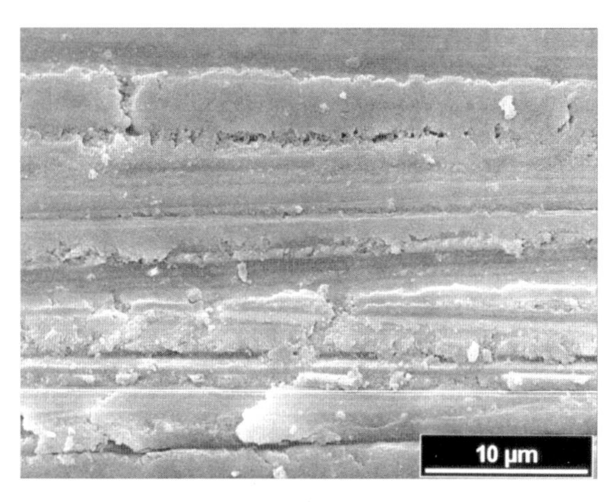

Figure 10.5 Smear layer following tooth preparation.

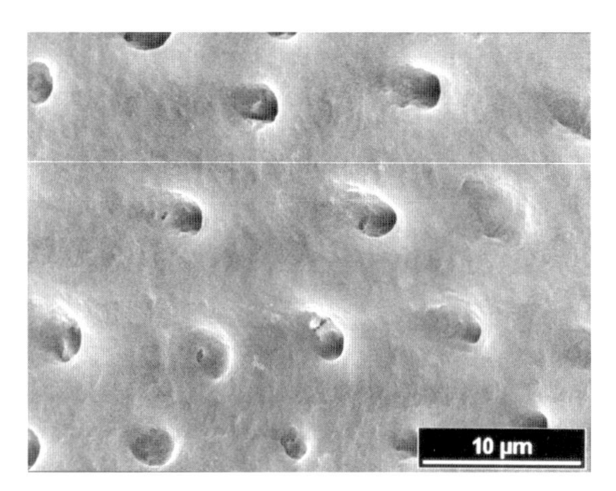

Figure 10.6 Exposed dentine tubules after removal of the smear layer.

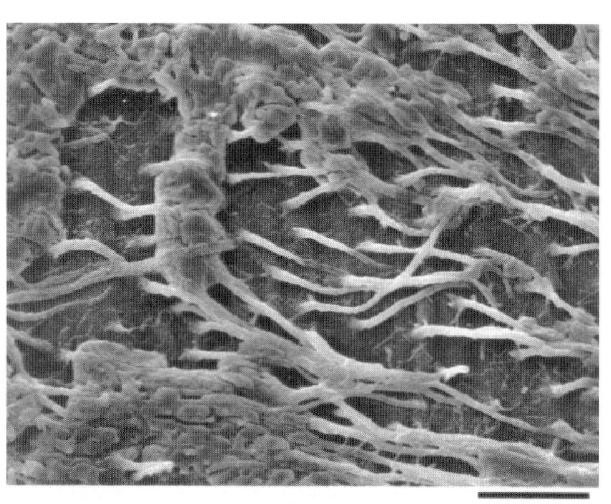

Figure 10.7 Exposed collagen fibres after removal of the smear layer.

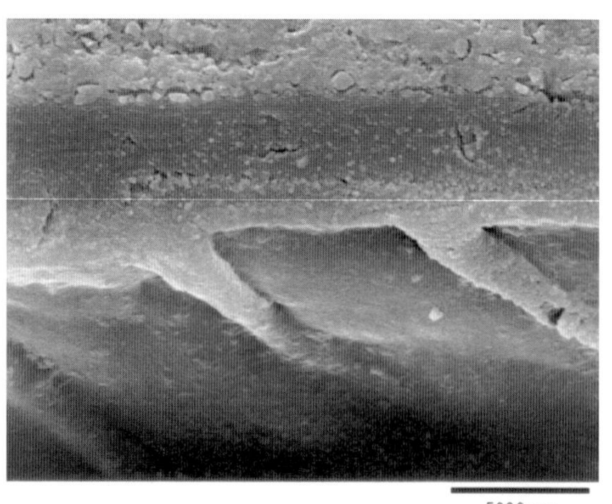

Figure 10.8 Formation of the hybrid layer with resin tags within the dentine tubules.

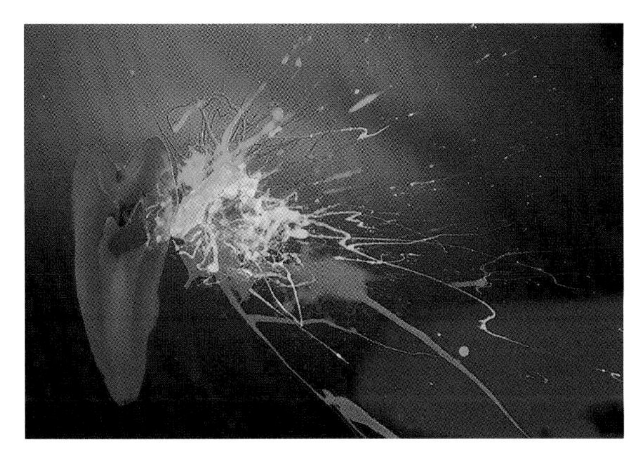

Figure 10.9 Multi-component (MC) bonding agents require application of individual chemicals to achieve the desired result. Firstly the etchant (green), secondly the primer (yellow) and finally the adhesive (red).

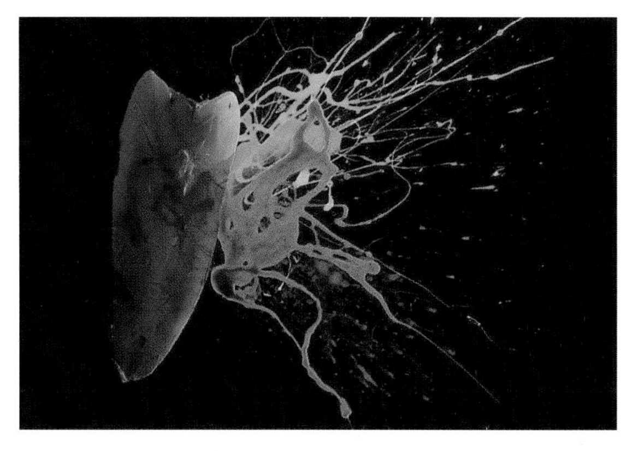

Figure 10.10 Single-component (SC) bonding agents require application of two chemicals to achieve the desired result. Firstly the etchant (green) and secondly the combined primer and adhesive (red).

The appearance, size, composition and quality of this hybrid layer have attracted much attention among researchers and clinicians. The dimension of this layer has wide variance, ranging from 2–10 μm, but even thin layers have been shown to produce very high immediate bond strengths.[33] It transpires that the thickness and morphology of the hybrid layer seems less important than its consistency and integrity (lack of gaps, porosity and voids), which are paramount for achieving efficacious and durable dentine sealing and bonding.[34]

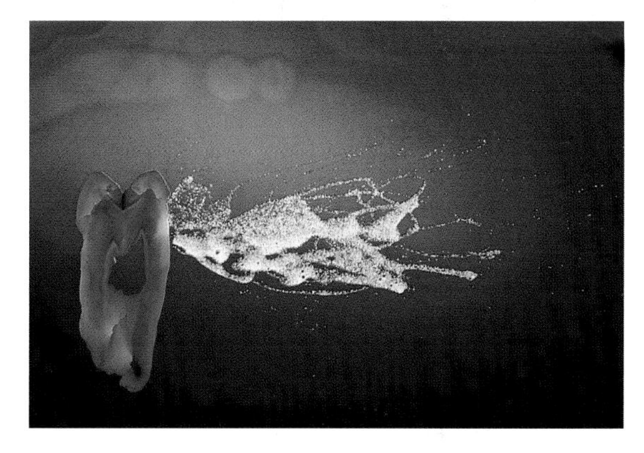

Figure 10.11 The self-etching (SE) bonding agents require application of only one chemical to achieve conditioning, priming and sealing/adhesion.

Generations

Achieving efficacious dentine bonding relies on an agent or agents to condition, prime and seal tubules and stabilise the collagen fibres, previously supported by the inorganic phase. DBAs are categorised into three types:

- Multi-component (MC) (Fig. 10.9)
- Single component (SC) (Fig. 10.10)
- Self-etching (SE) (Fig. 10.11)

The MCs require application of individual components for each bonding stage. Initially, the etchant, usually 37% phosphoric acid, is applied, rinsed and dried to remove the smear layer. A recent study concludes that a combination of phosphoric and hydrofluoric acid results in superior marginal seal at the cement–tooth interface.[35] The next stage is application of a primer that subsequently evaporates, and finally an adhesive resin is introduced to seal the tubules and form the hybrid layer. These multi-component systems show diversity in their presentation and make up, forming the first to fourth generations of dentine adhesives.

The SC systems combine the primer and adhesive into one component, but still require an initial total etching step and are termed fifth generation, e.g. Scotchbond 1, Syntac Single and Syntac Sprint. Finally, the SE agents obviate the need for etching by incorporating pyrophosphate initiators, e.g. Etch & Prime 3 (Dentsply, Germany), and iBond (Heraeus Kulzer, Germany) (Fig. 10.12), forming the sixth and seventh generations, respectively. A recently introduced SE, seventh generation dental adhesive is iBond GI (Heraeus Kulzer, Hanau, Germany). The 'i' is an abbreviation for 'intelligent' or 'innovative', as the need for mixing components before application has been eliminated, while 'GI' signifies inclusion of the Gluma desensitiser. The constituents of iBond include all three chemicals necessary for dentine bonding, i.e. etching, priming and adhesive resin. The solvent is a mixture of acetone (promoting evaporation) and water (facilitating hydration of the collagen fibres and the self-etching mechanism). Its properties boast a SBS to both dentine and enamel in excess of 20 MPa, and a marginal gap of almost zero.[36]

The clinical protocols are crucial for achieving an effective and successful bond, and the entire procedure is extremely technique sensitive. It is imperative that the components infiltrate, mingle with, and finally encapsulate the remaining collagen matrix. Failure at any of these stages results in a compromise, leading to deterioration by water, infestation by bacteria and a breakdown of the collagen fibres, no longer supported by the hydroxyapatite crystals. Therefore, the advantages of reducing the number of components are obvious. Fewer clinical steps ultimately reduce the scope for error. The SE agents are essentially 'automatic' DBAs, expediting dentine bonding. The clinician is no longer burdened with precise timings for application of etchant, primer and resin to prevent collapse and penetration of the collagen matrix, which is necessary when using MC systems.

Solvents

Solvents are significant constituents of primers, precursors of the adhesive resin. The function of solvents is to promote wetting of dentine, and to act as water chasers and monomer carriers for interaction with collagen fibres. The solvents currently used are hydrophilic, categorised as either organic (acetone and ethanol) or inorganic (water) (Figs. 10.13–10.15).

Acetone is frequently used as a solvent; it has a boiling point of 56.5°C, efficiently removes water from the substrate, facilitates resin penetrations and yields a superior bond with dentine.[37] However, it fails in preventing collapse of the collagen matrix if applied to dehydrated or arid dentine. Furthermore, acetone-based agents are more technique sensitive, requiring strict adherence to manufacturer's guidelines for use.

Water has a boiling point of 100°C and is therefore less volatile than acetone. This results in water retention, obscuring the collagen matrix, impeding infiltration of HEMA (adhesive resin) molecules, and therefore reducing the

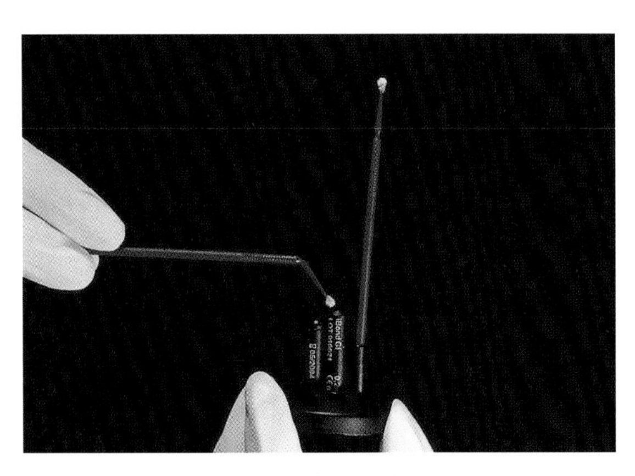

Figure 10.12 An example of a SE DBA is iBond (Heraeus Kulzer).

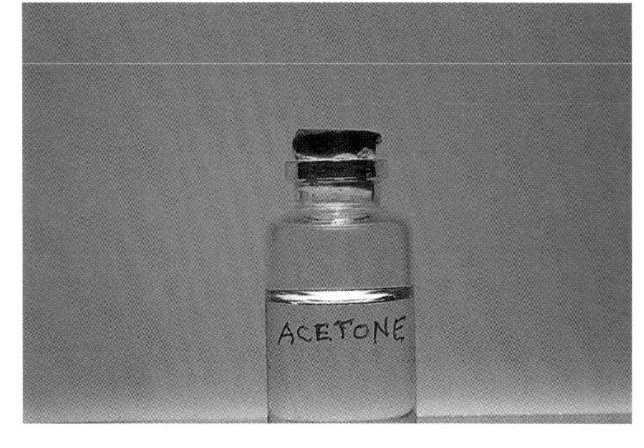

Figure 10.13 Organic solvent: acetone.

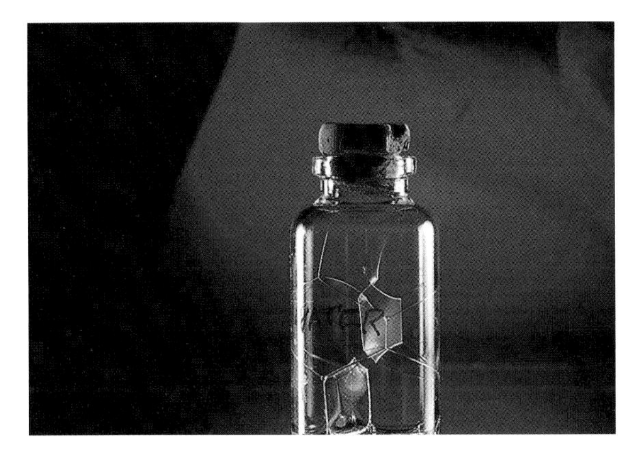

Figure 10.14 Inorganic solvent: water.

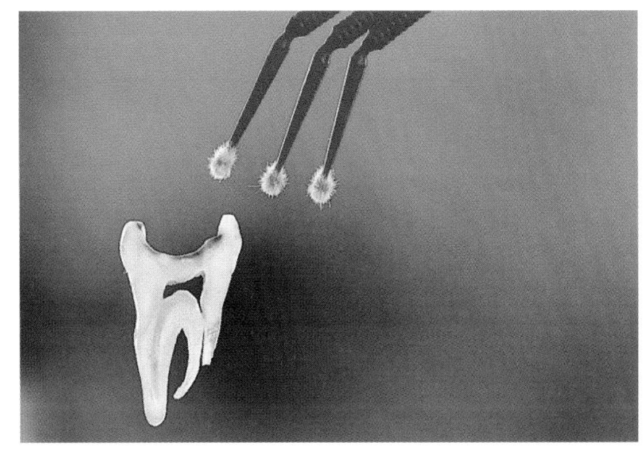

Figure 10.16 DBA application protocol: three coats of a SE bonding agent are successively applied to all cavity surfaces.

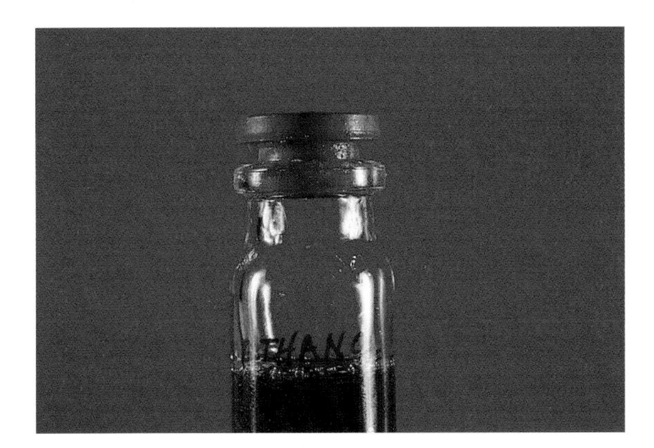

Figure 10.15 Organic solvent: ethanol.

quality of the hybrid layer. However, water does have the advantage of re-erecting collapsed collagen fibres favouring monomer penetration,[38] and eliminating the need for moist dentine.

Ethanol has a boiling point of 78.5°C, intermediate between acetone and water, and is present in many fifth generation bonding systems. Ethanol-based agents are less technique sensitive than acetone and more efficient at removing water than water-based systems. Many formulations on the market exploit the benefits of each solvent by using a combination to gain optimum results, e.g. in a mixture of acetone and water, the water stabilises acetone evaporation and promotes wetting of dentine, while the acetone encourages evaporation of water, facilitating monomer and resin penetration.[39]

Efficacy

Bonding efficacy is usually assessed by two parameters, the marginal gap at the cement–tooth interface and the SBS. As a comparison, mean SBSs to enamel are in the range of 23–25 MPa. Assessing dentine SBS is erratic, often dependent on the in vitro experimental model and measurement criteria. The SBS for dentine ranges from as little as 3.5 MPa to as large as 25 MPa, equalling that of enamel.[40] These figures should be viewed with caution since they do not represent a clinical environment; further research and in vivo trials will eventually reveal credible values.

The second factor used for assessing bonding efficacy is the marginal opening (MO) at the cement–tooth interface. Again, no definitive values are ascribed, ranging from 0–10 μm,[41] but minimising this gap is essential for success and longevity. Large MOs result in caries, pulpal pathologies, discolouration and, ultimately, deterioration of the resin luting agent. However, marginal integrity is not solely influenced by the bonding agent, but also by clinical procedures, such as preparation design, adequate isolation (retraction cord or rubber dam), application techniques and modes of light polymerisation (Figs. 10.16–10.18).

Numerous studies have reported that the newer SC and SE agents, even with thin hybrid

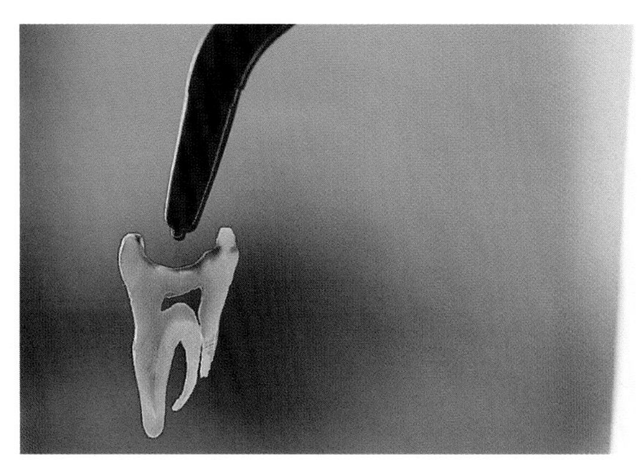

Figure 10.17 DBA application protocol: air is used to evaporate the acetone solvent from the bonding agent.

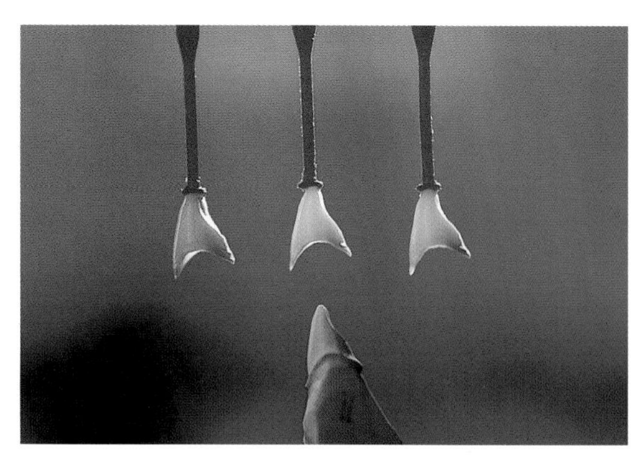

Figure 10.19 The intaglio surfaces of Procera copings have inherent surface roughness.

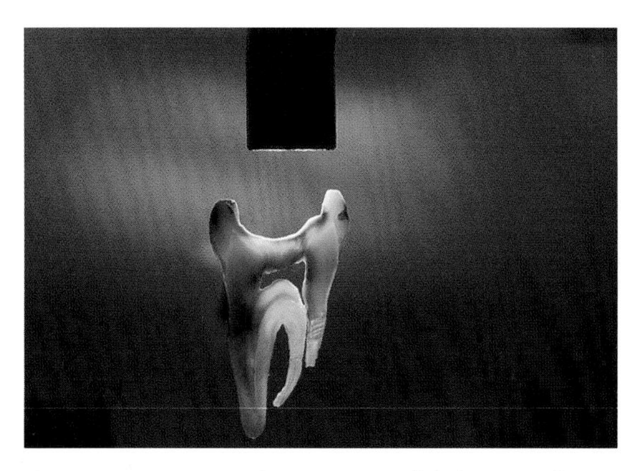

Figure 10.18 DBA application protocol: light curing for 30 seconds completes the bonding process.

layers (0.5 μm), show similar bonding capabilities to those of traditional MC systems.[42,43,44,45]

Pre-treatment of intaglio surface

After pre-treatment of the abutment tooth, the next step before cementation is pre-treatment of the intaglio of the restoration. Pre-treatment of the adherent surface varies according to the restorative material of the prosthesis, and can be categorised into mechanical and chemical.

The aim of any mechanical roughening is enhancing adhesion by micro-mechanical retention. Prostheses fabricated by CAD/CAM and milling processes have inherent surface roughness due to the manufacturing process (Fig. 10.19). This is analogous to etching silica-based ceramics with hydrofluoric acid to increase micro-mechanical interlocking. Surface roughening with diamond burs and aluminium oxide discs is useful for metallic surfaces, but excess or indiscriminate roughening of ceramics initiates crack formation causing weakening or fractures. Micro-etching surface roughening with air abrasion using aluminum oxide particles (50–100 μm) has a similar effect to rotary instruments for fragile ceramics, initiating microfractures and therefore compromising physical resilience. This is particularly significant with weaker feldspathic or leucite-reinforced glass ceramics, but less important for high-strength ceramics such as alumina or zirconia. Nevertheless, luting agents have proven successful for sealing these micro-flaws while significantly enhancing adhesion.[46]

Chemical pre-treatment achieves either micromechanical interlocking, or true chemical bonding. For silica-based ceramics, phosphoric acid (37%) only decontaminates with no effect on intaglio surface topography, but hydrofluoric acid (5–9.5%) for 5 minutes decontaminates and etches porcelain, creating pronounced surface relief and tunnel-like undercuts, and, in conjunction with a silane-coupling agent, forms chemical bonds at the cement–restoration interface. The SBS (approx. 22 MPa), irrespective of the resin luting agent and DBA, is highest when the intaglio surface is treated with a combination of hydrofluoric acid and silane.[47]

Using hydrofluoric acid for high-strength ceramics, such as alumina and zirconia, has no effect on surface roughening for micro-mechanical interlocking. The application of silane for high-strength ceramics is controversial. Theoretically, since the pure alumina or zirconia lack silica, the formations of chemical silane–silica bonds are absent. However, some studies advocate use of silane as it increases wettability.[48] One study has reported the highest initial SBS (21 MPa) and after artificial ageing (16 MPa), using air particle abrasion, silane and an SAAR cement.[49]

Ceramic primers (CP) and self-adhesive cements are another way for achieving chemical bonding at the cement–restoration interface. The newer multi-component CP can be used as a substitute for hydrofluoric acid and silane pre-treatment for silica-based ceramics, expediting procedures without compromising bond strength or integrity.[50] Using a CP in conjunction with SADR and SAAR cements is a pre-requisite for a chemical bond with alumina and zirconia ceramics. Some studies advocate airborne aluminum oxide (Al_2O_3) particle abrasion[51] and a silane coupling agent in combination with a MDP-containing resin luting agent (Clearfil SE Bond and Clearfil Porcelain Bond Activator, Kuraray Tokyo, Japan) to increase the SBS, even after ageing of zirconia-based ceramics.[52] It is important to note that the chemical composition and manufacturing of specific zirconia substructures with different intaglio morphologies is unique for each commercial product. Hence, conclusions derived from a single study may not be applicable to every zirconia prosthesis. In addition, the significant factor for yielding high-bond strengths to zirconia is application of a MDP-containing bonding/silane coupling agent, irrespective of the resin cement. The latter is confirmed when using a bonding/silane coupling agent without a MDP, which results in weaker bonds to both alumina and zirconia ceramics.[53]

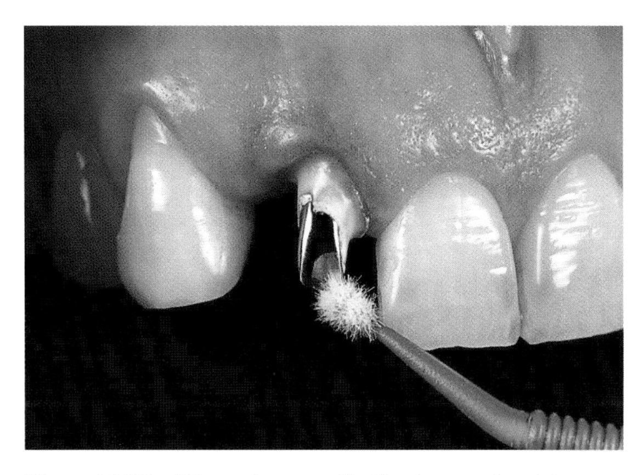

Figure 10.20 Alloy primer application to a cast metal core.

Table 10.3 summarises pre-treatment of different intaglio surfaces for optimal adhesion.

CLINICAL PRACTICE

Cementation should not be considered the final stage for the provision of artificial dental prostheses. In fact, it is the penultimate stage, preceding periodic maintenance and review to ensure survival and compatibility of the prosthesis with the surrounding hard and soft tissues. The following is a clinical sequence for cementation:

(1) Remove therapeutic temporary restoration (Fig. 10.21)
(2) Isolate tooth abutment with retraction cord (Fig. 10.22) (Hint 10.1). Isolation of the tooth before bonding has recently become a point of contention. Some studies have stated that presence of ambient humidity[54] and contamination by saliva has no adverse effect on bond strength.[55,56] However, these new concepts require further validation, and, in the author's opinion, it is probably prudent to isolate for a reliable dentine bond and inadvertent spillage on to the soft tissues, avoiding transient and reversible acidic burns. The cord functions as a

barrier between the epithelial attachment and the luting agent, ensuring integrity of the biologic width, as well as allowing clear visualisation of the tooth margins and maintaining a moisture- and contaminant-free environment (Hint 10.2)

(3) Rinse abutment with water to remove remnants of provisional cement
(4) Clean abutment with pumice mixed with 0.2% chlorhexidine paste, rinse and dry (not desiccate) with a gentle stream of warm air (Fig. 10.23)
(5) Place definitive prostheses on to abutment to verify fit, correct seating and occlusion (Hints 10.3 and 10.4)
(6) Pre-treatment of the intaglio surface of prosthesis. The type of pre-treatment will depend on the restorative material of the prosthesis (see Table 10.3) (Hint 10.5)
(7) Pre-treatment of abutment. Use DBA of choice, according to manufacturer's instructions. If using a SE all-in-one DBA (Hint 10.5), etch uncut enamel and sclerotic dentine with 37% phosphoric acid for 20 seconds, rinse and dry (not desiccate), apply SE agent. Alternately, if using a fifth generation DBA, etch entire abutment with 37% phosphoric acid for 20 seconds, rinse and dry (not desiccate) before successively applying primer and adhesive (Hint 10.7). The highest SBS (15–20 MPa) to dentine is achieved using light-cured or chemical-cured DBAs; dual-cured DBAs achieve SBS of 8–12 MPa. This is because the dual-cured DBAs have additives to their solvents, which dilute the desired mixture of primer and adhesive necessary for forming a viable hybrid layer[57] (Fig. 10.24) (Hint 10.8)
(8) Choose appropriate cement from Table 10.2 for specific restoration, and mix according to manufacturer's instructions
(9) Load cement into the prosthesis, and seat passively on to abutment (Fig. 10.25)
(10) Once correctly seated, gently ease retraction cord from gingival sulcus together with extruded excess cement (Fig. 10.26) (Hint 10.9)
(11) Use dental floss, tape or Super Floss (Oral-B) to mop interproximal excess cement
(12) Apply oxygen-blocking gel (Oxyguard II, Kuraray, Osaka, Japan) around margins to minimise oxygen inhibition layer
(13) Apply gentle pressure to the prosthesis until cement is completely set, or polymerise with a curing light if using dual-cured cements (Fig. 10.27)
(14) Remove oxygen-blocking gel with cotton wool swabs
(15) Cut set excess cement around margins with a #12 scalpel blade (Fig. 10.28)
(16) Irrigate gingival sulcus with a 0.2% chlorhexidine solution to remove set cement remnants and promote gingival health (Fig. 10.29).

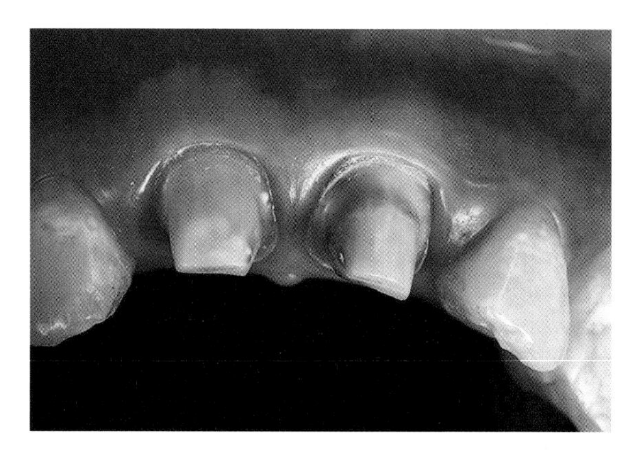

Figure 10.21 Cementation protocol: remove temporary restoration.

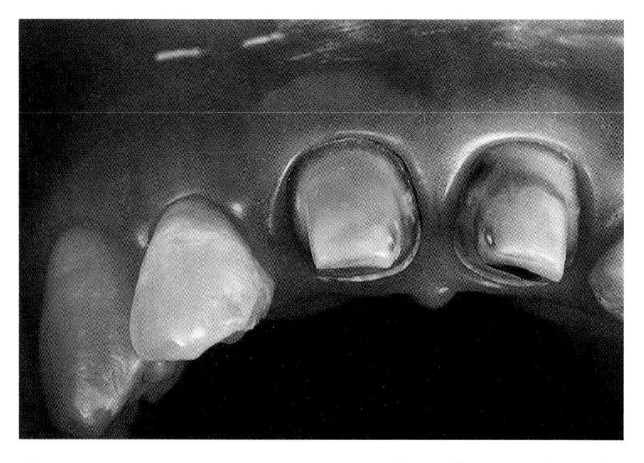

Figure 10.22 Cementation protocol: isolate tooth with retraction cord (right central incisor).

Table 10.3 Intaglio surface pre-treatment.

Material/ pre-treatment	Acrylic or composite (temporary crown)	High-gold alloy	Semi- or non-precious alloy	Silica ceramics[i]	Alumina ceramics[ii]	Zirconia ceramics[iii]	Implant-supported prostheses
Rotary instruments	N	Y	Y	N	N	N	N
Al_2O_3 air abrasion	Y[iv]	Y[iv]	Y[iv]	N	Y[iv]	Y[iv]	N
Alcohol	Y	N	N	N	N	N	N[v]
Tin plating	N	N	Y[vi]	N	N	N	N
Phosphoric acid (37%)	Y	N	N	N	N	N	N
Hydrofluoric acid (5–9.5%)	N	N	N	Y	N	N	N
Silane	N	N	N	Y[vii]	Y[vii]	Y[vii]	N
Ceramic primer	N	N	N	Y[viii]	Y	Y	N

Y – Yes.
N – No.
[i] Silica-ceramics – e.g. feldspathic, leucite reinforced glass ceramic (Empress 1, Ivoclar-Vivadent, Liechtenstein), lithium disilicate glass ceramic (Empress 2, Ivoclar-Vivadent, Liechtenstein).
[ii] Alumina ceramics – e.g. densely sintered pure aluminum oxide ceramic (Procera, Nobel Biocare, Sweden), glass infiltrated alumina (In-Ceram, Vita, Germany).
[iii] Zirconia ceramics – e.g. Cercon (Dentsply, Germany), Lava (3M-ESPE, Germany), Procera Zircon (Nobel Biocare, Sweden).
[iv] Following air abrasion, clean restoration in an ultra-sonic bath to remove all traces of the aluminum oxide powder.
[v] Traces of alcohol after cleaning the intaglio surface of the prosthesis may cause necrosis of the epithelial cells of the trans-mucosal attachment, or cuff, around an implant abutment.
[vi] Pre-treatment of the intaglio surface with an alloy primer (e.g. Alloy Primer, Kuraray, Osaka, Japan) negates tin plating (Fig. 10.20).
[vii] Silane has a relatively short self-life, and is most effective when warm. Ensure silane is not used beyond expiry date, and that the intaglio surface is heated (e.g. with a hair drier) before application of the silane.
[viii] As a substitute for hydrofluoric acid and silane.

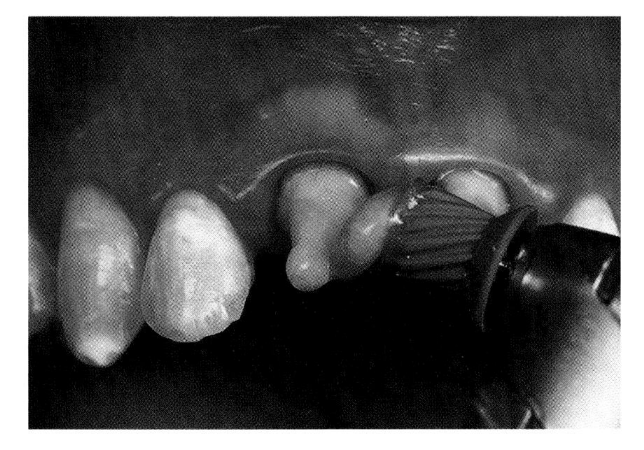

Figure 10.23 Cementation protocol: clean abutment with pumice and chlorhexidine paste.

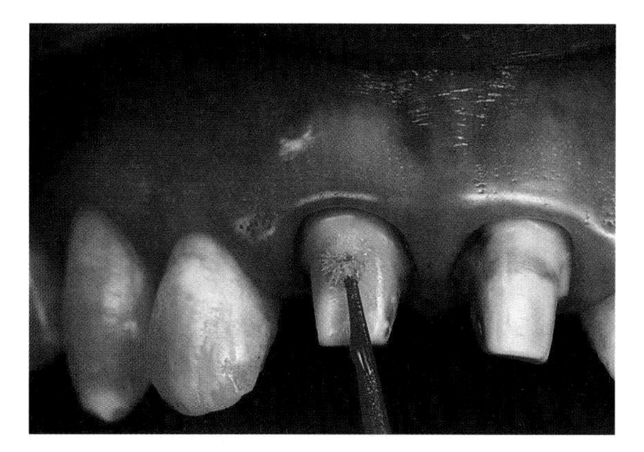

Figure 10.24 Cementation protocol: apply DBA.

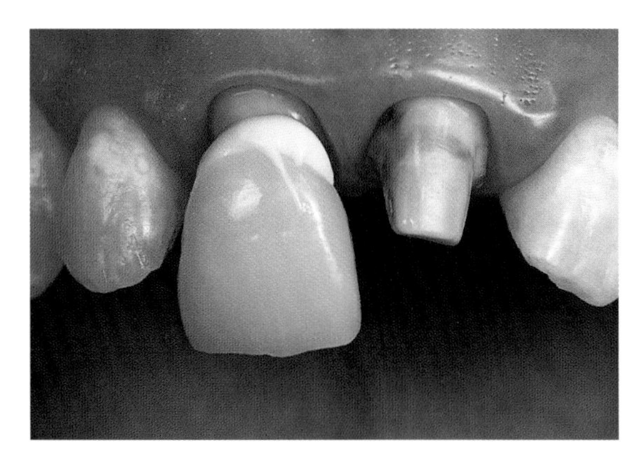

Figure 10.25 Cementation protocol: seat cement-loaded crown on to abutment.

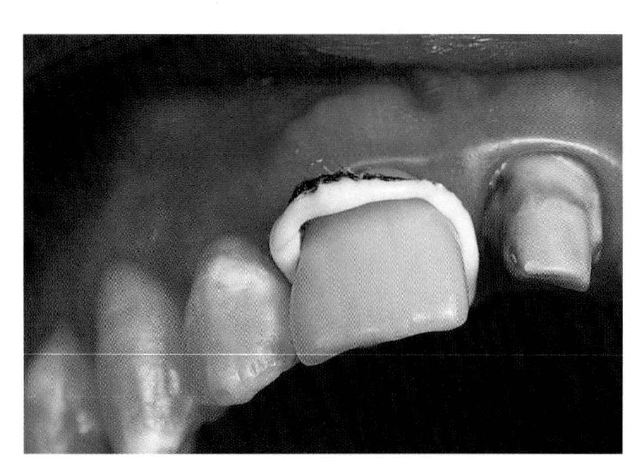

Figure 10.26 Cementation protocol: remove retraction cord.

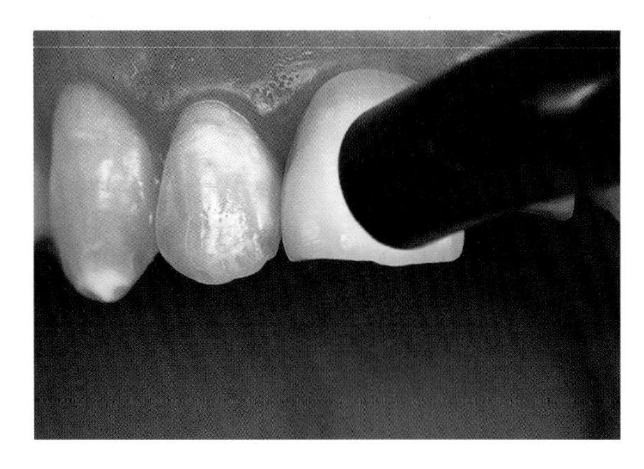

Figure 10.27 Cementation protocol: light polymerisation if using dual- or light-cured luting agents.

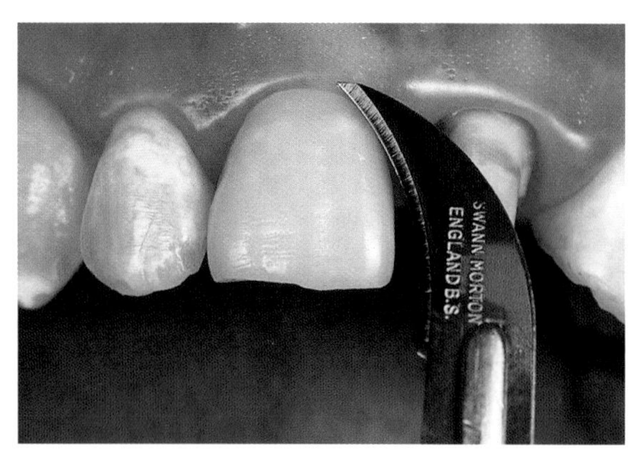

Figure 10.28 Cementation protocol: remove set cement with a #12 scalpel blade.

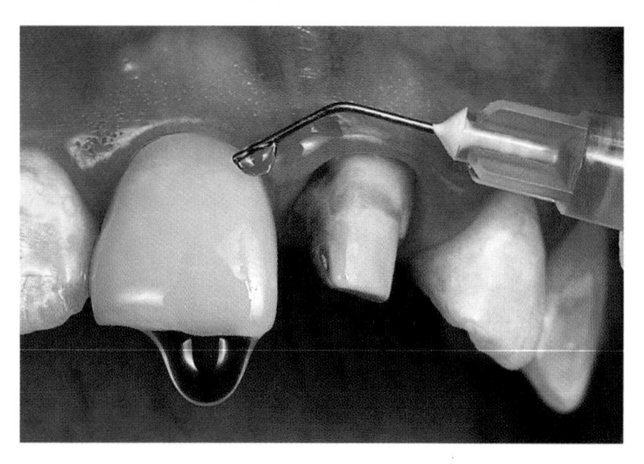

Figure 10.29 Cementation protocol: irrigate with chlorhexidine solution.

Hints and tips

- Hint 10.1 – Use dry, non-impregnated retraction cord to absorb crevicular fluid
- Hint 10.2 – Avoid using retraction cord around implant abutments, because the trauma from cord placement damages the epithelial attachment of the transmucosal cuff. This results in undesirable gingival recession, and possible apical migration of the biologic width with ensuing bone loss around the implant fixture. The latter is particularly relevant with a thin, scalloped periodontal biotype
- Hint 10.3 – If crown margins are subgingival or indiscernible, use a silicone try-in paste, such as Fit Checker (GC, Tokyo, Japan), to confirm fit and seating
- Hint 10.4 – The occlusion should have been finalised with the therapeutic temporary restoration(s) and at the try-in stage. However, minor adjustments can be performed with appropriate rotary instruments with copious irrigations and meticulously polished to close surface irregularities (micro-fractures) by using fine diamond burs (less than 20 μm grit), tungsten carbide finishing burs (20 to 30 fluted), silicone tips and diamond polishing pastes
- Hint 10.5 – Pre-treatment of the intaglio surface can be delegated to the dental assistant, and performed either before or concurrently with pre-treatment of the abutment. This ensures that the pre-treated tooth after DBA application is not left unattended, avoiding detrimental contamination with oral fluids
- Hint 10.6 – It is recommended to use corresponding DBA from the same manufacturer as the luting agent, ensuring chemical compatibility of the DBA with the luting agent
- Hint 10.7 – The following points should be followed prior to using a DBA. Many solvents in DBAs are extremely volatile, and sealing the bottle after dispensing is mandatory, avoiding unwanted evaporation. Next, the solution should be refrigerated (4–10°C), ensuring consistency of the components, and brought to room temperature 1 hour before use. In addition, stagnant containers have an undesirable phase separation of the solvent and active ingredients, and shaking the bottle before use is essential to re-mix these components, ensuring that the adhesive functions as intended. Finally, a uni-dose rather than bottle dispensers are preferred, ensuring sterility, ease of use and chemical consistency
- Hint 10.8 – Most failures with DBA occur due to insufficient evaporation of the solvent. After application and dwell time, dry DBA with a gentle stream of air until no liquid movement is detected and the surface has a glossy appearance; depending on the surface area of the abutment, this usually takes 10–15 seconds
- Hint 10.9 – Avoid using auto-cured cements with SE DBAs, since the latter form an 'acidic inhibition' layer, which interferes with complete setting of auto-cured cements

References

[1] Piwowarczyk, A., Lauer, H.-C. and Sorensen, J.A. (2004) In vitro shear bond strength of cementing agents to fixed prosthodontic restorative materials. *J Prosthet Dent*, **92**, 265–273

[2] Diaz-Arnold, A.M., Vargas, M.A. and Haselton, D.R. (1999) Current status of luting agents for fixed prosthodontics. *J Prosthet Dent*, **81(2)**, 135–141

[3] Knobloch, L.A., Kerby, R.E., Seghi, R., Berlin, J.S. and Lee, J.S. (2000) Fracture toughness of resin-based luting cements. *J Prosthet Dent*, **83**, 204–209

[4] Komine, F., Tomic, M., Gerds, T. and Strub, J.R. (2004) Influence of different adhesive resin cements on the fracture strength of aluminum oxide ceramic posterior crowns. *J Prosthet Dent*, **92**, 359–364

[5] Kern, M. and Thompson, V.P. (1995) Bonding to glass infiltrated alumina ceramic: adhesive methods and their durability. *J Prosthet Dent*, **73**, 240–249

[6] Wegner, S.M. and Kern, M. (2000) Long-term resin bond strength to zirconia ceramic. *J Adhes Dent*, **2**, 139–147

[7] Tay, F.R., Suh, B.I., Pashley, D.H. *et al.* (2003) Factors contributing to the incompatibility between simplified-step adhesives and the self-cured or dual cured composites. Part II. Single bottle, total-etch adhesives. *J Adhes Dent*, **5(2)**, 91–105

[8] Nikaido, T., Kunzelmann, K.H., Chen, H. *et al.* (2002) Evaluation of thermal cycling and mechanical loading on the bond strength of a self-etching primer system to dentine. *Dent Mater*, **18**, 269–275

[9] Sorensen, J.A. and Munksgaard, E.C. (1996) Relative gap formation adjacent to ceramic inlays with combination of resin cements and dentine bonding agents. *J Prosthet Dent*, **76**, 472–476

[10] Strub, J.R. and Beschnidt, M. (1998) Fracture strengths of five different all-ceramic crown systems. *Int J Prosthodont*, **11**, 602–609

[11] Morena, R., Lockwood, P.E. and Fairhurst, C.W. (1986) Fracture toughness of commercial porcelains. *Dent Mater*, **2**, 58–62

[12] Attia, A and Kern, M. (2004) Fracture strength of all-ceramic crowns luted using two bonding methods. *J Prosthet Dent*, **91**, 247–252

[13] Romao, W. Jr, Miranda, W.G. Jr, Cesar, P.F. and Braga, R.P. (2004) Correlation between microleakage and the cement thickness in three Class II inlay ceramic systems. *Oper Dent*, **29(2)**, 212–218

[14] Tay, F.R., Pashley, D.H., Yiu, C.K. *et al.* (2003) Factors contributing to the incompatibility between simplified-step adhesives and the chemically-cured or dual cured composites. Part I. Single-step, self-etching adhesives. *J Adhes Dent*, **5(1)**, 27–40

[15] Ettinger, R.L., Kambhu, P.P., Asmussen, C.M. and Damiano, P.C. (1998) An in vitro evaluation of the integrity of stainless steel crown margins cemented with different luting agents. *Spec Care Dent*, **18**, 78–83

[16] Xin-Hua, G. and Kern, H. (2003) Marginal discrepancies and leakage of all-ceramic crowns: Influence of luting agents and aging conditions. *Int J Prosthodont*, **16**, 109–116

[17] Goodcare, C.J., Campagni, W.V. and Aquilino, S.A. (2001) Tooth preparation for complete crowns: an art form based on scientific principles. *J Prosthet Dent*, **85**, 363–376

[18] Smith, C.T., Gary, J.J., Conkin, J.E. and Franks, H.L. (1999) Effective taper criterion for the full veneer crown preparation in preclinical prosthodontics. *J Prosthodont*, **8**, 196–200

[19] Zidan, O. and Ferguson, G.C. (2003) The retention of complete crowns prepared with different tapers and luted with four different cements. *J Prosthet Dent*, **89**, 565–571

[20] Sorensen, J.A., Kang, S.K. and Avera, S.P. (1991) Porcelain-composite interface microleakage with various porcelain surface treatments. *Dent Mater*, **7**, 118–123

[21] Burke, F.J. (1996) Fracture resistance of teeth restored with dentine-bonded crowns: the effect of increased tooth preparation. *Quintessence Int*, **27**, 115–121

[22] el-Mowaft, O. (2001) The use of resin cements in restorative dentistry to overcome retention problems. *J Can Dent Assoc*, **67**, 97–102

[23] Ozturk, N. and Aykent, F. (2003) Dentin bond strengths of two ceramic inlay systems after cementation with three different techniques and one bonding system. *J Prosthet Dent*, **89**, 275–281

[24] Uno, S. and Finger, W.J. (1995) Function of the hybrid layer as a stress-absorbing layer in resin-dentine bonding. *Quintessence Int*, **26**, 733–738

[25] Attia, A. and Kerm, M. (2004) Influence of cyclic loading and luting agents on the fracture load of two all-ceramic crown systems. *J Prosthet Dent*, **92**, 551–556

[26] Buonocore, M. (1955) A simple method of increasing the adhesion of acrylic filling materials to enamel surfaces. *J Dent Res*, **34**, 849–853

[27] Fusayama, T., Nakamura, M., Kurosaki, N. and Iwaku, M. (1979) Non-pressure adhesion of a new adhesive restorative resin. *J Dent Res*, **58**, 1364–1370

[28] Nakabayashi, N., Ashizawa, M. and Nakamura, M. (1992) Identification of a resin-dentine hybrid layer in vital human dentine created in vivo: Durable bonding to dentine. *Quintessence Int*, **23**, 135–141

[29] Finger, W.J., Lee, K.S. and Podsum, W. (1996) Monomers with low oxygen inhibition as enamel dentine adhesives. *Dent Mater*, **12**, 256

[30] Perdigao, J., Lambrechts, P., van Meerebeek, B., Tome, A.R., VanHerle, G. and Lopes, A. (1996) Morphological field emission-SEM study of effect of six phosphoric acid etching agents on human dentine. *Dent Mater*, **12**, 262

[31] van Meerebeek, B., Dhem, A., Goret-Nicaise, M., Braem, M., Lambrechts, P. and VanHerle, G. (1993) Comparative SEM and TEM examination of the ultrastructure of the resin-dentine interdiffusion zone. *J Dent Res*, **72**, 495–501

[32] Prati, C., Chersoni, S., Mongiorgi, R. and Pashley, D.H. (1998) Resin-infiltrated dentine layer formation of new bonding system. *Operative Dent*, **23**, 185–194

[33] Prati, C., Chersoni, S., Mongiorgi, R. Pashley, D.H. (1998) Resin-infiltrated dentine layer formation of new bonding system. *Operative Dent*, **23**, 185–194

[34] Yoshiyama, M., Carvalho, R., Sano, H., Horner, J., Brewer, P. and Pashley, D.H. (1995) Interfacial morphology and strength of bonds made to superficial versus deep dentine. *Am J Dent*, **8**, 279–302

[35] Szep, S., Langner, N., Bayer, S., Bornichen, D., Schulz, C., Gerhardt, T., Schriever, A., Becker, J. and Heidemann, D. (2003) Comparison of microleakage on one composite with phosphoric acid or a combination of phosphoric and hydrofluoric acid and bonded with several systems. *J Prosthet Dent*, **89**, 161–169

[36] Dunn, J.R. (2003) iBond: the seventh generation, one bottle dental bonding agent. *Compendium*, **24(2)**, 14–18

[37] Kanca, J. (1992) Resin bonding to wet substrate. 1. Bonding to dentine. *Quintessence Int*, **23**, 39–41

[38] Manhart, J., Weber, K., Mehl, A. and Hickel, R. (1999) Marginal quality of dentine adhesives/composites in mixed class V cavities. *J Dent Res*, **78**, 444–447

[39] Abate, P.F., Rodriguez, V.I. and Macchi, R.L. (2000) Evaporation of solvent in one-bottle adhesives. *J Dent*, **8**, 437–440

[40] Finger, W.J., Lee, K.S. and Podsum, W. (1996) Monomers with low oxygen inhibition as enamel dentine adhesives. *Dent Mater*, **12**, 256

[41] Hanning, M., Reinhardt, K.J. and Bott, B. (1999) Self-etching primer vs phosphoric acid: an alternative concept for composite-to-enamel bonding. *Oper Dent*, **24**, 172–180

[42] Tani, C. and Finger, W.J. (2002) Effect of smear layer thickness on bond strength mediated by three all-in-one self etching priming adhesives. *J Adhes Dent*, **4**, 283–289

[43] Ernst, C.P., Holzmeier, M. and Willershausen, B. (2003) In vitro shear bond strength of self etching adhesives. Abstract IADR Goteborg, Paper 29757

[44] Vargas, M.A., Cobb, D.S. and Denehy, G.E. (1997) Interfacial micromorphology and shear bond strength of single-bottle primer/adhesives. *Dent Mater*, **13**, 316–324

[45] Geirsson, J., Ritter, A.V., Heymann, H.O. and Swift, E.J. (2001) Enamel and dentine bond strengths of a new self-etching dental adhesive. *Compend Contin Educ Dent*, **22(12)**, 8–11

[46] Burke, F.J., Fleming, G.J., Nathanson, D. and Marquis, P.M. (2002) Are adhesive technologies needed to support ceramics? An assessment of the current literature. *J Adhes Dent*, **4**, 7–22

[47] Stewart, G.P., Jain, P. and Hodges, J. (2002) Shear bond strength of resin cements to both ceramic and dentine. *J Prosthet Dent*, **88**, 277–284

[48] Madani, M., Chu, F.C., McDonald, A.V. and Smalkes, R.J. (2000) Effects of surface treatments on shear bond strengths between a resin cement and an alumina core. *J Prosthet Dent*, **83**, 644–647

[49] Blatz, M.B., Sadan, A., Arch, G.H. and Lang, B.R. (2003) In vitro evaluation of long-term bonding of Procera AllCeram alumina restorations with a modified resin luting agent. *J Prosthet Dent*, **89**, 381–387

[50] Attia, A. and Kern, M. (2004) Fracture strength of all-ceramic crowns luted using two bonding methods. *J Prosthet Dent*, **91**, 247–252

[51] Wegner, S.M. and Kern, M. (2000) Long-term resin bond strength to zirconia ceramic. *J Adhes Dent*, **2**, 139–147

[52] Blatz, M.B., Sadan. A., Martin, J. and Lang, B. (2004) In vitro evaluation of shear bond strength of resin to densely-sintered high-purity zirconium-oxide ceramic after long-term storage and thermal cycling. *J Prosthet Dent*, **91**, 356–362

[53] Wegner, S.M., Gerdes, W. and Kern, M. (2002) Effect of different artificial ageing conditions on ceramic–composite bond strengths. *Int J Prosthodont*, **15**, 267–272

[54] Finger, W.J. and Tani, C. (2002) Effect of humidity on bonding strength of self-etching adhesives to dentine. *J Adhes Dent*, **4**, 277–282

[55] El-Kalla, I.H. (1999) Saliva contamination and resin micromorpholgical adaptation to cavity walls using single-bottle adhesives. *Am J Dent*, **12(4)**, 172–176

[56] Taskonak, B. and Sertgoz, A. (2002) Shear bond strength of saliva contaminated ‘one-bottle’ adhesives. *J Oral Rehab*, **29**, 559–564

[57] Stewart, G.P., Jain, P. and Hodges, J. (2002) Shear bond strength of resin cements to both ceramic and dentine. *J Prosthet Dent*, **88**, 277–284

Index

W

Y

Z